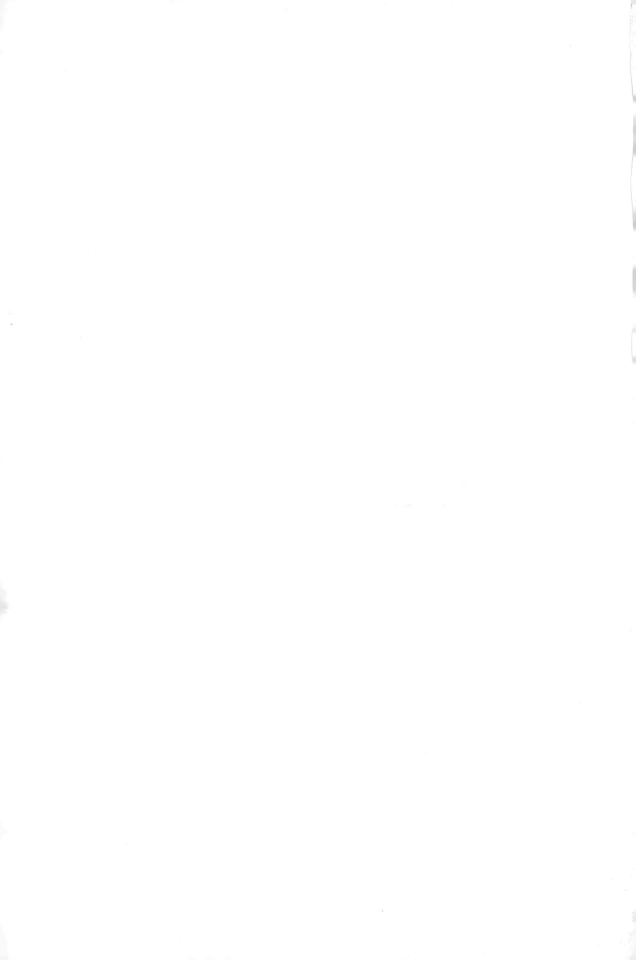

Cardiac Conduction System Disorders

Editors

ERIC N. PRYSTOWSKY
BENZY J. PADANILAM

CARDIOLOGY CLINICS

www.cardiology.theclinics.com

August 2023 • Volume 41 • Number 3

ELSEVIER

1600 John F. Kennedy Boulevard • Suite 1800 • Philadelphia, Pennsylvania, 19103-2899

http://www.theclinics.com

CARDIOLOGY CLINICS Volume 41, Number 3
August 2023 ISSN 0733-8651, ISBN-13: 978-0-443-18312-6

Editor: Joanna Gascoine
Developmental Editor: Karen Justine S. Dino

Cardiology Clinics (ISSN 0733-8651) is published quarterly by Elsevier Inc., 360 Park Avenue South, New York, NY 10010-1710. Months of issue are February, May, August, and November. Business and Editorial Offices: 1600 John F. Kennedy Blvd., Ste. 1800, Philadelphia, PA 19103-2899. Customer Service Office: 3251 Riverport Lane, Maryland Heights, MO 63043. Periodicals post-age paid at New York, NY and additional mailing offices. Subscription prices are $377.00 per year for US individuals, $743.00 per year for US institutions, $100.00 per year for US students and residents, $468.00 per year for Canadian individuals, $932.00 per year for Canadian institutions, $490.00 per year for international individuals, $932.00 per year for international institutions, $100.00 per year for Canadian students/residents and $220.00 per year for international students/residents. To receive student/resident rate, orders must be accompanied by name of affiliated institution, data of term, and the *signature* of program/residency coordinator on institution letterhead. Orders will be billed at individual rate until proof of status is received. Foreign air speed delivery is included in all *Clinics* subscription prices. All prices are subject to change without notice. **POSTMASTER:** Send address changes to *Cardiology Clinics*, Elsevier Health Sciences Division, Subscription Customer Service, 3251 Riverport Lane, Maryland Heights, MO 63043. **Customer Service: 1-800-654-2452 (U.S. and Canada); 314-447-8871 (outside U.S. and Canada). Fax: 314-447-8029. E-mail: journalscus-tomerservice-usa@elsevier.com (for print support); journalsonlinesupport-usa@elsevier.com (for online support).**

Reprints. For copies of 100 or more, of articles in this publication, please contact the Commercial Reprints Department, Elsevier Inc., 360 Park Avenue South, New York, NY 10010-1710. Tel.: 212-633-3874; Fax: 212-633-3820; E-mail: reprints@elsevier.com.

Cardiology Clinics is also published in Spanish by McGraw-Hill Interamericana Editores S. A., P.O. Box 5-237, 06500, Mexico D. F., Mexico; in Portuguese by Reichmann and Alfonso Editores Rio de Janeiro, Brazil; and in Greek by Dimitrios P. Lagos, 8 Pondon Street, GR115-28 Ilissia, Greece.

Cardiology Clinics is covered in *MEDLINE/PubMed (Index Medicus), Excerpta Medica, The Cumulative Index to Nursing and Allied Health Literature* (CINAHL).

Printed in the United States of America.

Contributors

BRADLEY A. CLARK, DO
Cardiac Electrophysiologist, St. Vincent
Hospital, Indianapolis, Indiana, USA

EMANUEL EBIN, MD
Cardiac Arrhythmia Service, Cardiovascular
Division, Cardiovascular Medicine, University
of Minnesota Medical School, Minneapolis,
Minnesota, USA

KENNETH A. ELLENBOGEN, MD
Kimmerling Professor of Cardiology,
Department of Cardiac Electrophysiology, VCU
School of Medicine, Richmond, Virginia,
USA

FATIMA M. EZZEDDINE, MD
Department of Cardiovascular Medicine, Mayo
Clinic College of Medicine, Rochester,
Minnesota, USA

DAVID S. FRANKEL, MD
Associate Professor of Medicine, Program
Director, Cardiac Electrophysiology
Fellowship, Cardiovascular Division, Perelman
School of Medicine, University of
Pennsylvania, Philadelphia, Pennsylvania,
USA

PHILIP GEORGE, MD
Assistant Professor of Medicine, University of
Florida College of Medicine, Gainesville,
Florida, USA

EDWARD P. GERSTENFELD, MD, MS
Section of Cardiac Electrophysiology, Division
of Cardiology, University of California
San Francisco, San Francisco, California,
USA

JASEN L. GILGE, MD
Cardiac Electrophysiologist, St. Vincent
Hospital, Indianapolis, Indiana, USA

LARRY R. JACKSON II, MD, MHS
Division of Cardiovascular Medicine, Duke
University Medical Center, Duke Clinical
Research Institute, Duke University School of
Medicine, Durham, North Carolina,
USA

ROSHAN KARKI, MBBS
Department of Cardiovascular Medicine, Mayo
Clinic College of Medicine, Rochester,
Minnesota, USA

SHAAN KHURSHID, MD, MPH
Clinical Electrophysiology Fellow, Division of
Cardiology and Cardiovascular Research
Center, Massachusetts General Hospital,
Boston, Massachusetts, USA

WILLIAM M. MILES, MD, FACC, FHRS
Professor of Medicine, Silverstein Chair for
Cardiovascular Education, University of Florida
College of Medicine, Gainesville, Florida,
USA

LLUÍS MONT, MD, PhD
Arrhythmia Section, Cardiology Department,
Institut Clínic Cardiovascular, Hospital Clínic
de Barcelona, Universitat de Barcelona, Institut
d'Investigacions Biomédiques August Pi i
Sunyer, Barcelona, Catalonia, Spain; Centro de
Investigación Biomédica en Red
Enfermedades Cardiovasculares, Madrid,
Spain

SHUMPEI MORI, MD, PhD
UCLA Cardiac Arrhythmia Center, University of
California Los Angeles, Center of the Health
Science, Los Angeles, California, USA

SANTOSH K. PADALA, MD
Assistant Professor of Cardiology, Department
of Cardiac Electrophysiology, VCU School of
Medicine, Richmond, Virginia, USA

BENZY J. PADANILAM, MD
Director, Electrophysiology Lab, Ascension St.
Vincent Hospital, Indianapolis, Indiana, USA

CHIARA PAVONE, MD
Cardiovascular Sciences Department,
Fondazione Policlinico Universitario Agostino
Gemelli IRCCS, Rome, Italy

GEMMA PELARGONIO, MD, PhD
Cardiovascular Sciences Department,
Fondazione Policlinico Universitario Agostino
Gemelli IRCCS, Cardiology Institute, Catholic
University of the Sacred Heart, Rome, Italy

ANDREU PORTA-SÁNCHEZ, MD, PhD
Cardiologia Molecular, Fundación Centro
Nacional de Investigaciones Cardiovasculares
Carlos III (CNIC), Departamento de
Cardiología, Unidad de Arritmias, Hospital
Universitario Quironsalud Madrid, Spain;
Departamento de Medicina, Universidad
Europea de Madrid, Madrid, Spain

SILVIA GIULIANA PRIORI, MD, PhD
Cardiologia Molecular, Fundación Centro
Nacional de Investigaciones Cardiovasculares
Carlos III (CNIC), Molecular Medicine
Department, University of Pavia, Istituti
Clinici Scientifici Maugeri, IRCCS, Pavia,
Italy

ERIC N. PRYSTOWSKY, MD
Director, Cardiac Arrhythmia Service,
Ascension St. Vincent Hospital, Indianapolis,
Indiana; Consulting Professor of
Medicine, Duke University Medical
Center, Durham, North Carolina,
USA

MARGARIDA PUJOL-LÓPEZ, MD
Arrhythmia Section, Cardiology Department,
Institut Clínic Cardiovascular, Hospital Clínic
de Barcelona, Universitat de Barcelona, Institut
d'Investigacions Biomédiques August Pi I
Sunyer, Barcelona, Catalonia, Spain

ANVI RAINA, MD
Department of Cardiovascular Medicine, Mayo
Clinic College of Medicine, Rochester,
Minnesota, USA

SYED RAFAY A. SABZWARI, MBBS, MD
Clinical Cardiac Electrophysiology Fellow,
University of Colorado Anschutz Medical
Campus, Aurora, Colorado, USA

NEERAJ SATHNUR, MD
Cardiac Arrhythmia Service, Cardiovascular
Division, Cardiovascular Medicine, University
of Minnesota Medical School, Cardiac
Electrophysiology, Park-Nicollet Medical
Center, St Louis Park, Minneapolis, Minnesota,
USA

LEONARD STEINBERG, MD, BS
Pediatric Cardiology, Children's Heart Center,
Ascension St. Vincent, Indianapolis, Indiana,
USA

JOSÉ M. TOLOSANA, MD, PhD
Arrhythmia Section, Cardiology Department,
Institut Clínic Cardiovascular, Hospital Clínic
de Barcelona, Universitat de Barcelona, Institut
d'Investigacions Biomédiques August Pi I
Sunyer, Barcelona, Catalonia, Spain; Centro de
Investigacio' n Biomédica en Red
Enfermedades Cardiovasculares, Madrid,
Spain

RODERICK TUNG, MD
Center for Arrhythmia Care, Pritzker School of
Medicine, University of Chicago, The University
of Chicago Medicine, Heart and Vascular
Center, Chicago, Illinois, USA; Division of
Cardiology, Banner Cardiovascular Center,
The University of Arizona College of Medicine,
Banner University Medical Center, Phoenix,
Arizona, USA

WENDY S. TZOU, MD, FHRS, FACC
Director, Cardiac Electrophysiology, Associate
Professor of Medicine, University of Colorado
Anschutz Medical Campus, Aurora, Colorado,
USA

FRANCIS UGOWE, MD
Duke University Medical Center, Duke
University School of Medicine, Durham, North
Carolina, USA

GAURAV A. UPADHYAY, MD
Center for Arrhythmia Care, Pritzker School of
Medicine, University of Chicago, The University
of Chicago Medicine, Heart and Vascular
Center, Chicago, Illinois, USA

Contents

Supernormal conduction may explain unusual conduction phenomena in patients with abnormal His-Purkinje function or poorly conducting accessory pathways.

The peculiar electrophysiological properties of the sinoatrial node and the cardiac conduction system are key components of the normal physiology of cardiac impulse generation and propagation. Multiple genes and transcription factors and metabolic proteins are involved in their development and regulation. In this review, we have summarized the genetic underlying causes, key clinical findings, and the latest available clinical evidence. We will discuss clinical diagnosis and management of the genetic conditions associated with conduction disorders that are more prevalent in clinical practice, for this reason, very rare genetic diseases presenting sinus node or cardiac conduction system abnormalities are not discussed.

Sinus node dysfunction (SND) is a multifaceted disorder most prevalent in older individuals, but may also occur at an earlier age. In most cases, the SND diagnosis is ultimately established by documenting its ECG manifestations. EPS has limited utility. The treatment strategy is largely dictated by symptoms and ECG manifestations. Not infrequently, both bradycardia and tachycardia coexist in the same patients, along with other diseases common in the elderly (e.g., hypertension, coronary artery disease), thereby complicating treatment strategy. Prevention of the adverse consequences of both bradyarrhythmia and tachyarrhythmia is important to reduce susceptibility to syncope, falls, and thromboembolic complications.

PR prolongation is defined primarily as delayed conduction through the AV node, but can also signify delayed electrical impulse propagation through any part of the conduction system. The prevalence of PR prolongation ranges from 1% to 5% in patients younger than 50 years, with increasing prevalence, after the sixth decade of life and in patients with organic heart disease. Contemporary studies have documented increased risk of atrial arrhythmias, heart failure, and mortality in patients with PR prolongation. Future studies are needed to more accurately risk stratify elderly patients with PR prolongation who may be at increased risk of adverse outcomes.

Left bundle branch block (LBBB) is not just a simple electrocardiogram alteration. The intricacies of this general terminology go beyond simple conduction block. This review puts together current knowledge on the historical concept of LBBB, clinical significance, and recent insights into the pathophysiology of human LBBB. LBBB is an entity that affects patient diagnosis (primary conduction disease, secondary to underlying pathology or iatrogenic), treatment (cardiac resynchronization therapy or conduction system pacing for heart failure), and prognosis. Recruiting the left bundle branch with conduction system pacing depends on the complex interaction between anatomy, site of pathophysiology, and delivery tools.

Left bundle branch block (LBBB) and right bundle branch block (RBBB) are classic manifestations of bundle branch conduction disorders. However, a third form that is uncommon and underrecognized may exist that has features and pathophysiology of both: bilateral bundle branch block (BBBB). This unusual form of bundle branch block exhibits an RBBB pattern in lead V1 (terminal R wave) and an LBBB pattern in leads I and aVL (absence of S wave). This unique conduction disorder may confer an increased risk of adverse cardiovascular events. BBBB patients may be a subset of patients that respond well to cardiac resynchronization therapy.

Congenital complete heart block (CCHB) defines atrioventricular conduction abnormalities diagnosed in utero or within the first 27 days of life. Maternal autoimmune disease and congenital heart defects are most commonly responsible. Recent genetic discoveries have highlighted our understanding of the underlying mechanism. Hydroxychloroquine shows promise in preventing autoimmune CCHB. Patients may develop symptomatic bradycardia and cardiomyopathy. The presence of these and other specific findings warrants placement of a permanent pacemaker to relieve symptoms and prevent catastrophic events. The mechanisms, natural history, evaluation, and treatment of patients with or at risk for CCHB are reviewed.

Atrioventricular blocks may be caused by a variety of potentially reversible conditions, such as ischemic heart disease, electrolyte imbalances, medications, and infectious diseases. Such causes must be always ruled out to avoid unnecessary pacemaker implantation. Patient management and reversibility rates depend on the underlying cause. Careful patient history taking, monitoring of vital signs, electrocardiogram, and arterial blood gas analysis are crucial elements of the diagnostic workflow during the acute phase. Atrioventricular block recurrence after the reversal of the underlying cause may pose an indication for pacemaker implantation, because reversible conditions may actually unmask a preexistent conduction disorder.

Iatrogenic atrioventricular (AV) block can occur in the context of cardiac surgery, percutaneous transcatheter, or electrophysiologic procedures. In cardiac surgery, patients undergoing aortic and/or mitral valve surgery are at the highest risk for developing perioperative AV block requiring permanent pacemaker implantation. Similarly, patients undergoing transcatheter aortic valve replacement are also at increased risk for developing AV block. Electrophysiologic procedures, including catheter ablation of AV nodal re-entrant tachycardia, septal accessory pathways, para-Hisian atrial tachycardia, or premature ventricular complexes, are also associated with risk of AV conduction system injury. In this article, we summarize the common causes for iatrogenic AV block, predictors for AV block, and general management considerations.

Systemic diseases can cause heart block owing to the involvement of the myocardium and thereby the conduction system. Younger patients (<60) with heart block should be evaluated for an underlying systemic disease. These disorders are classified into infiltrative, rheumatologic, endocrine, and hereditary neuromuscular degenerative diseases. Cardiac amyloidosis owing to amyloid fibrils and cardiac sarcoidosis owing to noncaseating granulomas can infiltrate the conduction system leading to heart block. Accelerated atherosclerosis, vasculitis, myocarditis, and interstitial inflammation contribute to heart block in rheumatologic disorders. Myotonic, Becker, and Duchenne muscular dystrophies are neuromuscular diseases involving the myocardium skeletal muscles and can cause heart block.

Pacing-Induced Cardiomyopathy

Shaan Khurshid and David S. Frankel

Right ventricular (RV) pacing-induced cardiomyopathy (PICM) is typically defined as left ventricular systolic dysfunction resulting from electrical and mechanical dyssynchrony caused by RV pacing. RV PICM is common, occurring in 10-20% of individuals exposed to frequent RV pacing. Multiple risk factors for PICM have been identified, including male sex, wider native and paced QRS durations, and higher RV pacing percentage, but the ability to predict which individuals will develop PICM remains modest. Biventricular and conduction system pacing, which better preserve electrical and mechanical synchrony, typically prevent the development of PICM and reverse left ventricular systolic dysfunction after PICM has occurred.

Pacing of Specialized Conduction System

Santosh K. Padala and Kenneth A. Ellenbogen

Right ventricular pacing for bradycardia remains the mainstay of pacing therapy. Chronic right ventricular pacing may lead to pacing-induced cardiomyopathy. We focus on the anatomy of the conduction system and the clinical feasibility of pacing the His bundle and/or left bundle conduction system. We review the hemodynamics of conduction system pacing, the techniques to capture the conduction system and the electrocardiogram and pacing definitions of conduction system capture. Clinical studies of conduction system pacing in the setting of atrioventricular block and after AV junction ablation are reviewed and the evolving role of conduction system pacing is compared with biventricular pacing.

CARDIOLOGY CLINICS

SERIES OF RELATED INTEREST

Heart Failure Clinics
Available at: https://www.heartfailure.theclinics.com/
Cardiac Electrophysiology Clinics
Available at: https://www.cardiacep.theclinics.com/
Interventional Cardiology Clinics
Available at: https://www.interventional.theclinics.com/

Preface
Cardiac Conduction System Disorders

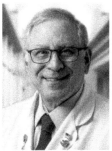 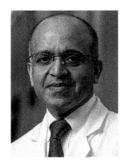

Eric N. Prystowsky, MD   Benzy J. Padanilam, MD

Editors

I (E.N.P.) was asked to guest edit an issue of *Cardiology Clinics* on "Cardiac Conduction System Disorders." My partner and colleague, Dr Benzy Padanilam, coedited this with me. There are many parts of the conduction system and diseases that affect it, and we developed 15 separate articles on this subject. Carefully selected authors were asked to provide state-of-the-art information for clinicians on topics of their expertise. They have focused not just on a pure academic review but also on the clinical applications important to the practicing physicians. We cannot thank them enough for their outstanding contributions. In the end, we feel this issue of the *Cardiology Clinics* will be a valuable resource for health care providers from students to clinicians.

The first 5 articles focus on more broad-based topics. The article by Karki and colleagues is a thorough review of the anatomy and pathology of the conduction system, followed by the article by Prystowsky and Gilge that discusses in detail the physiology of atrioventricular (AV) conduction and the effects of the autonomic nervous system on it. The article by Clark and Prystowsky shows the electrocardiographic representation of various conduction patterns, and the article by Miles and George informs on the variants of AV

conduction, for example, gap and aberrancy. The article by Porta-Sanchez and Giuliana Priori details genetic abnormalities of sinus node and AV conduction.

The next 5 articles are more focused on a specific abnormality of the conduction system. The article by Sathnur and colleagues discusses sinus node abnormalities, and the article by Jackson and Ugowe discusses the epidemiology of prolonged PR interval. The article by Pujol Lopez and colleagues updates our knowledge of left bundle branch block, and the article by Gilge and Padanilam reviews bilateral bundle branch block. The article by Steinberg is an in-depth discussion of congenital heart block.

The last 5 articles focus on a variety of causes of AV conduction disorders and pacemaker therapy for them. The article by Pelargonio and Pavone discusses reversible causes of heart block, and the article by Cheung and colleagues informs on iatrogenic AV block. Systemic diseases that cause heart block are covered in the article by Sabzwari and Tzou, and pacemaker-induced cardiomyopathy is covered in the article by Khurshid and Frankel. The article by Padala and Ellenbogen reviews the latest data on conduction system pacing for patients with heart block.

Cardiol Clin 41 (2023) xiii–xiv
https://doi.org/10.1016/j.ccl.2023.05.001
0733-8651/23/© 2023 Published by Elsevier Inc.

We hope you enjoy this issue of *Cardiology Clinics*.

Eric N. Prystowsky, MD
Cardiac Arrhythmia Service
Ascension St. Vincent Hospital
Indianapolis, IN 46260, USA

Duke University Medical Center
Durham, NC, USA

Benzy J. Padanilam, MD
Electrophysiology Lab
Ascension St. Vincent Hospital
Indianapolis, IN 46260, USA

E-mail addresses:
enprysto@ascension.org (E.N. Prystowsky)
bjpadani@ascension.org (B.J. Padanilam)

Anatomy and Pathology of the Cardiac Conduction System

Roshan Karki, MBBS[a], Anvi Raina, MD[a], Fatima M. Ezzeddine, MD[a],
Melanie C. Bois, MD[b], Samuel J. Asirvatham, MD[a],*

KEYWORDS

- Sinus node • Atrioventricular node • His bundle • Left bundle • Right bundle • Purkinje fibers

KEY POINTS

- The Human cardiac conduction system has unique anatomic features.
- Understanding the normal and variant anatomy of the cardiac conduction system is vital to an interventional electrophysiologist.

INTRODUCTION

Although atrioventricular (AV) conduction was first described independently by Kent and His in 1893, the landmark work of Sunao Tawara,[1] published in 1906, formed the basis of what we know about the human conduction system. In this review, we have sought to describe the normal and developmental anatomy of the conduction system and its variation in normal and congenitally abnormal hearts, the understanding of which is critical to an interventional electrophysiologist.

THE SINUS NODE
Normal and Developmental Anatomy

The sinus or sinoatrial node (SAN), the principal cardiac pacemaker, was first described in 1907 by Keith and Flack.[2] Sinus node embryogenesis begins in the sinus venosus of the early heart tube as mesodermal cells differentiate into cardiomyocytes with automaticity and fast conduction properties.[3] Key gene transcription factors differentiate these pacemaker cells from the surrounding myocardium with specialized ion channels.[3] In adults, this tadpole-like structure has nodal extensions in multiple directions and measures 10 to 22 mm in length and 2 to 3 mm in width.[4] The head

and proximal body of the sinus node (**Fig. 1**) are usually subepicardial in location at the junction of the superior vena cava and the right atrial appendage. The distal body and tail penetrate inferiorly and obliquely into the musculature of the crista terminalis and toward the eustachian ridge.[3,5]

The blood supply of the SAN comes from its namesake artery, which branches off the right coronary artery in roughly 60% of patients (**Fig. 2**). In the other 40%, the sinoatrial (SA) nodal artery originates from the left circumflex artery as a branch of the left anterior or left lateral atrial artery.[5] A few instances of dual origins from both arteries have also been reported.[6] When branching from the right system, the right anterior atrial artery climbs the anterior interatrial groove to give rise to the SA nodal artery. Rarely, the SA nodal artery can originate from the distal right lateral atrial artery, which takes a more inferior course to reach the SAN. The SA nodal artery can take variable courses to reach the SAN; it can enter via the cavoatrial junction in a precaval or postcaval fashion or divide and form an arterial circle as it approaches the node at the cavoatrial junction.[5] The SA nodal artery, when branching from the left system, courses over the roof of the left atrium. Regardless of its origin

This article originally appeared in *Cardiac Electrophysiology Clinics*, Volume 13 Issue 4, December 2021.
[a] Department of Cardiovascular Medicine, Mayo Clinic College of Medicine, Rochester, MN 55905, USA;
[b] Department of Laboratory Medicine and Pathology, Mayo Clinic, Rochester, MN 55905, USA
* Corresponding author. Mayo Clinic College of Medicine, 200 First Street Southwest, Rochester, MN 55905.
E-mail address: asirvatham.samuel@mayo.edu

Cardiol Clin 41 (2023) 277–292
https://doi.org/10.1016/j.ccl.2023.03.016

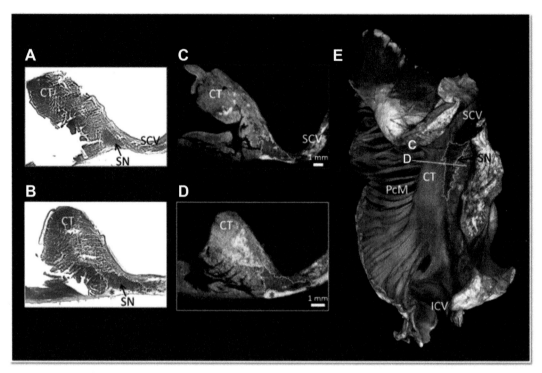

Fig. 1. Anatomy of the human sinus node (*C, D*) as seen on histology (*A, B*) and on microcomputed tomographic sections with 3D volume rendering (*E*). CT, crista terminalis; ICV, inferior caval vein; SCV, superior caval vein; PcM, pectinate muscles; SN, sinus node. *Epicardial fat pad. (*From* Stephenson RS, Boyett MR, Hart G, Nikolaidou T, Cai X, Corno AF, et al. (2012) Contrast Enhanced Micro-Computed Tomography Resolves the 3-Dimensional Morphology of the Cardiac Conduction System in Mammalian Hearts. PLoS ONE 7(4): e35299. https://doi.org/10.1371/journal.pone.0035299)

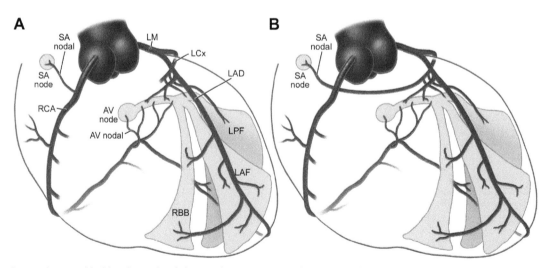

Fig. 2. The variable blood supply of the conduction system. The sinus node is supplied by the SA nodal artery, a branch of the right coronary artery in 60% of patients (*A*) and the left circumflex artery in 40% of patients (*B*). The AV node is supplied by the AV nodal artery, which branches from the right coronary artery. Note the dual supply of the left and right bundle branches (RBB). See text for further explanations. RCA, right coronary artery; LAD, left anterior descending artery; LAF, left anterior fascicle; LCx, left circumflex artery; LM, left main artery; LPF, left posterior fascicle.

and course, the SA nodal artery has an extensive collateral network that preserves SA nodal function in the event of proximal atherosclerotic lesions.[5]

Histologically, the SAN comprises weakly coupled, densely packed specialized myocytes called pacemaker (P) cells and nonpacemaker cells embedded in a dense supporting connective tissue. The pacemaker activity is not confined to a single cell in the SAN. Instead, P cells are electrically coupled and discharge synchronously owing to mutual entrainment.[4] The concept of a "pacemaker hierarchy" is used to explain heart rate variability of the SAN with cells that depolarize at a higher frequency and generate faster heart rates being located superiorly in the SAN. In contrast, slower firing cells that generate slower heart rates are situated inferiorly in the tail of the node.[3,4]

The sinus node is the most richly innervated component of the conduction system.[7] The dense distribution of parasympathetic and sympathetic nerves and ganglia allow for the regulation and sensitive responsiveness of the SAN by paired yet opposite autonomic influences.[3] Parasympathetic fibers innervate the SAN via the vagus nerve, and the sympathetic innervation occurs via the T1 to T4 spinal nerves. At rest, the parasympathetic system governs the SAN and slows the heart rate through acetylcholine and nitric oxide release. In contrast, the sympathetic system increases the heart rate generated by the SAN during exercise or stress through adrenergic stimulation of β-receptors.[3] This autonomic interplay between the sympathetic and parasympathetic systems determines the leading pacemaker site within the SAN; increasing sympathetic stimulation shifts the leading site of activation cranially, whereas an increase in vagal input migrates the site inferiorly.[3]

Normal Variation of the Sinus Node

A common SAN variant, present in 10% of individuals, is situated anteriorly and extends over the crest of the right atrial appendage into the interatrial groove in a horseshoe-like pattern.[8] The variation of origin and course of the SA nodal artery has been discussed elsewhere in this article.

Congenital Anomalies of the Sinus Node

The sinus node may be absent, double, or displaced in patients with some forms of congenital heart defects. In left juxtaposed atrial appendages, the sinus node is displaced inferior and more anterior to the crista terminalis leading to increased risk of trauma and dysfunction following cardiac surgery or an electrophysiologic procedure.[9]

Atrial septal defects (ASD) of secundum and sinus venosus types (**Fig. 3**) are most frequently associated with sinus node dysfunction (SND), particularly with late age of repair and large shunt size.[10] Although the defect in secundum ASDs are remote from the sinus node, SND has also been reported preprocedurally in a small subset of patients. Two possible mechanisms have been suggested. ASDs with chronic left-to-right shunts can lead to structural and electrical remodeling of atrial myocytes and interstitial fibrosis by pressure and volume overload, resulting in SA exit block.[10] Remarkably, these changes may be reversible with early surgical intervention.[11] Another possibility for preprocedural SND in this population is the simultaneous development of the atrial septum and nodal tissue. The SAN and AV node develop from rings of specialized tissue that lie between the primordial chambers of the early heart tube. The sinus ring lies in a loop between the superior and inferior vena cava, touching the AV ring tissue.[12] A defect in atrial septal development at this time could influence SAN and AV node development and result in altered morphogenesis, which may present as SND in this cohort.[12] Superior sinus venosus ASDs involve the posterior and superior portion of the atrial septum and often override the superior vena cava.[10] The proximity of the septal defect to the sinus node presents a higher risk of developing

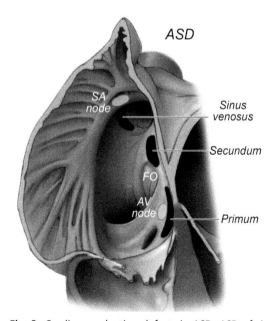

Fig. 3. Cardiac conduction defects in ASD. ASD of sinus venosus type is associated with SND. ASD of primum type is associated with AV block. ASD of secundum type is physically remote from both sinus and AV nodes, making their dysfunction less common.

SND as a complication of surgical intervention, with SND rates as high as 10% to 15%.[10] More recent surgical techniques such as the Warden procedure or modified double patch technique, avoid an incision across the cavoatrial junction and thus trauma to the SA nodal artery, resulting in a much lower incidence of SND (1%–2%).[10]

Heterotaxy syndromes are rare congenital defects characterized by bilateral mirror-image symmetry (or isomerism) of the atria. Typically, much of the atrial septum is absent and atrial symmetry is defined by the anatomic landmarks of the atrial free walls.[13] For example, the morphologic right atrium consists of crista terminalis and pectinate muscles, compared with the smooth-walled vestibule of the left atrium. Patients with right atrial isomerism have a mirror image right atrium, may have twin SA nodes, AV nodes, or infranodal systems, and often present with 2 distinct atrial or ventricular rhythms (**Figs. 4** and **5**).[9] Furthermore, this can be exacerbated by reentrant arrhythmias if a concomitant swing bundle is present (**Fig. 5**).[9] In patients with left atrial isomerism, SND is common (16%–50%); the usual right-sided sinus node may be absent or hypoplastic (see **Fig. 4**). About 79% of these patients have the tachycardia–bradycardia syndrome from concomitant supraventricular tachycardia and SND.[9]

Pathology of the Sinus Node

SND refers to a spectrum of abnormalities involving the sinus node and its neighboring architecture leading to variable presentation, including sinus bradycardia, SA exit block, sinus arrest, chronotropic incompetence, or tachycardia-bradycardia syndrome. The SND is often degenerative, and there are many other etiologies that have been listed in **Table 1**.

Key Points for the Proceduralist

Although rare, acute nonreversible SND requiring pacemaker implantation can result from ablation of atrial arrhythmias.[14] The patients who undergo perisuperior vena cava ablation are more likely to develop SND. The mechanism for sinus arrest can be the isolation of the SAN owing to extensive ablation in the context of prior atrial surgery. It can also result from the injury of the SA nodal artery (with an origin from the left circumflex artery) during the left atrial roof ablation.[14] Preablation planning with a careful review of surgical history and review of the computed tomography angiogram can help to avoid such complications.

Sinus node modification or ablation as the treatment for inappropriate sinus tachycardia has been out of favor owing to the risk for pacemaker implantation and limited efficacy.[15] Therefore, it should be reserved only for highly symptomatic, refractory patients.[16] It behooves the proceduralist to appreciate the variability in SAN and SA nodal artery location when preparing for this ablation and treat the entire cavoatrial junction with the utmost respect. In most hearts, the nodal body is relatively shallow with a distance of 0.1 to 1.0 mm, and the distance of SAN from the

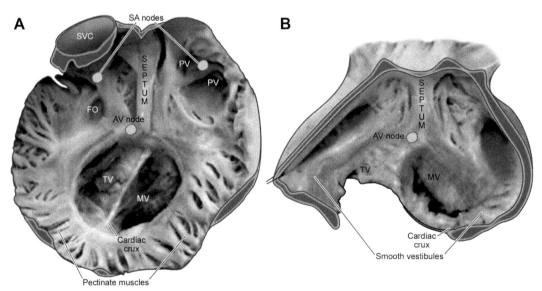

Fig. 4. Sinus and AV nodes in heterotaxy syndromes. (*A*) Right atrial isomerism (mirror-imaged right atria with pectinate muscles) with twin sinus nodes. (*B*) Left atrial isomerism (the mirror-imaged left atria with smooth vestibule) with an absent SA node. FO, fossa ovalis; MV, mitral valve; PV, pulmonary valve; TV, tricuspid valve.

HETEROTAXY

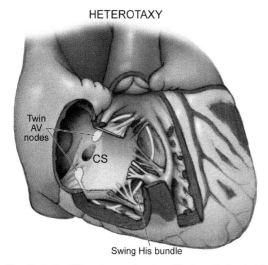

Fig. 5. Twin AV nodes and swing His bundle in right atrial isomerism. CS, coronary sinus.

Table 1 Causes of sinus node dysfunction	
Pathogenesis	**Examples**
Ischemic	Acute myocardial infarction
Degenerative	Idiopathic or age related, atrial arrhythmias, hypertension
Congenital	Heterotaxy syndrome, atrial septal defects, juxtaposition of atrial appendages
Infiltrative	Sarcoidosis, amyloidosis, hemochromatosis, tumors
Familial causes	*SCN5A, HCN4, CASQ2, RYR2, EMD, ANK2, GJA5* gene mutations
Infectious	Myocarditis/pericarditis, rheumatic fever, Lyme's disease, legionella, Chagas disease, typhoid fever, dengue, leptospirosis
Neuromuscular disorders	Friedreich's ataxia, myotonic dystrophy, Emery–Dreifuss muscular dystrophy
Endocrine	Hypothyroidism
Metabolic	Hyperkalemia, hypothermia, Cushing response (increased intracranial pressure), hypoxia, hypercapnia
Drug induced	Beta-blockers, calcium channel blocking agents, ivabradine, digoxin, clonidine, antiarrhythmics, lithium, methyldopa, cisplatin
Iatrogenic	Mustard, Senning, Glenn, and Fontan procedures ASD closure, cardiac transplant (especially atrial–atrial anastomosis)

endocardium ranges from 2.3 to 4.6 mm.[17] In roughly 30% of patients, the distance from the endocardium was 7 mm thick, and the nodal tail was 3.3 to 5.8 mm distant from the endocardial surface.[17] This variability in depths from endocardial and epicardial surfaces and a heat sink effect from the SA nodal artery may cause difficulties in targeting lesions with higher energy and longer application times required to achieve success.[15] It is also prudent to note that the location of the SAN in the lateral and anterolateral quadrants of the cavoatrial junction may coincide with the course of descent of the right phrenic nerve in some patients, making phrenic nerve injury a possibility during this procedure.

INTERNODAL AND INTERATRIAL CONDUCTION

The SAN is separated from its surrounding myocardium by an indistinct and irregular border called the transition zone of loosely packed cells with histologic and electrophysiologic characteristics intermediate between sinus node cells and atrial myocytes.[3] However, no specialized conduction tissue connections between the nodes (internodal tracts) have been uncovered to date.[18] Instead, the internodal conduction occurs by depolarizing atrial myocardial bundles formed by continuous longitudinal fibers of similarly orientated myocytes.[18] Electroanatomic analysis has shown reproducible craniocaudal right atrial activation, which starts at the SAN and splits into 2 wave fronts running simultaneously along the interatrial septum and the lateral wall of the right atrium.[19] The 2 wave fronts fuse at the inferoseptal right atrium, slightly below the AV node and anterior to the coronary sinus ostium.[19]

For synchronized contraction between 2 atria, 3 distinct muscular bundles (**Fig. 6**) have been described.[18] The most prominent of these is the interatrial or Bachmann's bundle that cross the anterior septal raphe between the atria and have bifurcating branches that encircle the respective atrial appendages.[18] The septopulmonary bundle arises underneath Bachmann's bundle from the interatrial groove and fans out superiorly over the dome to the posterior wall of the left atrium and then around the left and right pulmonary veins. The septoatrial bundle is the deepest

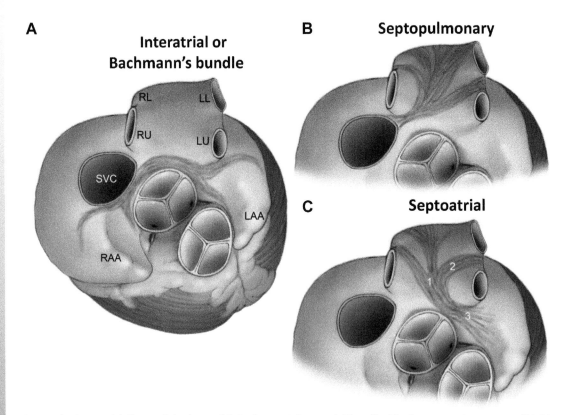

Fig. 6. The interatrial fibers of the heart. (*A*) Bachmann's interatrial bundle: The largest and most superficial interatrial bundles. (*B*) Septopulmonary bundle: Just superficial to Bachmann's bundle, this bundle runs from the interatrial groove and fans out posteriorly to the pulmonary veins. (*C*) Septoatrial bundle: It is the deepest of the interatrial bundles and runs anterior to posterior and further divides into 3 fascicles which run toward the pulmonary veins and the left atrial appendage. LAA, left atrial appendage; LL, left lower; LU, left upper; RL, right lower; RU, right upper; RAA, right atrial appendage; SVC, superior vena cava.

(subendocardial) layer with fibers that ascend from the anterior septal raphe and divide into 3 fascicles, 2 of which continue over the dome to combine with the septopulmonary bundle and insert around the pulmonary veins on either side.[18] The third fascicle is circumferential, passing leftward to surround the mouth of the left atrial appendage and then combining with the subepicardial circular fibers in the inferior wall.[18] These bundles, mainly Bachmann's and the septoatrial bundle, induce early contraction of the left atrial appendage relative to the left atrium and therefore improve left atrial emptying and hemodynamics.[5] In addition, several smaller interatrial fibers run alongside these bundles and play a supplementary role in interatrial conduction.

ATRIOVENTRICULAR NODE AND ATRIOVENTRICULAR CONNECTIONS
Normal and Developmental Anatomy

The AV node receives atrial impulses and acts as a gatekeeper to reduce the transmission of rapid atrial rhythms to the ventricles. It also provides delay of conduction for optimum hemodynamics. The subsidiary pacemaker cells in the AV node can fire at a rate lower than the SAN rate providing a backup rhythm in case of SND. Tawara[1] first described the AV node in 1906 as a compact spindle-shaped structure connected to the His bundle. In adults, it measures approximately 5.0 mm in length, 5.0 mm in width, and 0.8 mm in thickness.[4] It is a right atrial structure located variably within the triangle of Koch (**Fig. 7**) that is defined by the tendon of Todaro, the septal leaflet of the tricuspid valve, and the floor of the coronary sinus ostium.[20] The AV node has rightward and leftward posterior extensions, initially described by Inoue and Becker and recently reevaluated by Anderson and colleagues.[21,22] These extensions provide the anatomic basis of the slow pathway limb of the reentrant circuit in AV nodal reentrant tachycardia.[21] Histologically, these extensions have been identified by examining the distribution of connexin gap channels. The right nodal extension is connexin-43 positive, whereas the left

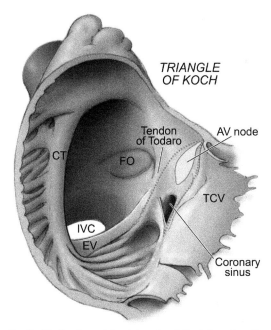

TRIANGLE
OF KOCH

Tendon
of Todaro   AV node

CT   FO

TCV

IVC
EV

Coronary
sinus

Fig. 7. Illustration of the triangle of Koch housing the AV node. CT, crista terminalis; EV, eustachian valve; FO, fossa ovalis; IVC, inferior vena cava; TCV, tricuspid valve.

nodal extension is connexin-43 negative.[23] In contrast with the slow pathway, the anatomic substrate of the fast pathway is not well-defined. It is thought to be made of transitional cells located on the anterior interatrial septum and directed superiorly toward the tendon of Todaro and foramen ovale.[24]

The AV node blood supply is provided by the AV nodal artery, which runs between the 2 posterior extensions of the AV node. The AV nodal artery is most commonly (in 80%–90% of the cases) derived from the right coronary artery (see **Fig. 2**).[25] In the rest of the cases, it originates from the left coronary artery.[25] The AV node is richly innervated with sympathetic and parasympathetic nerves. It is more affected by the left sympathetic and vagus nerves than the right sympathetic and vagus nerves.[26] In addition to vagal innervation, the AV node receives parasympathetic nerves from an epicardial fat pad located at the junction of the right inferior pulmonary vein and inferior left atrium.[27] During embryogenesis, the AV node and AV junction are derived from the AV canal myocardium.[28,29] The left inferior extension is also derived from the AV canal myocardium. The right inferior extension is derived from the primary ring of specialized cardiomyocytes surrounding the interventricular foramen.[30] BMP2 protein is involved in the early stages of the AV canal myocardium differentiation.[31,32]

Several transcription factors, including T-box transcription factors (Tbx2 and Tbx5), are essential for AV canal and AV node formation, as well as AV insulation.[33] The mutations involving BMP-Tbx pathway can lead to AV conduction disorders and AV septal defects (eg, Holt Oram syndrome).[34]

Congenital Anomalies of the Atrioventricular Node

In certain congenital heart diseases, the AV node may be absent, double, or displaced. In heterotaxy, patients with right atrial isomerism may have twin AV nodes (see **Fig. 5**), whereas those with left atrial isomerism have an absent or defective AV node.[35] Twin AV nodes may also be associated with congenitally corrected transposition of great arteries and double inlet left ventricle.

Displacement of the AV node is noted mostly in septal defects. Generally, the location of the AV node is determined by the morphology of AV junction and its alignment with trabecular interventricular septum. In AV septal defects, the AV node is posteroinferiorly displaced (**Fig. 8**).[36] The triangle of Koch is well formed but does not house the AV node. Another triangle is used as an anatomic landmark to locate the AV node in these patients. This triangle is defined by the lower rim of the atrial septum, the posterior attachment of the AV valve, and the coronary sinus.[37] The AV node forms the penetrating His bundle at the apex of this triangle. In patients with AV septal defect and ventricular shunt alone, the AV node is closer to the apex of the triangle of Koch compared with patients with atrial or AV involvement.[36] Other congenital anomalies in which the AV node is abnormally located include congenitally corrected transposition (anterior node), univentricular connection to left ventricle (anterior node), ambiguous AV connection with left-hand architecture (anterior node), and straddling tricuspid valve (lateral node).[37] In patients with perimembranous ventricular septal defects, the conduction axis is close to part of the septal defect borders and is at risk for damage during surgical repair (see **Fig. 8**). To avoid damaging the conduction system, it is recommended to place the sutures through the tricuspid valve leaflet tissue rather than through its attachment.[37]

Pathology of the Atrioventricular Node

The AV node can be affected by several disease processes resulting in AV conduction abnormalities. A list of common AV node pathologies is summarized in **Table 2**. The most common cause of acquired AV block is fibrous degeneration of the conduction system.[38] Another common cause of

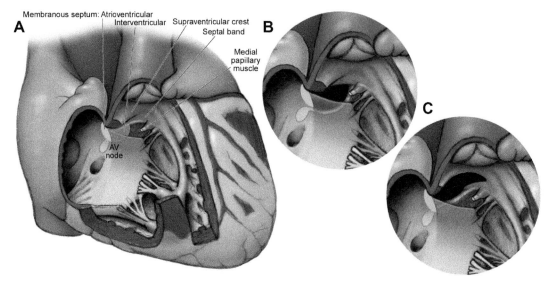

Fig. 8. Displacement of the AV node in AV septal defects. (*A*) Illustration of the normal ventricular septum. Note the proximity of the conduction axis to the lower rim of the septal defect in central perimembranous defects (*B*) and outlet perimembranous defects (*C*).

AV block is ischemia, which accounts for around 40% of AV blocks.[38] Complete AV block after an inferior myocardial infarction tends to be AV nodal owing to either the Bezold-Jarisch reflex or ischemia involving the AV nodal artery. The AV block usually resolves within few days and rarely requires permanent pacing. In contrast, complete AV block after anterior infarction is infranodal and often warrants permanent pacing.[39] AV block associated with ventricular arrhythmias in young patients should raise concern for cardiac sarcoidosis. In cardiac sarcoidosis, conduction disturbances are mainly due to noncaseating granulomatous infiltration of the conduction system.

Key Points for the Proceduralist

Damage to the AV node and/or its blood supply can occur in electrophysiologic procedures such as ablation of AV nodal reentrant tachycardia,

Table 2
Causes of acquired AV block

Pathogenesis	Examples
Ischemic	Acute myocardial infarction
Fibrodegenerative	Lev's disease, Lenegre's disease
Infectious	Bacterial endocarditis (owing to perivalvular extension of an aortic abscess), myocarditis, Lyme's disease, syphilis, rheumatic fever
Infiltrative	Sarcoidosis, amyloidosis, hemochromatosis, carcinoid, malignancy
Connective tissue diseases	Rheumatoid arthritis, systemic lupus erythematosus, systemic scleroderma, ankylosing spondylitis
Neuromuscular disorders	Myotonic dystrophy, Kearns–Sayre syndrome, Friedreich's ataxia
Endocrine	Hypothyroidism
Metabolic	Hyperkalemia
Drug induced	AV nodal blocking agents (beta blockers, calcium channel blocking agents, digoxin), lithium, clonidine
Iatrogenic	Radiation, cardiac surgeries (coronary artery bypass grafting, aortic valve replacement and/or aortic root replacement, surgical repair of AV defects, septal myectomy or alcohol ablation of the interventricular septum).

septal accessory pathways, and septal mitral annular ventricular tachycardia. Knowledge of the exact AV node location is crucial to avoid the risk of causing AV block during these procedures especially given the inability to record electrograms from the AV node. Although the risk of AV block with a slow pathway has been variably reported to be about 1% to 2.3%,[40] an electrophysiologist is expected to keep the risk at less than 1%. During slow pathway ablation, the triangle of Koch is delineated using the His bundle as the apex of the triangle and the coronary sinus as its base. The AV node should be visualized as midseptal within the triangle of Koch. Ablation is then performed inferior to this approximated location of the AV node while maintaining good contact against the septum.[41] AV nodal block can occur anywhere in the septum, even near the coronary sinus ostium, especially near the roof. A safe approach would be to perform a linear ablation from the septal tricuspid annulus to the anterior lip of the coronary sinus at the level of the floor and move up gradually if needed. In septal accessory pathway ablations, ablation of midseptal accessory pathways is associated with a higher risk of AV block (10.4%) as compared with ablation of the anteroseptal (2.7%) and posteroseptal accessory pathways (1%).[42] Owing to the higher risk of AV block in the mid-septal area, cryoablation should be favored over radiofrequency ablation.[43] When radiofrequency ablation is considered in that location, more ventricular ablation would have a theoretically lower risk of AV block.[43]

THE HIS BUNDLE AND BUNDLE BRANCHES
Normal and Developmental Anatomy

The His bundle is a 20-mm long, cord-like ventricular structure, about 4 mm in diameter, extending from the AV node and penetrating the membranous interventricular septum.[44] The collagenous tissue in the membranous septum that forms the central fibrous body encapsulates the His bundle and renders electrical insulation. The His bundle mostly runs on the left of the membranous septum and bifurcates into the left and the right bundle branches at the interventricular crest (**Fig. 9**).

The right bundle branches off at an obtuse angle with an initial intramyocardial course before it becomes more superficial in its distal third in the septomarginal trabecula. It then crosses the right ventricular septum in the moderator band and attaches to the anterior papillary muscle on the right ventricular parietal wall. The left bundle emerges from the base of the interleaflet triangle between the noncoronary and the right sinuses of Valsalva

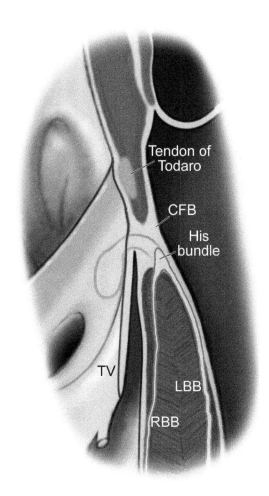

Fig. 9. Penetrating His bundle in the membranous septum giving rise to the left and right bundle branches at the interventricular crest. CFB, central fibrous body; LBBB, left bundle branch; RBB, right bundle branch; TV, tricuspid valve.

(**Fig. 10**).[44] The left bundle is a direct continuation of the His bundle, carrying most of its fibers. It is initially superficial before it becomes slightly deeper in the subendocardial myocardium.

The His bundle has a dual arterial supply from the AV nodal artery and septal perforator of the left anterior descending artery (see **Fig. 2**). The left bundle has a dual blood supply from the right coronary and left anterior descending arteries, and the right bundle is perfused by the septal perforators alone (see **Fig. 2**).

Variations in the Normal Heart

Although the His bundle resides in the lower border of the membranous septum (type 1 anatomy), an autopsy study describes other variations.[45] In about one-third of cases, the His

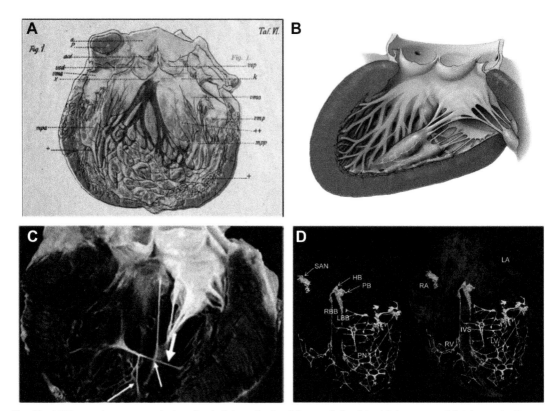

Fig. 10. (*A*) Tawara's monograph showing left bundle, fascicles, and distal Purkinje system. (*B*) Schematic diagram of fan-like fascicular branches of the left bundle. (*C*) False tendons that may house Purkinje fibers. (*D*) Computed tomography micrograph of the conduction system. IVS, interventricular septum; PN, purkinjie network. (*From* Stephenson RS, Boyett MR, Hart G, Nikolaidou T, Cai X, Corno AF, et al. (2012) Contrast Enhanced Micro-Computed Tomography Resolves the 3-Dimensional Morphology of the Cardiac Conduction System in Mammalian Hearts. PLoS ONE 7(4): e35299. https://doi.org/10.1371/journal.pone.0035299)

bundle runs intramyocardially in the interventricular septum (type 2 anatomy). The His bundle has a subendocardial course away from the muscular interventricular septum (type 3 anatomy, also called a naked AV bundle) in about one-fourth of cases.[45] Dandamudi and colleagues[46] propose these anatomic variations as an explanation to why some patients have selective or nonselective His bundle capture only irrespective of high or low pacing outputs.

Congenital Anomalies of the His Bundle

In isolated ventricular septal defects, the AV node and the His bundle are located in usual locations with reference to Koch's triangle.[37] However, patients with a perimembranous ventricular septal defect are at high risk of injury to His bundle if the ventricular septal defect is sutured at the attachment of the tricuspid valve leaflet.[37] In an AV septal defect, the AV node is displaced posteriorly and not in Koch's triangle. The His bundle is located at the apex of a nodal triangle formed by

the lower rim of the atrial septum, posterior attachment of the AV valve, and the coronary sinus.[37] Like AV nodes, a twin His bundle (see **Fig. 5**) may be present in patients with congenitally corrected transposition of great arteries and right atrial isomerism.

Pathology of the His Bundle and Bundle Branches

The causes of AV block have been summarized in **Table 2**. Transcatheter aortic valve replacement has been associated with AV block requiring pacemaker implantation. However, gross anatomic variation of the aortic root and membranous septum is not predictive of pacemaker implantation or new left bundle branch block.[47] Among the familial cardiomyopathies, lamin A/C–related cardiomyopathy is associated with a very high risk for the early development of conduction disorders and sudden cardiac death. Conduction system pacing (**Fig. 11**) is being used increasingly to prevent or treat dyssynchrony from right

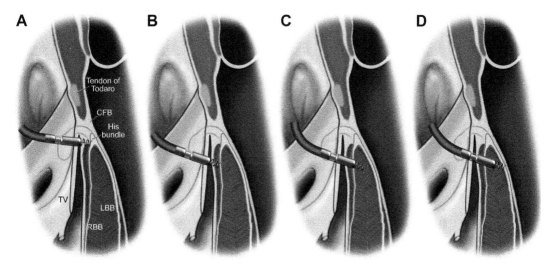

Fig. 11. Conduction system pacing. (*A*) His bundle pacing and (*B–D*) the relative positions of the tip of the lead from the right septum, through deep septum to left bundle area. CFB, central fibrous body.

ventricular pacing or left bundle branch block. It has been demonstrated that pacing at the level of His bundle or proximal left bundle can lead to activation of the conduction system past the presumed level of the block in the distal left bundle. This phenomenon has been attributed to longitudinally dissociated predestined fibers, an idea that was initially proposed by Kaufmann and Rothberger[48] and demonstrated histologically by James and Sherf.[49] However, the presence of longitudinal dissociation has been challenged. Alternative explanations for recruitment of distal fibers with conduction system pacing include (1) modulation of the source-sink relationship and (2) virtual electrode polarization effect.[50] The location of His bundle in the membranous septum in the commissure between septal and anterior tricuspid leaflets allows for selective His bundle pacing and decreased risk of tricuspid regurgitation.[51] However, there is a potential risk conduction system injury during the procedure and a Gerbode-type right atrial–left ventricular defect from membranous septal perforation during implantation or extraction. Although the risk of perforation would be expected to be lower with left bundle area pacing, an attempt to selectively engage the proximal left bundle, which is relatively superficial, may pose such risk as well.

Key Points for the Proceduralist

The membranous septum where the His bundle resides is a confluence of the commissures between the anterior and septal leaflets of the tricuspid valve on the right and between the noncoronary and right coronary sinus of Valsalva on the left.

These structures serve as landmarks for an electrophysiologist during mapping and ablation at or near the His bundle and help to avoid inadvertent His bundle injury and AV block. The right sinus of Valsalva can serve as a vantage point for ablation of para-Hisian premature ventricular contractions and noncoronary sinus of Valsalva for para-Hisian accessory pathways and atrial tachycardia.

Because of the insulation around the His bundle extending into the bundle branches and the fascicles, para-Hisian pacing causes a differential ventriculoatrial conduction time, depending on whether the His bundle is captured or not. Para-Hisian pacing cannot be interpreted in the presence of a fasciculoventricular pathway in which the insulation is breached.

During ablation of bundle branch reentry ventricular tachycardia, the right bundle is preferred as a target because the left bundle is broader and has variable branching pattern and interconnections.[52]

FASCICLES AND THE DISTAL PURKINJE SYSTEM
Normal and Developmental Anatomy

The left bundle gives rise to anterior and posterior fascicles that head toward anterior and posterior papillary muscles (see **Fig. 10**). The posterior fascicle is thicker and shorter compared with the anterior fascicle. There can be a septal or median fascicle that usually arises from the posterior fascicle. The fibers in the fascicles may have intraventricular connections via false tendons (see **Fig. 10**). The fascicular system finally terminates in a mesh-like subendocardial network of noninsulated Purkinje fibers that penetrate about a third of the myocardial thickness.[1] The Purkinje fibers are nonuniformly distributed with a predilection for papillary muscle and midventricle compared with the ventricle base.[1]

Variations in the Normal Heart

As demonstrated by Demoulin and Kulbertus,[53] the left bundle has a variable branching pattern. The branching of the left bundle into discrete anterior and posterior fascicles in human has also been questioned.

Pathology of the Fascicular and Distal His–Purkinje System

The distal Purkinje system has been implicated in the genesis of ventricular arrhythmias owing to its unique properties.[54,55] The redundancy within the Purkinje system allows for reentry even in structurally normal hearts causing fascicular ventricular tachycardia.[56] The Purkinje fibers are relatively resistant to ischemia and may predispose to both automatic and reentrant postinfarction ventricular tachycardia.[57,58] The ventricular ectopy arising from the Purkinje system can trigger idiopathic or long QT-related ventricular fibrillation.[59,60]

Key Points for the Proceduralist

The site of earliest ventricular activation in fascicular ventricular tachycardia may not be a successful site of ablation because it may represent the exit site and true origin may be at a distant site. If the earliest activation is mapped to multiple disparate sites, upstream Purkinje or fascicular signals should be sought during mapping to localize the origin of a fascicular arrhythmia.[52] Similar considerations apply to mapping and ablation of ventricular arrhythmias arising from the endocavitary structures such as the papillary muscles, moderator band, and false tendons. The use of intracardiac echocardiography is of immense importance to allow real-time visualization of these structures.

RETROAORTIC NODE AND BLIND-END TRACT

The AV node in animals has been demonstrated to have right and left inferior extensions with histologic and immunohistochemical characteristics (connexin-43 negative and HCN4 positive) of cardiac conduction tissue.[61] These extensions traverse around the vestibule of the tricuspid valve and the mitral annulus, and unite superiorly in the atrial myocardium behind the aortic root to form the retroaortic node (**Fig. 12**).[61] These specialized cells, derived from embryologic AV ring, are believed

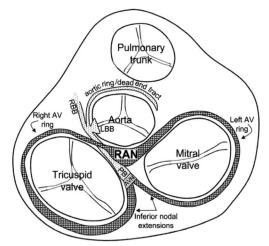

Fig. 12. The retroaortic node (RAN) is formed by the combination of left and right AV rings in the atrial tissue behind the nonsinus of Valsalva. The blind end tract is an extension of the AV conduction axis and fades into the superior intermuscular septum between the aortic and pulmonic valve. (*From* Yanni J, Boyett MR, Anderson RH, Dobrzynski H. The extent of the specialized atrioventricular ring tissues. Heart Rhythm. 2009;6(5):672-680. https://doi.org/10.1016/j.hrthm.2009.01.021, with permission)

to be sequestered in discrete fashion and cause arrhythmias.

Apart from bundle branches, the AV conduction axis is described, in neonates, to have a third extension that forms an aortic ring and fades into the summit of the interventricular septum called the blind-end tract (see **Fig. 12**).[62] These tracts are believed to be remnants of specialized embryologic conduction tissue, and have been implicated in idiopathic ventricular arrhythmias and AV nodal reentrant tachycardia.

INTRAVENTRICULAR CONDUCTION

The conduction of electrical impulses in the ventricular myocardium is based on its complex fiber orientation described elegantly by Torrent-Gausp.[63] In his model, the ventricular myocardium is formed by the folding of a single muscular band from pulmonary artery to aorta in a double-loop helical orientation (**Fig. 13**). Such fiber orientation is responsible for isotropic conduction leading to helical twist during left ventricular contraction.[63] This may have implication in why patients have different responses to cardiac resynchronization therapy, depending on the location of the left ventricular lead. An immediate postimplantation improvement of the left ventricular twist has been shown to predict reverse remodeling with cardiac resynchronization therapy.[64]

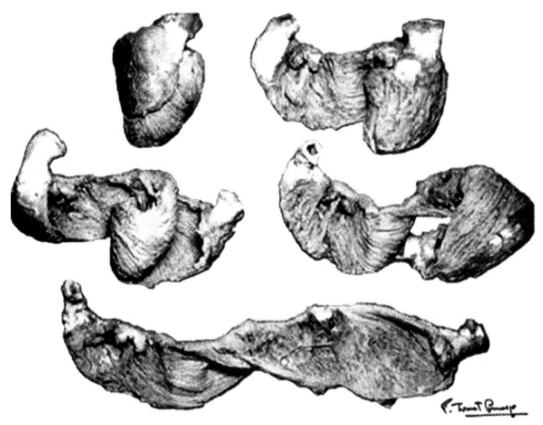

Fig. 13. Torrent–Gausp's model of the helical ventricular myocardial band in bovine hearts. (*Courtesy of* Francisco Torrent-Gausp, MD, Denia, Spain via torrent-guasp.com; with permission.)

SUMMARY

The human conduction system is complex and understanding its normal anatomy and variations both in normal and abnormal hearts is critical to treat patients with arrhythmias related to the conduction system.

CLINICS CARE POINTS

- Ablation of atrial arrhythmias can result in SND. Therefore, preablation planning with a careful review of surgical history and review of computed tomography angiogram can help avoid such complication.
- The sinus and AV nodes can be displaced, duplicate or absent in the presence of congenital anomalies such as septal defects, heterotaxy syndromes and congenitally corrected transposition of great arteries.
- The AV node is located in the triangle Koch, which is defined by the tendon of Todaro, the septal leaflet of the tricuspid valve and the floor of the coronary sinus ostium. Knowledge of the AV node location is crucial to avoid the risk of causing AV block during ablation of AV nodal reentry, septal accessory pathways, and septal mitral annular ventricular tachycardia.
- The His bundle resides in the membranous septum between the anterior and septal leaflets of the tricuspid valve on the right and between the noncoronary and right coronary sinus of Valsalva on the left. Knowledge of these anatomic landmarks help to avoid inadvertent His bundle injury when mapping and ablating at or near the His bundle.
- The earliest activation site may or may not represent the true origin of fascicular ventricular tachycardia. If the earliest activation is mapped to multiple sites, upstream Purkinje or fascicular signals should be mapped to localize the origin of a fascicular arrhythmia.

DISCLOSURE

S.J. Asirvatham receives honoraria or speaker fees from Abiomed, Atricure, Biotronik, Blackwell

Futura, Boston Scientific, Medtronic, Medtelligence, Spectranetics, St. Jude, and Zoll. All other authors have no conflicts of interest to disclose relevant to the content of this article.

REFERENCES

1. Tawara S. Das Reizleitungssystem des Säugetierherzens: eine anatomisch-histologische Studie über das Atrioventrikularbündel und die Purkinjeschen Fäden. Jena: Fischer; 1906.
2. Keith A, Flack M. The form and nature of the muscular connections between the primary divisions of the vertebrate heart. J Anat Physiol 1907;41(Pt 3): 172–89.
3. Murphy C, Lazzara R. Current concepts of anatomy and electrophysiology of the sinus node. J Interv Card Electrophysiol 2016;46(1):9–18.
4. Issa Z, Miller JM, Zipes DP. Clinical Arrhythmology and Electrophysiology: A Companion to Braunwald's Heart Disease E-Book: Expert Consult: Online and Print. Philadelphia PA: Elsevier Health Sciences; 2012.
5. Ho SY, Sánchez-Quintana D. Anatomy and pathology of the sinus node. J Interv Card Electrophysiol 2016;46(1):3–8.
6. Busquet J, Fontan F, Anderson RH, et al. The surgical significance of the atrial branches of the coronary arteries. Int J Cardiol 1984;6(2):223–36.
7. Crick SJ, Sheppard MN, Ho SY, et al. Localisation and quantitation of autonomic innervation in the porcine heart I: conduction system. J Anat 1999; 195(Pt 3):341–57.
8. Hudson RE. The human pacemaker and its pathology. Br Heart J 1960;22(2):153–67.
9. Carlson SK, Patel AR, Chang PM. Bradyarrhythmias in Congenital Heart Disease. Card Electrophysiol Clin 2017;9(2):177–87.
10. Williams MR, Perry JC. Arrhythmias and conduction disorders associated with atrial septal defects. J Thorac Dis 2018;10(Suppl 24):S2940–4.
11. Karpawich PP, Antillon JR, Cappola PR, et al. Pre- and postoperative electrophysiologic assessment of children with secundum atrial septal defect. Am J Cardiol 1985;55(5):519–21.
12. Clark EB, Kugler JD. Preoperative secundum atrial septal defect with coexisting sinus node and atrioventricular node dysfunction. Circulation 1982; 65(5):976–80.
13. Ware AL, Miller DV, Porter CB, et al. Characterization of atrial morphology and sinus node morphology in heterotaxy syndrome: an autopsy-based study of 41 cases (1950-2008). Cardiovasc Pathol 2012; 21(5):421–7.
14. Killu AM, Fender EA, Deshmukh AJ, et al. Acute Sinus Node Dysfunction after Atrial Ablation: Incidence, Risk Factors, and Management. Pacing Clin Electrophysiol 2016;39(10):1116–25.
15. Yasin OZ, Vaidya VR, Chacko SR, et al. Inappropriate Sinus Tachycardia: Current Challenges and Future Directions. J Innov Card Rhythm Manag 2018;9(7):3239–43.
16. Shabtaie SA, Witt CM, Asirvatham SJ. Efficacy of medical and ablation therapy for inappropriate sinus tachycardia: A single-center experience. J Cardiovasc Electrophysiol 2021;32(4):1053–61.
17. Sánchez-Quintana D, Doblado-Calatrava M, Cabrera JA, et al. Anatomical Basis for the Cardiac Interventional Electrophysiologist. Biomed Res Int 2015;2015:547364.
18. Ho SY, Anderson RH, Sánchez-Quintana D. Atrial structure and fibres: morphologic bases of atrial conduction. Cardiovasc Res 2002;54(2):325–36.
19. De PR, Ho SY, Salerno-Uriarte JA, et al. Electroanatomic analysis of sinus impulse propagation in normal human atria. J Cardiovasc Electrophysiol 2002;13(1):1–10.
20. Koch W. Welche Bedeutung kommt dem Sinusknoten zu. Med Klinik 1911;7:447–52.
21. Inoue S, Becker AE. Posterior extensions of the human compact atrioventricular node: a neglected anatomic feature of potential clinical significance. Circulation 1998;97(2):188–93.
22. Anderson RH, Sanchez-Quintana D, Mori S, et al. Re-evaluation of the structure of the atrioventricular node and its connections with the atrium. Europace 2020;22(5):821–30.
23. Temple IP, Inada S, Dobrzynski H, et al. Connexins and the atrioventricular node. Heart Rhythm 2013; 10(2):297–304.
24. Keim S, Werner P, Jazayeri M, et al. Localization of the fast and slow pathways in atrioventricular nodal reentrant tachycardia by intraoperative ice mapping. Circulation 1992;86(3):919–25.
25. Pejković B, Krajnc I, Anderhuber F, et al. Anatomical aspects of the arterial blood supply to the sinoatrial and atrioventricular nodes of the human heart. J Int Med Res 2008;36(4):691–8.
26. Ng GA, Brack KE, Coote JH. Effects of direct sympathetic and vagus nerve stimulation on the physiology of the whole heart–a novel model of isolated Langendorff perfused rabbit heart with intact dual autonomic innervation. Exp Physiol 2001;86(3):319–29.
27. Quan KJ, Lee JH, Van Hare GF, et al. Identification and characterization of atrioventricular parasympathetic innervation in humans. J Cardiovasc Electrophysiol 2002;13(8):735–9.
28. Virágh S, Challice CE. The development of the conduction system in the mouse embryo heart. Dev Biol 1977;56(2):397–411.
29. Moorman AF, Christoffels VM. Cardiac chamber formation: development, genes, and evolution. Physiol Rev 2003;83(4):1223–67.
30. Anderson RH, Sánchez-Quintana D, Mori S, et al. Unusual variants of pre-excitation: from anatomy to

ablation: part I-understanding the anatomy of the variants of ventricular pre-excitation. J Cardiovasc Electrophysiol 2019;30(10):2170–80.

31. Gaussin V, Morley GE, Cox L, et al. Alk3/Bmpr1a receptor is required for development of the atrioventricular canal into valves and annulus fibrosus. Circ Res 2005;97(3):219–26.

32. Yamada M, Revelli JP, Eichele G, et al. Expression of chick Tbx-2, Tbx-3, and Tbx-5 genes during early heart development: evidence for BMP2 induction of Tbx2. Dev Biol 2000;228(1):95–105.

33. Moskowitz IP, Pizard A, Patel VV, et al. The T-Box transcription factor Tbx5 is required for the patterning and maturation of the murine cardiac conduction system. Development 2004;131(16):4107–16.

34. Postma AV, van de Meerakker JB, Mathijssen IB, et al. A gain-of-function TBX5 mutation is associated with atypical Holt-Oram syndrome and paroxysmal atrial fibrillation. Circ Res 2008;102(11):1433–42.

35. Smith A, Ho SY, Anderson RH, et al. The diverse cardiac morphology seen in hearts with isomerism of the atrial appendages with reference to the disposition of the specialised conduction system. Cardiol Young 2006;16(5):437–54.

36. Adachi I, Uemura H, McCarthy KP, et al. Surgical anatomy of atrioventricular septal defect. Asian Cardiovasc Thorac Ann 2008;16(6):497–502.

37. Anderson RH, Ho SY, Becker AE. The surgical anatomy of the conduction tissues. Thorax 1983;38(6):408–20.

38. Zoob M, Smith KS. The aetiology of complete heartblock. Br Med J 1963;2(5366):1149–53.

39. Kusumoto FM, Schoenfeld MH, Barrett C, et al. 2019 2018 ACC/AHA/HRS guideline on the evaluation and management of patients with bradycardia and cardiac conduction delay: executive summary: a report of the American College of Cardiology/American Heart Association Task Force on Clinical Practice Guidelines, and the Heart Rhythm Society. J Am Coll Cardiol 2019;74(7):932–87.

40. Clague JR, Dagres N, Kottkamp H, et al. Targeting the slow pathway for atrioventricular nodal reentrant tachycardia: initial results and long-term follow-up in 379 consecutive patients. Eur Heart J 2001;22(1):82–8.

41. Asirvatham SJ, Stevenson WG. Atrioventricular nodal block with atrioventricular nodal reentrant tachycardia ablation. Circ Arrhythm Electrophysiol 2015;8(3):745–7.

42. Schaffer MS, Silka MJ, Ross BA, et al. Inadvertent atrioventricular block during radiofrequency catheter ablation. Results of the Pediatric radiofrequency ablation Registry. Pediatric Electrophysiology Society. Circulation 1996;94(12):3214–20.

43. Macedo PG, Patel SM, Bisco SE, et al. Septal accessory pathway: anatomy, causes for difficulty, and an approach to ablation. Indian Pacing Electrophysiol J 2010;10(7):292–309.

44. Elizari MV. The normal variants in the left bundle branch system. J Electrocardiol 2017;50(4):389–99.

45. Kawashima T, Sasaki H. A macroscopic anatomical investigation of atrioventricular bundle locational variation relative to the membranous part of the ventricular septum in elderly human hearts. Surg Radiol Anat 2005;27(3):206–13.

46. Dandamudi G, Vijayaraman P. The complexity of the his bundle: understanding its anatomy and physiology through the lens of the past and the present. Pacing Clin Electrophysiol 2016;39(12):1294–7.

47. Tretter JT, Mori S, Anderson RH, et al. Anatomical predictors of conduction damage after transcatheter implantation of the aortic valve. Open Heart 2019;6(1):e000972.

48. Kaufmann R, Rothberger CJ. Beiträge zur Entstehungsweise extrasystolischer Allorhythmien. Z F D G Exp Med 1920;11(1):40–88.

49. James TN, Sherf L. Fine structure of the his bundle. Circulation 1971;44(1):9–28.

50. Sharma PS, Huizar J, Ellenbogen KA, et al. Recruitment of bundle branches with permanent His bundle pacing in a patient with advanced conduction system disease: what is the mechanism? Heart Rhythm 2016;13(2):623–5.

51. Mulpuru SK, Cha YM, Asirvatham SJ. Synchronous ventricular pacing with direct capture of the atrioventricular conduction system: functional anatomy, terminology, and challenges. Heart Rhythm 2016;13(11):2237–46.

52. Munoz FDC, Buescher TL, Asirvatham SJ. Teaching points with 3-Dimensional mapping of cardiac arrhythmias. Circ Arrhythmia Electrophysiol 2011;4(2):e11–4.

53. Demoulin JC, Kulbertus HE. Left hemiblocks revisited from the histopathological viewpoint. Am Heart J 1973;86(5):712–3.

54. Syed FF, Hai JJ, Lachman N, et al. The infrahisian conduction system and endocavitary cardiac structures: relevance for the invasive electrophysiologist. J Interv Card Electrophysiol 2014;39(1):45–56.

55. Scheinman MM. Role of the His-Purkinje system in the genesis of cardiac arrhythmia. Heart Rhythm 2009;6(7):1050–8.

56. Kapa S, Gaba P, DeSimone CV, et al. Fascicular ventricular arrhythmias. Circ Arrhythmia Electrophysiol 2017;10(1):e002476.

57. Szumowski L, Sanders P, Walczak F, et al. Mapping and ablation of polymorphic ventricular tachycardia after myocardial infarction. J Am Coll Cardiol 2004;44(8):1700–6.

58. Bogun F, Good E, Reich S, et al. Role of Purkinje fibers in post-infarction ventricular tachycardia. J Am Coll Cardiol 2006;48(12):2500–7.

59. Haïssaguerre M, Shah DC, Jaïs P, et al. Role of Purkinje conducting system in triggering of idiopathic ventricular fibrillation. Lancet 2002;359(9307):677–8.

60. Haïssaguerre M, Extramiana F, Hocini M, et al. Mapping and ablation of ventricular fibrillation associated with long-QT and Brugada syndromes. Circulation 2003;108(8):925–8.

61. Yanni J, Boyett MR, Anderson RH, et al. The extent of the specialized atrioventricular ring tissues. Heart Rhythm 2009;6(5):672–80.

62. Kurosawa H, Becker AE. Dead-end tract of the conduction axis. Int J Cardiol 1985;7(1):13–20.

63. Torrent-Guasp F. [Structure and function of the heart]. Rev Esp Cardiol 1998;51(2):91–102.

64. Bertini M, Marsan NA, Delgado V, et al. Effects of cardiac resynchronization therapy on left ventricular twist. J Am Coll Cardiol 2009;54(14):1317–25.

Atrioventricular Conduction
Physiology and Autonomic Influences

Eric N. Prystowsky, MD[a,b,*], Jasen L. Gilge, MD[c]

KEYWORDS

- AV node • His-Purkinje system • Autonomic nervous system • AV node reentry • WPW reentry
- Parasympathetic • Sympathetic • Conduction

KEY POINTS

- Changes in the autonomic nervous system can lead to substantial alterations of atrioventricular (AV) nodal conduction.
- The direct effects of increasing heart rate during activity that prolong AV nodal conduction are offset by vagal withdrawal and enhanced sympathetic tone resulting in minimal change in the PR interval.
- Termination of AV and atrioventricular node (AVN) reentry with vagal maneuvers relates to vagal effects on the vulnerable part of the AVN function curve, which is present during tachycardia.
- Heart block during activity is likely in the His-Purkinje system.

INTRODUCTION

Atrioventricular (AV) conduction typically starts with a sinus impulse that activates the atria and subsequently conducts through the atrioventricular node (AVN) and His-Purkinje system (HPS) before activation of the ventricles. The PR interval on the electrocardiogram (ECG) represents the total conduction time through these tissues (**Fig. 1**).[1] This article focuses mainly on AVN conduction, represented by the atrio-His (AH) interval in the figure, but also discusses important aspects of HPS conduction, represented by the His-ventricle (HV) interval in the figure. The influences of the autonomic nervous system (ANS) tone on AV conduction and AVN-dependent arrhythmias also are discussed in depth.

ATRIOVENTRICULAR NODE
Structure

Anatomically, the AVN is located in the right atrium anteriorly at the base of the interatrial septum in the apex of the triangle of Koch.[1–4] It is a complex structure anatomically and electrophysiologically. The compact node has right and left posterior extensions,[5] which may play a role in AVN reentry. Initial microelectrode studies of the AVN subdivided it into 3 functional zones: the atrionodal (AN), nodal (N), and nodo-His (NH) zones,[1] whereas more recent observations suggest 6 different cell types.[6] Cells in the N region seem to correlate with the compact AVN, where block in the AVN typically occurs. Action potentials in the AVN are mediated primarily by calcium channels (slow-channel-dependent) and have fewer intercalated disks, both of which lead to reductions in nodal conduction velocity.[7] Surrounding the compact AVN are transitional cell types, with intermediate histology between atrial myocardium and compact nodal cells. Thus, slow and decremental conduction through the AVN (**Fig. 2**) is multifactorial, depending on factors, such as complex anatomy, reduced electrical cellular coupling, and action potentials dependent on the slow inward calcium current.

This article originally appeared in *Cardiac Electrophysiology Clinics*, Volume 13 Issue 4, December 2021.
[a] Cardiac Arrhythmia Service, St. Vincent Hospital, 8333 Naab Road, Indianapolis, IN 46260, USA; [b] Duke University Medical Center, Durham, NC, USA; [c] St.Vincent Hospital, 8333 Naab Road, Indianapolis, IN 46260, USA
* Corresponding author.
E-mail address: enprysto@ascension.org

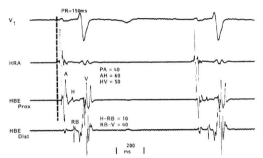

Fig. 1. Intracardiac conduction intervals during the PR interval. Simultaneous recordings from ECG lead V1, high right atrium (HRA), His bundle proximal (HBE prox), and distal (HBE dist) electrode pairs. Sinus impulses conduct to the AVN (PA interval), through the AVN measured as the AH interval, and then to the ventricles by way of the His and the right and left bundles, which comprise the HV interval. The PR interval represents the time it takes to conduct through all these tissues. H-RB, his to right bundle; RB-V, right bundle to ventricle. (*From* Prystowsky EN, Klein GJ, Daubert JP. Cardiac Arrhythmias: Interpretation, Diagnosis, and Treatment, 2nd edition. New York: McGraw Hill; 2020; with permission).

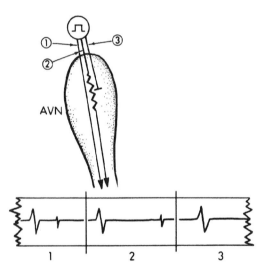

Fig. 2. Wenckebach AV nodal block at electrophysiologic study during incremental atrial pacing. (*top*) The AVN and the impulses conducting through it during pacing. (*bottom*)The AH interval for each beat. The AH interval in beat 1 is relatively short, but the second beat conducts with an increased AH interval. The third atrial paced complex blocks in the AVN. This progressive increase in the AH interval (decremental conduction) is the cause of the increase in PR interval when block occurs in the AVN. (*From* Prystowsky EN, Klein GJ, Daubert JP. Cardiac Arrhythmias: Interpretation, Diagnosis, and Treatment, 2nd edition. New York: McGraw Hill; 2020; with permission).

There appears to be 2 distinct atrial inputs to the AVN, an anterior one via the interatrial septum, and posteriorly by the crista terminalis.[3] The anterior input seems to favor conduction over the "fast" AVN pathway, or the usual mode of AVN conduction, and the posterior input leads to conduction over the "slow" AVN pathway (**Fig. 3**). Although this is likely too simplistic, observations from catheter ablation of AVN reentry generally support this hypothesis.[3]

Induction of the usual form of slow/fast AVN reentry occurs with anterograde block over the fast AVN pathway, conduction over the slow AVN pathway, and retrograde conduction over the fast pathway that has recovered excitability (**Fig. 4**). The initial approach was to ablate the fast pathway inputs in the anterior septum, and this resulted in a marked prolongation of the AH interval supposedly via conduction through the AVN from the posterior atrial AVN inputs. Alternatively, ablation in the posterior right atrial septum cures AVN reentry without any significant change in the AH interval (assuming no damage to the AVN).

Autonomic Inputs

Autonomic innervation of the AVN has been well demonstrated and seems to change with age.[4,8] In a study of 24 human hearts, Chow and colleagues[8] used immunohistochemical and histochemical analysis to analyze the sympathetic and parasympathetic nerve inputs to the AVN. They found an initial sympathetic dominance in infancy,

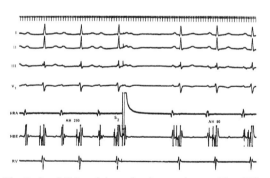

Fig. 3. Dual AV nodal conduction pathways. The ECGs and intracardiac tracings are recorded simultaneously. Note on the first 3 complexes the PR interval is long as is the AH interval (290 milliseconds) because of conduction over the slow AV nodal pathway. A premature atrial stimulus is given that blocks in the AVN. The fourth and subsequently conducted P waves now have normal PR intervals and AH intervals (80 milliseconds) because conduction is over the fast AV nodal pathway. RV, right ventricle. (*From* Prystowsky EN, Klein GJ, Daubert JP. Cardiac Arrhythmias: Interpretation, Diagnosis, and Treatment, 2nd edition. New York: McGraw Hill; 2020; with permission).

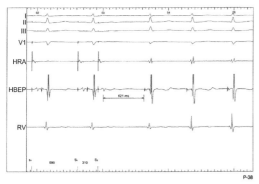

Fig. 4. Initiation of slow-fast AVN reentry at EPS. The atrium is paced, and the third paced beat is premature. There is block in the fast AVN pathway with conduction over the slow pathway (AH 621 milliseconds). The previously blocked anterograde fast pathway has recovered excitability for retrograde conduction allowing AVN reentry to occur. HBEP, proximal his bundle electrogram; RV, right ventricle.

but a more balanced parasympathetic and sympathetic neural input in adulthood. Furthermore, there was a reduction in density of innervation with aging.

Parasympathetic and sympathetic tone exerts negative and positive dromotropic effects, respectively, on AVN conduction. Acetylcholine shortens nodal action potentials, but prolongs post-repolarization refractoriness, with a net effect to slow AVN conduction.[4] In contrast, catecholamine-mediated phosphorylation of L-type calcium channels has a marked effect to enhance inward calcium currents, which leads to an increase in AV nodal conduction velocity.[4] In humans, alterations in autonomic tone can either facilitate or impede AVN conduction (**Fig. 5**).

HIS-PURKINJE SYSTEM

Impulses leave the AVN and enter the HPS, a ventricular specialized conduction system composed of the His bundle, left and right bundle branches, and the peripheral network of Purkinje fibers.[1] The HPS has more rapid conduction properties, and the action potentials are initiated by the fast-acting sodium current. A normal HPS does not usually demonstrate decremental conduction as heart rate increases, because it has rapid accommodation to changes in rate. Thus, when block in the HPS occurs during incremental atrial pacing, it is an abnormal response and signifies a diseased HPS[9] (**Fig. 6**). It is important that evaluation of HPS conduction be done with an incremental atrial pacing run, not by the sudden onset of atrial pacing that can lead to shortening of the atrial cycle length (CL), resulting in a "long-short" sequence with block below the HPS (**Fig. 7**). Block in the HPS in this context is a physiologic, not a pathologic event.[1]

Autonomic Inputs

Autonomic innervation of the HPS has been demonstrated,[8] although the direct effects of the ANS on HPS conduction are generally small in a normal HPS in humans.[1] Changes in autonomic tone can have a direct effect on sinus rate and thereby an indirect effect on HPS conduction, and which predominates is not always clear. Markel and colleagues[10] studied the effects of intravenous atropine, propranolol, or isoproterenol in 4 patients with documented Mobitz II block clinically and below the His at electrophysiologic study. In 2 of 3 patients, propranolol prolonged the atrial pacing cycle length (PCL) with block below the His compared with control; in contrast, in 3 of 4

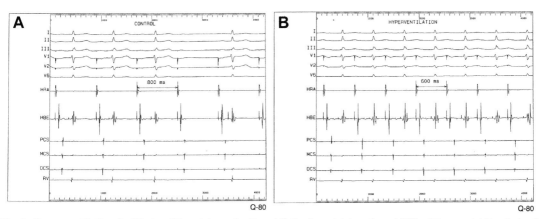

Fig. 5. Hyperventilation facilitates AV nodal conduction. (*A*) During atrial pacing at 800 milliseconds Wenckebach block occurs in the AVN. (*B*) Hyperventilation changes the autonomic inputs to the AVN to facilitate conduction, and even at 600 milliseconds 1:1 AV nodal conduction occurs.

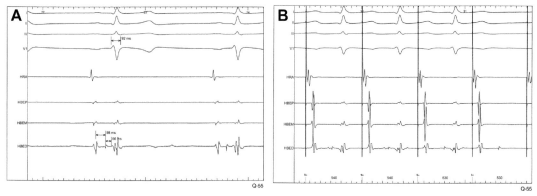

Fig. 6. Diseased HPS with block below the His during incremental atrial pacing. (*A*) HV interval is essentially normal during sinus rhythm. (*B*) During atrial pacing the fourth paced beat blocks below the His recording.

patients, atropine in the presence of propranolol shortened the PCL of block below the His. Isoproterenol in 1 patient improved HPS conduction. Thus, it appears that beta-adrenergic blockers may worsen, whereas atropine can improve dynamic HPS conduction.

Clinical Correlates

Fig. 8 demonstrates the complex interaction of direct and indirect effects of changes in autonomic tone on HPS conduction. During sinus rhythm at rest, there is 1:1 conduction with a prolonged HV interval of 70 milliseconds (see **Fig. 8**A). Atropine 1 mg was given, and the sinus rate increases as does the HV interval with maintenance of 1:1 conduction (see **Fig. 8**B). The heart rate substantially increases with 1.5 mg of atropine, and 2:1 block occurs below the His potential (see **Fig. 8**C).

Maneuvers to alter heart rate may be used to aid in the diagnosis of intra-His or infra-His block. In **Fig. 9**, Mobitz II block is present in a patient who was recovering from cardiac surgery (see **Fig. 9**A). Carotid sinus massage slows the heart rate and restores 1:1 conduction. In **Fig. 9**B at electrophysiology study, block below the His potential is confirmed.

Exercise testing under careful observation can also aid in diagnosing HPS block. **Fig. 10**A shows

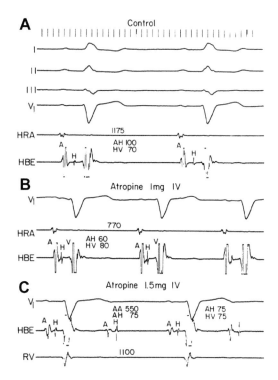

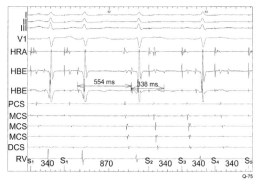

Fig. 7. Physiologic block in the HPS. The first 2 atrial paced beats (S$_1$) conduct to the ventricle. The stimulator is turned off to give a pause of 554 milliseconds. Then, pacing resumes at the same cycle as in the first 2 beats, but 2:1 block below the His recording occurs because of the long-short sequence (554 to 338 milliseconds); this is a physiologic response, not a pathologic one as seen in **Fig. 6**. CS, coronary sinus; DCS, distal CS, MCS, mid CS; PCS, proximal CS.

Fig. 8. The effects of atropine on the HPS with increased heart rate. IV, intravenous. See text for details. (*From* Prystowsky EN, Klein GJ, Daubert JP. Cardiac Arrhythmias: Interpretation, Diagnosis, and Treatment, 2nd edition. New York: McGraw Hill; 2020; with permission).

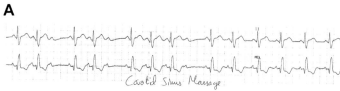

A

Carotid Sinus Massage.

L-77

Fig. 9. Slowing of the heart rate with carotid sinus massage (CSM) improves AV conduction. (*A*) Mobitz II block occurs on the left side of the figure, but CSM slows the sinus rate and restores 1:1 conduction on the right side of the figure. (*B*) Block below the His bundle deflection is noted at EPS.

B

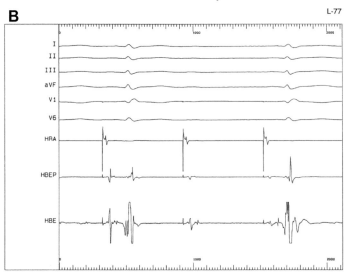

L-77

an ECG with 2:1 AV block. A narrow QRS normally implies the level of block is in the AVN. However, note that the PR interval is normal at about 180 milliseconds. It is relatively rare for 2:1 block to occur in the AVN with a normal PR interval, so one must consider block in the His bundle in this circumstance. The patient was exercised, and the block worsened (**Fig. 10**B). Typically, the PR interval

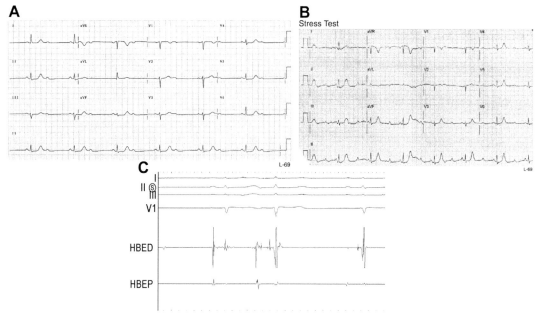

Fig. 10. Block in the His bundle. (*A*) 2:1 AV block. (*B*) AV block worsens during exercise. (*C*) Second complex shows a split His potential, and block would always occur after the first His recording. See text for details. ([*A, C*] *From* Prystowsky EN, Klein GJ, Daubert JP. Cardiac Arrhythmias: Interpretation, Diagnosis, and Treatment, 2nd edition. New York: McGraw Hill; 2020; with permission).

does not change much with exercise, where the effect of increased rate is countered by vagal withdrawal and increased sympathetic tone. At electrophysiology study, intra-His block was demonstrated (**Fig. 10**C), and the patient received a permanent pacemaker.

ATRIOVENTRICULAR NODE CONDUCTION
Atrioventricular Nodal Function Curves

In the 1970s, the concept of enhanced AVN conduction was proposed for a subset of patients who had an AH interval during sinus rhythm of ≤60 milliseconds; 1:1 conduction during atrial PCL to ≤300 milliseconds; and at atrial PCL 300 milliseconds an AH interval ≤100 milliseconds longer than the AH during sinus rhythm.[11] Various theories were proposed as the mechanism of enhanced AVN conduction, including conduction over an atrio-Hisian pathway. The authors studied 160 patients to determine if such a subgroup of patients existed, or whether those with rapid AVN conduction characteristics were merely part of the overall spectrum of AVN behavior.[11] They concluded that patients with these rapid conduction criteria were not a unique subgroup, but rather the lower end of a continuous spectrum of normal AVN physiology.

An important observation on AVN conduction curves was identified by the study of Jackman and colleagues[11] (**Fig. 11**). For each patient, AH measurements were made at atrial PCLs 600, 500, 400, and 300 milliseconds, and at each of the 5- to 10-millisecond intervals before AVN block. The slopes of the segments of each curve were calculated. Importantly, regardless of the shortest PCL with 1:1 conduction, the shape of each curve was similar, as was the slope at the

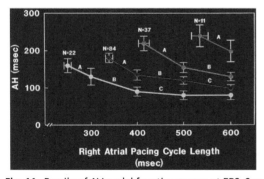

Fig. 11. Family of AV nodal function curves at EPS. See text for details. (*From* Jackman WM, Prystowsky EN, Naccarelli GV, et al. Reevaluation of enhanced atrioventricular nodal conduction: evidence to suggest a continuum of normal atrioventricular nodal physiology. Circulation 1983;67:441-448; with permission).

stressed end of each curve (labeled A). Thus, the shape of this AVN conduction curve during incremental atrial pacing represents a fundamental property of the AVN.

Autonomic Blockade and Atrioventricular Nodal Conduction

In humans, the parasympathetic nervous system predominates over the sympathetic nervous system on sinus rate.[12] Whether this is similar for AVN conduction was investigated by Prystowsky and colleagues.[13] In 13 patients, atrial pacing to assess 1:1 AVN conduction was evaluated in the control state, in the presence of either intravenous propranolol (0.15 mg/kg) or atropine (0.03 mg/kg) alone, and with both drugs (autonomic blockade). The doses of drugs used have been shown to block effectively ANS influences on sinus nodal automaticity in humans.[12] As expected, propranolol increased and atropine decreased the shortest atrial PCL sustaining 1:1 AVN conduction. However, there was no significant difference in atrial PCL with 1:1 conduction at control versus propranolol plus atropine (386 ± 109 to 372 ± 74 milliseconds). Thus, it appears that in contrast to the prepotent effect of the parasympathetic nervous system on sinus nodal automaticity at rest, vagal and adrenergic tone have a more balanced effect on resting AV nodal conduction.

In a follow-up study, the authors evaluated the effect of autonomic blockade in patients with normal and abnormal AV nodal function.[14] To define a normal atrial PCL with 1:1 conduction, 168 patients without ECG AVN conduction abnormalities were studied. Using the 95th percentile, normal was defined as a shortest atrial PCL with 1:1 conduction less than 505 milliseconds. In 14 patients with normal AVN conduction, atrial PCL with 1:1 conduction did not change from control to autonomic blockade (361 ± 16 to 359 ± 14 milliseconds). However, in the 9 patients with abnormal AVN conduction, atrial PCL with 1:1 conduction shortened from control to autonomic blockade (610 ± 33 to 493 ± 20 milliseconds). If one considers AVN conduction in the presence of autonomic blockade as the intrinsic AV nodal conduction, then the patients with abnormal AVN conduction at rest also had significantly longer atrial PCL with 1:1 conduction versus those in the normal AVN conduction group. There was a clear predominance of vagal tone on AVN conduction in patients with intrinsically abnormal AV nodal conduction.

All patients had normal PR intervals, so there would be no way of knowing which ones had an intrinsic abnormality of AVN conduction. This has several potential clinical consequences. It may explain why some people are more prone to vagal-mediated heart block during sleep. Furthermore, patients with an abnormal intrinsic AVN may demonstrate exaggerated responses to drugs, such as beta-adrenergic blockers or slow-channel blockers, especially during atrial fibrillation. Further research is needed in this area.

Isoproterenol and Atrioventricular Nodal Conduction

Increased sympathetic tone can accelerate sinus rate and improve AV nodal conduction. It is important to keep the heart rate constant to determine the effects of increased adrenergic tone on AV nodal conduction. Because AV nodal function curves do not depend on the shortest atrial PCL with 1:1 conduction,[11] one can study the effects of isoproterenol in patients by comparing the same parts of the curve before and after isoproterenol infusion. **Fig. 12** shows the results from such a study in patients with normal PR intervals (Eric N. Prystowsky, MD, unpublished data). Atrial pacing was performed before and after isoproterenol was given at 1 ug/min constant infusion. At the longest mean atrial PCL of 650 milliseconds, the AH interval shortened by a mean of 34 milliseconds. However, there was a significant and marked 63-millisecond shortening of the AH interval at the atrial PCL (414 milliseconds) near the steep slope of the curve. This was the authors' first observation that alterations in autonomic tone appear to have a differential effect on AV nodal conduction depending on whether they occur during the flat or stressed part of the functional AV nodal curve.

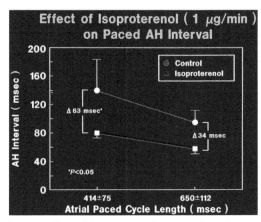

Fig. 12. Effect of isoproterenol on paced AH interval at different points on the AVN function curve. See text for details. (*From* Prystowsky EN, Klein GJ, Daubert JP. Cardiac Arrhythmias: Interpretation, Diagnosis, and Treatment, 2nd edition. New York: McGraw Hill; 2020; with permission).

Enhanced Vagal Tone and Atrioventricular Node Conduction

Page and colleagues[15] investigated the effect of enhanced vagal tone on AV nodal conduction and sinus nodal automaticity. To augment reflex vagal tone, a constant intravenous infusion of phenylephrine (0.74 ± 0.41 ug/kg/min) was given to 10 patients. The mean diastolic blood pressure increased during the infusion from 76 to 89 mm Hg. This technique allowed the authors to study the enhanced vagal effects in a new steady state. Incremental atrial pacing was performed before and during the infusion, and AH intervals for each patient were measured at the long (845 ± 132 milliseconds) and short (575 ± 209 milliseconds) atrial PCLs (**Fig. 13**). The AH interval during sinus rhythm was not significantly prolonged with enhanced vagal tone. The shortest atrial PCL with 1:1 conduction significantly increased during phenylephrine infusion from 412 ± 120 to 575 ± 211 milliseconds. There was a significant increase in the mean AH interval at both the longer and the shorter atrial PCLs. However, the mean increase in AH interval of 59 milliseconds at the shorter PCL was significantly greater than the 18 milliseconds at the longer PCL. Thus, the effect of enhanced vagal tone was greater on the stressed or steeper part of the functional AV nodal curve.

A comparison was done of the magnitude of changes in sinus nodal automaticity with AV nodal conduction during phenylephrine infusion. Importantly, although enhanced vagal tone significantly increased sinus CL and the shortest atrial PCL with 1:1 conduction, there was a lack of correlation between the two. This has important clinical implications, because one cannot judge the magnitude of enhanced vagal tone on the AVN, and likely other cardiac tissues, by the degree of sinus slowing.

Combined heart rate and autonomic nervous system effects on atrioventricular nodal conduction

The above data demonstrate that in a resting state, increasing the heart rate with atrial pacing will yield a progressive lengthening of the AH interval until AV nodal block occurs. However, during normal daily activity, increases in heart rate are accompanied by predictable changes in autonomic tone, with enhanced sympathetic and reduced parasympathetic effects on the AVN. **Fig. 14** illustrates how these opposing changes affect the AH interval and therefore the PR interval in a person without HPS disease.

Note that the resulting PR interval is nearly the same as the heart rate increases, and one need

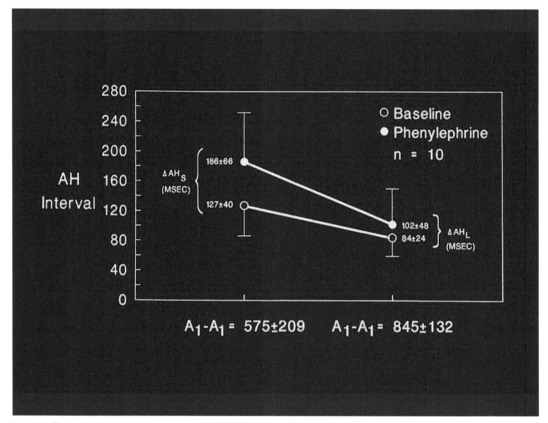

Fig. 13. Effect of enhanced reflex parasympathetic tone during intravenous phenylephrine infusion on AH interval at different points of the AV node function curve. See text for details. (*From* Page RL, Tang AS, Prystowsky EN. Effect of continuous enhanced vagal tone on atrioventricular nodal and sinoatrial nodal function in humans. Circulation Research 1991;68:614-620; with permission).

merely measure the PR interval during a treadmill examination to confirm this observation. If there is a marked increase in the PR interval, or block occurs, consider disease in the HPS, even if the

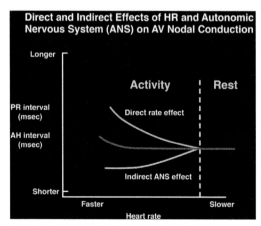

Fig. 14. Direct and indirect effects of heart rate and ANS on AV nodal conduction and the PR interval. See text for details.

QRS is normal (see **Fig. 10**). A constant PR interval improves hemodynamics, and if the PR increased enough that the P wave fell within the T wave at faster heart rates, a pacemaker-like syndrome may occur. Thus, the system works amazingly well!

A clinical pearl from all of this is to measure the PR interval on rhythm strips when trying to decide whether an atrial tachycardia or sinus tachycardia is present. An atrial tachycardia is like pacing the atrium without the advantage of the autonomic changes that occur with sinus tachycardia. Thus, if the PR during sinus rhythm is shorter than during the tachycardia, consider the possibility of an atrial tachycardia; if it is the same, sinus tachycardia is usually present.

SUPRAVENTRICULAR TACHYCARDIA AND AUTONOMIC NERVOUS SYSTEM
Atrioventricular Reentry

Atrioventricular reentry (AVRT) comprises several tissue types in its circuit (**Fig. 15**). However, the

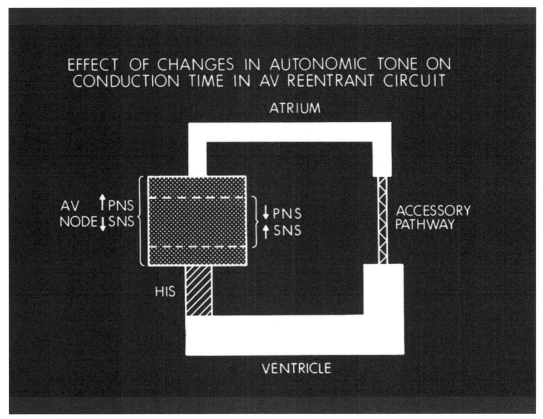

Fig. 15. The components of the AV reentry circuit, and the effects of changes in autonomic tone on it. Changes in CL are mainly due to ANS effects on AV nodal conduction. The AVN acts like an accordion "opening and closing" with alterations of parasympathetic (PNS) and sympathetic (SNS) nervous system tone on it. See text for details.

CL of tachycardia is usually decided by the anterograde properties of the AVN, a dramatic example of which is the change in AVRT CL when anterograde conduction over the fast AV nodal pathway switches to the slow AV nodal pathway.[16]

Increased adrenergic tone can shorten atrial and ventricular refractoriness to some degree, as well as the accessory pathway (AP),[17] but the effects on the AVN usually predominate. Enhanced vagal tone shortens atrial refractoriness,[18] whereas resting vagal tone increases ventricular refractoriness,[13] but has minimal effect on AP conduction and refractoriness.[19] As noted above, changes in vagal tone can have marked effects on AV nodal refractoriness and conduction. Thus, alterations in ANS tone primarily affect AVRT CL by its effect on the AVN.

Autonomic Changes and Atrioventricular Reentry Cycle Length

As described above, changes in autonomic tone have their greatest effect on the stressed part of the AV nodal function curve. The authors (Eric N. Prystowsky, MD, unpublished data) studied a group of patients with AVRT using a concealed AP for retrograde conduction to determine if AV nodal conduction during AVRT was at the stressed part of the curve. They further evaluated the effects of vagal withdrawal and adrenergic enhancement on the AVRT circuit (**Fig. 16**). The term "electrophysiologic reserve" is used to calculate

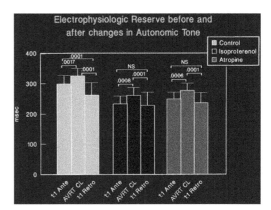

Fig. 16. Electrophysiologic reserve before and after changes in autonomic tone. Ante, anterograde; Retro, retrograde. NS, non significant. See text for details.

how close the 1:1 conduction over the AP and AVN are to the AVRT CL.

Patients were studied first in the control state; then, after constant intravenous infusion of isoproterenol to increase sinus rate by about 20%, and after washout of isoproterenol, intravenous atropine was given in graded doses to approximate the sinus rate during isoproterenol infusion. The authors recognized that the changes in sinus rate by both agents do not necessarily mirror alterations of AV nodal conduction. At control and ANS perturbations, atrial and ventricular pacing were performed to assess 1:1 conduction over the AVN and AP, and AVRT was induced.

At control, the 1:1 AVN conduction was typically about 30 milliseconds shorter than the AVRT CL, placing it on the stressed area of the AVN function curve. Note that there was more "reserve" with retrograde conduction over the AP. Both isoproterenol and atropine shorted the AVRT CL. Retrograde 1:1 conduction over the AP shortened with isoproterenol, but unexpectedly also with atropine. Note that the 1:1 AVN conduction still was within 30 milliseconds of the AVRT CL, again on the stressed part of the AVN conduction curve. The more pronounced effect of vagal withdrawal and adrenergic enhancement on AV nodal conduction lessened the electrophysiologic reserve of the AVRT circuit, as 1:1 AP conduction was now closer to the AVRT CL.

These observations demonstrate the AVRT CL "finds" its fastest rate at various levels of autonomic tone. The AH interval during AVRT is on the steep slope of its curve, and at faster rates would lengthen the AVRT CL.

Clinical Correlates

AV nodal conduction is most vulnerable at the stressed part of its function curve, and this explains why enhanced vagal tone can terminate AVRT yet exert minimal effect on AVN conduction in sinus rhythm. **Fig. 17** shows an example of enhanced vagal tone during breath-holding in a patient with AVRT induced at electrophysiologic study. Note that it terminates tachycardia, yet the returning sinus impulse conducts with a normal AH interval along with preexcitation. Similar examples are seen with carotid sinus massage, and this also explains why intravenous verapamil and adenosine can terminate paroxysmal supraventricular tachycardias but minimally prolong PR interval during sinus rhythm.

Autonomic Changes and Atrioventricular Nodal Reentry

Changes in ANS can affect AV nodal reentry. At electrophysiologic study, isoproterenol or

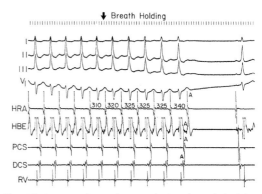

Fig. 17. Increased vagal tone during breath holding terminates AVRT at electrophysiologic study. See text for details. (*From* Prystowsky EN, Klein GJ, Daubert JP. Cardiac Arrhythmias: Interpretation, Diagnosis, and Treatment, 2nd edition. New York: McGraw Hill; 2020; with permission).

epinephrine may be needed to facilitate induction of AVN reentry by exerting positive effects on AV nodal conduction and refractoriness.[20] In contrast, enhanced vagal tone has a negative dromotropic effect on AV nodal conduction. Chiou and colleagues[19] studied 10 patients with AVN reentry at control and during enhanced parasympathetic tone using constant phenylephrine infusion. Enhanced vagal tone prolonged 1:1 conduction time over the anterograde fast and slow pathways, and retrograde fast pathway. However, phenylephrine prolonged the effective and functional refractory periods of the anterograde fast pathway but had no effect on the refractoriness of the anterograde slow or retrograde fast pathway. Such disparate results in vagal-induced refractoriness on these pathways may explain the common occurrence of AVN reentry occurring at rest and during sleep. One could imagine a premature atrial complex during increased vagal tone blocking over the fast AVN pathway but being able to conduct over both the anterograde slow pathway and the retrograde fast pathway, allowing AVN reentry to occur.

Clinical Correlate

Hyperventilation can have substantial effects on autonomic tone, with vagal withdrawal and sympathovagal imbalance.[21] Chen and colleagues[21] studied the effects of hyperventilation on AV nodal function in patients with AVRT and AVN reentry. In patients with slow-fast AVN reentry, hyperventilation significantly improved 1:1 conduction over the anterograde fast and slow pathways, and over the retrograde fast pathway. In 7 of 9 patients without AVNRT induced at baseline state, initiation occurred during hyperventilation (**Fig. 18**). Patients

Hyperventilation Facilitates Induction of AVN Reentry

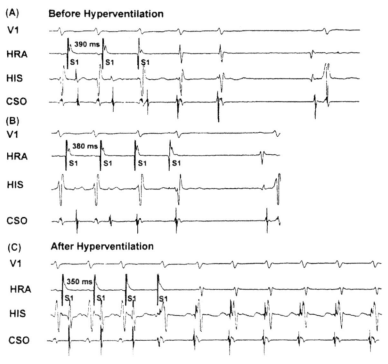

Fig. 18. Hyperventilation facilitates induction of AV nodal reentry at electrophysiologic study. See text for details. (*From* Chen CC, Chen SA, Tai CT, et al. Hyperventilation facilitates induction of supraventricular tachycardia: a novel method and the possible mechanism. J Cardiovasc Electrophysiol 2001;12:1242-1246. doi:10.1046/j.1540-8167.2001.01242.x; with permission).

diagnosed with panic disorders can have PSVT that is undiagnosed.[22] It is possible that hyperventilation, which is common in this disorder, can help to initiate AVNRT or AVRT in these individuals.

Atrial Flutter

Fig. 19 demonstrates increased AVN block in atrial flutter during left carotid massage. Concealed conduction occurs during atrial flutter, and Page and colleagues[23] evaluated the effect of vagal

enhancement on concealed conduction in the AVN.

Enhanced reflex vagal tone was produced using constant intravenous phenylephrine infusion. Page and colleagues[23] found that enhanced vagal tone could magnify the effects of concealed AVN conduction. They further hypothesized that the common occurrence of 4:1 block during atrial flutter often seen during times of increased vagal tone, such as sleep, might be explained by augmentation of concealed conduction (**Fig. 20**).

Left CSM

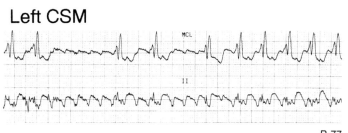

Fig. 19. Left CSM increases level of block in atrial flutter. See text for details.

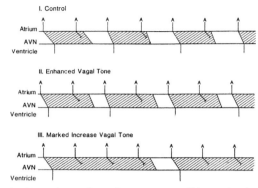

Fig. 20. Enhanced vagal tone as a possible mechanism for 4:1 AV block in atrial flutter. (*top*) 2:1 AV block occurs, and the blocked flutter complex occurs near the end of AVN refractoriness (shaded area). (*middle*) Increased vagal tone that prolongs AVN refractoriness, and the blocked beat is now further away from the end of refractoriness. (*bottom*) Marked vagal tone that causes such an increase in refractoriness that the third beat is blocked, and the concealed conduction from that beat prolongs refractoriness even more, resulting in block of the fourth beat, with a 4:1 conduction pattern in the AVN. (*From* Page RL, Wharton, JM, Prystowsky EN. Effect of continuous vagal enhancement on concealed conduction and refractoriness within the atrioventricular node. Am J Cardiol 1996;77:260-265. doi:10.1016/s0002-9149(9789390-3) with permission)

Clinical Examples of Autonomic Nervous System Effects on Atrioventricular Node Conduction

Fig. 21 shows heart block during sleep. Note that the third PP interval suddenly lengthens and is associated with the first nonconducted P wave. When there is a concomitant increase in the PP interval and heart block, the mechanism is increased parasympathetic tone. Remember, the magnitude of the vagal effect may be different on the sinus and AV nodes, and thus the degree of PP increase is not as important as the fact that it does lengthen.

Fig. 22 is taken during an episode of sleep apnea in a patient with an implantable loop recorder. As in **Fig. 21**, the PP interval lengths but the effect on AV nodal conduction is more pronounced. Treating the sleep apnea eliminated the heart block in this patient.

Fig. 23 occurred during swallowing in a patient with deglutition syncope. There is more than a 7-second pause of all electrical activity. In the absence of high vagal tone, one would have expected a junctional escape complex sooner. This demonstrates that extremely high levels of vagal tone can suppress not only the sinus and AV nodes, but also lower subsidiary pacemakers.

Fig. 24 occurred in a patient with atrial tachycardia. **Fig. 24**A is during rest with 3:1 conduction.

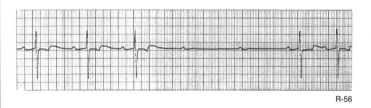

Fig. 21. Heart block during sleep owing to enhanced vagal tone. See text for details.

Sleep Apnea

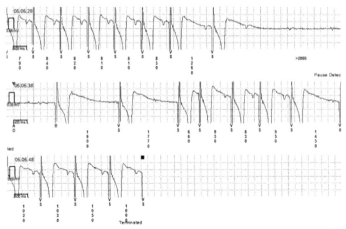

Fig. 22. Heart block during an episode of sleep apnea. See text for details.

Near Syncope While Swallowing

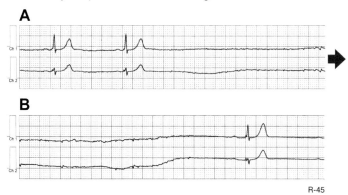

A

B

R-45

Fig. 23. Deglutation syncope. See text for details.

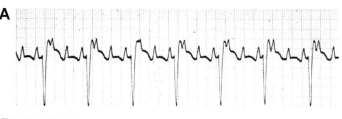

A

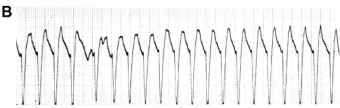

B

Fig. 24. Improvement in AVN conduction during atrial tachycardia from rest (*A*) to activity (*B*). See text for details. (*From* Prystowsky EN, Klein GJ, Daubert JP. Cardiac Arrhythmias: Interpretation, Diagnosis, and Treatment, 2nd edition. New York: McGraw Hill; 2020; with permission).

Fig. 24B was during activity and now shows 1:1 conduction. The increase in ventricular response results from vagal withdrawal and enhanced sympathetic tone. Such changes commonly occur during atrial fibrillation, and rate control should be assessed throughout the day to be sure adequate control is achieved.

DISCLOSURE

None.

REFERENCES

1. Prystowsky EN. Cardiac conduction. In: Prystowsky EN, Klein GK, Daubert JP, editors. Cardiac arrhythmias: interpretation, diagnosis, and treatment. 2nd edition. New York: McGraw Hill; 2020. p. 3–33.
2. Tawara S. Das Reizleitungssystem des Saugetierherzens: Eine Anatomisch-Histologische Studie uber das Atrioventrikurbundel und die Purkinjeschen Faden. Jena, Germany: Fischer; 1906.
3. Prystowsky EN. Atrioventricular node reentry: physiology and radiofrequency ablation. PACE 1997; 20(Pt. II):552–71.
4. Markowitz SM, Lerman BB. A contemporary view of atrioventricular nodal physiology. J Interv Card Electrophysiol 2018;52:271–9.
5. Inous S, Becker AE. Posterior extensions of the human compact atrioventricular node: a neglected anatomic feature of potential clinical significance. Circulation 1998;97:188–93.
6. Billette J. Atrioventricular nodal activation during periodic premature stimulation of the atrium. Am J Phys 1987;252:H163–73.
7. Temple IP, Inada S, Dobrzynski H, et al. Connexins and the atrioventricular node. Heart Rhythm 2013; 10:298–304.
8. Chow LTC, Chow SSM, Anderson RH, et al. Autonomic innervation of the human cardiac conduction system: changes from infancy to senility—an immunohistochemical and histochemical analysis. Anat Rec 2001;264:169–82.
9. Dhingra RC, Wyndham C, Baurenfeld R, et al. Significance of block distal to the His bundle induced by

atrial pacing in patients with chronic bifascicular block. Circulation 1979;60:1455–64.

10. Markel ML, Miles WM, Zipes DP, et al. Parasympathetic and sympathetic alterations of Mobitz type II heart block. J Am Coll Cardiol 1998;11:271–5.

11. Jackman WM, Prystowsky EN, Naccarelli GV, et al. Reevaluation of enhanced atrioventricular nodal conduction: evidence to suggest a continuum of normal atrioventricular nodal physiology. Circulation 1983;67:441–8.

12. Jose AD, Taylor RR. Autonomic blockade by propranolol and atropine to study intrinsic myocardial function in man. J Clin Invest 1969;48:2019–31.

13. Prystowsky EN, Jackman WM, Rinkenberger R, et al. Effect of autonomic blockade on ventricular refractoriness and atrioventricular nodal conduction in humans. Evidence supporting a direct cholinergic action on ventricular muscle refractoriness. Circ Res 1981;49:511–8.

14. Rahilly GT, Zipes DP, Naccarelli GV, et al. Autonomic blockade in patients with normal and abnormal atrioventricular nodal function. Am J Cardiol 1982;49(IV):898.

15. Page RL, Tang AS, Prystowsky EN. Effect of continuous enhanced vagal tone on atrioventricular nodal and sinoatrial nodal function in humans. Circ Res 1991;68:614–20.

16. Pritchett ELC, Prystowsky EN, Benditt DG, et al. Dual atrioventricular nodal pathways in patients with Wolff-Parkinson-White syndrome. Br Heart J 1980;43:7–13.

17. Wellens HJJ, Brugada P, Roy D, et al. Effect of isoproterenol on the anterograde refractory period of the accessory pathway in patients with the Wolff-Parkinson-White syndrome. Am J Cardiol 1982;50:180–4.

18. Prystowsky EN, Naccarelli GV, Jackman WM, et al. Enhanced parasympathetic tone shortens atrial refractoriness in man. Am J Cardiol 1983;51:96–100.

19. Chiou CW, Chen SA, Kung MH, et al. Effects of continuous enhanced vagal tone on dual atrioventricular node and accessory pathways. Circulation 2003;107:2583–8.

20. Patel PJ, Segar R, Patel JK, et al. Arrhythmia induction using isoproterenol or epinephrine during electrophysiology study for supraventricular tachycardia. J Cardiovasc Electrophysiol 2018. https://doi.org/10.1111/jce.13832.

21. Chen CC, Chen SA, Tai CT, et al. Hyperventilation facilitates induction of supraventricular tachycardia: a novel method and the possible mechanism. J Cardiovasc Electrophysiol 2001;12:1242–6.

22. Lessmeier TJ, Gamperling D, Johnson-Liddon V, et al. Unrecognized paroxysmal supraventricular tachycardia. Potential for misdiagnosis as panic disorder. Arch Intern Med 1997;157:537–43.

23. Page RL, Wharton JM, Prystowsky EN. Effect of continuous vagal enhancement on concealed conduction and refractoriness within the atrioventricular node. Am J Cardiol 1996;77:260–5.

Electrocardiography of Atrioventricular Block

Bradley A. Clark, DO[a],*, Eric N. Prystowsky, MD[b,c]

KEYWORDS

- Atrioventricular node • Atrioventricular delay • Dual atrioventricular node physiology
- Second degree type 1 atrioventricular block • Wenckebach
- Second degree type 2 atrioventricular block • Complete heart block
- Third degree atrioventricular block

KEY POINTS

- Atrioventricular (AV) conduction may be delayed in the atrium or His-Purkinje conduction system but is most commonly delayed in the AV node.
- Second degree type 1 AV block (Wenckebach; Mobitz 1) can occur at any level of the conduction system but most commonly occurs in the AV node with progressive PR prolongation prior to a blocked P wave along with other typical features.
- Second degree type 2 AV block (Mobitz 2) occurs without warning, as there is no PR prolongation preceding the blocked P wave.
- 2:1 AV block precludes the diagnosis of type 1 or type 2 second degree AV block, but clues from the baseline electrocardiogram may suggest the location of the block.

INTRODUCTION

Understanding normal cardiac conduction and common and uncommon anomalies is critical to interpreting both electrograms and intracardiac electrograms. Normal sinus rhythm begins in the sinoatrial node (SAN) at the superior and lateral aspect of the right atrium. This is recognized on the electrocardiogram (ECG) as the initiation of the P- wave, representing atrial depolarization that begins as the impulse exits the SAN. There is a wavefront of activation that progresses right to left and cranial to caudal across the atria and toward the atrioventricular (AV) node, where conduction is slowed and then enters the His-Purkinje system (HPS). The subsequent surface activation is represented by a QRS complex resulting from ventricular activation.[1]

ATRIOVENTRICULAR DELAYED CONDUCTION

Understanding various types of AV block requires knowledge of the normal flow of conduction through the cardiac electrical system as stated previously to understand better where delay or block may occur.

Delayed AV conduction will result in PR prolongation (PR interval >200 milliseconds). This is typically referred to as first degree AV block, but there is no actual block of impulses to the ventricle. The authors prefer first degree AV conduction delay, but realize that block is ingrained in ECG parlance and will not likely be changed. Delay can occur at any point from the atrium through the AV node and HPS up to the activation of the ventricles. The most common site of delay causing PR prolongation is within the AV node. This is demonstrated

This article originally appeared in *Cardiac Electrophysiology Clinics*, Volume 13 Issue 4, December 2021.

[a] St.Vincent Hospital, 10590 North Meridian Street, Suite 200, Indianapolis, IN 46290, USA; [b] Cardiac Arrhythmia Service, St. Vincent Hospital, 8333 Naab Road, Indianapolis, IN 46260, USA; [c] Duke University Medical Center, Durham, NC, USA

* Corresponding author.

E-mail address: bradley.clark@ascension.org

Cardiol Clin 41 (2023) 307–313
https://doi.org/10.1016/j.ccl.2023.03.007

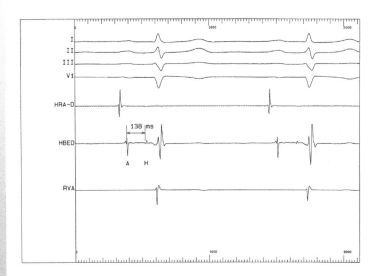

Fig. 1. First degree AV conduction delay with prolonged AH interval. Simultaneous tracings are from ECG leads I, II, III and V1. HBED, His-bundle distal electrogram, HRA, high right atrium, RVA, right ventricular apex.

on an intracardiac ECG by a prolonged AH interval as is evident in **Fig. 1**. When the QRS is normal as in **Fig. 1**, the delay is almost always in the AV node. However, when the QRS is wide, reflecting disease of the HPS, delay may be in the AV node, HPS, or both as detailed in the first chapter of the book "Cardiac Arrhythmias" by Prystowsky and colleagues.[1] This is also stated in Mark Josephson's text from 2016 with a wide QRS complex most compatible with infra-His disease but which may also occur with A-V nodal or intra-His disease in the presence of coexistent bundle branch block with an incidence ranging from 20% to 50%.[2]

Fig. 2 depicts a relatively rare form of AV conduction delay solely caused by slowing of conduction below the level of the His. In this case, the delay that caused PR prolongation was profound. Delay below the AV node is more concerning because of the elevated risk of progression to high grade AV block with an unstable and typically slow escape rhythm.[3]

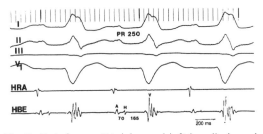

Fig. 2. First degree AV delay and left bundle branch block with normal AH interval and HV prolongation. HBED, His-bundle distal electrogram, HRA, high right atrium, RVA, right ventricular apex. (*From* Prystowsky EN, Klein GJ, Daubert JP. Cardiac Arrhythmias: Interpretation, Diagnosis, and Treatment, 2nd edition. New York: McGraw Hill; 2020; with permission.)

It is generally accepted that PR prolongation is a benign finding; however, this was refuted by a study out of Harvard in 2009 evaluating the Framingham population that suggested that PR prolongation is associated with increased risks of AF, pacemaker implantation, and all-cause mortality.[4] This remains controversial, however, as other studies including a large European study showed no increase in mortality or in hospitalizations because of coronary artery disease, heart failure, atrial fibrillation, or stroke associated with prolonged PR interval.[5]

DUAL ATRIOVENTRICULAR NODE PHYSIOLOGY

Many patients have dual inputs to the AV node with evidence of fast and slow pathway conduction. The exact mechanism by which conduction passes into and through the AV node has not been completely elucidated despite the existence of multiple theories.[6,7] However, with dual AV node physiology, there may be a normal PR interval at baseline, but pacing maneuvers can unmask slow pathway conduction with an increase in the AH interval. **Fig. 3** shows an uncommon occurrence where a baseline ECG shows minimal PR prolongation when conduction occurs over the fast AVN pathway, and at a different time marked PR prolongation with conduction occurring over the slow pathway. In panel B of **Fig. 3**, the fast pathway is refractory that allows for slow pathway conduction.

Another anomalous occurrence in patients with dual AV node physiology is seen when conduction occurs over both the fast and slow pathway with a subsequent two for one phenomenon. This is

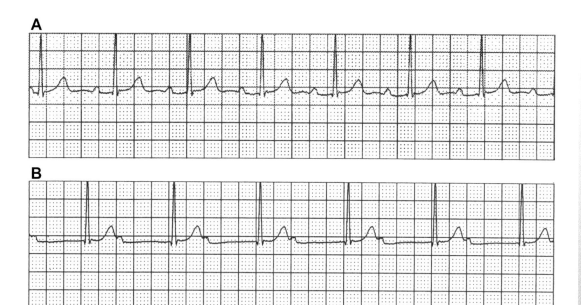

A

B

Fig. 3. (*A*) Tracing showing minimal PR interval prolongation in a patient with normal QRS interval. (*B*) The same person with a tracing showing marked PR prolongation consistent with slow pathway conduction consistent with dual AV node physiology.

represented by ventricular activation occurring twice for every atrial input. The mechanism by which this occurs has not been proven but is hypothesized to include a lack of retrograde concealed conduction into the slow pathway.[8] Sinus rhythm with a normal PR interval in a patient without this two for one response would typically lead to conduction over the fast pathway with retrograde conduction into the slow pathway preventing subsequent anterograde activation of the ventricle over the slow pathway.

SECOND DEGREE TYPE 1 ATRIOVENTRICULAR BLOCK (WENCKEBACH; MOBITZ 1)

Grouped beating is the hallmark of type 1 second degree AV block but is not diagnostic. Second

degree type 1 AV block typically begins as delay in the AV node, resulting in progressive PR prolongation followed by AV block with subsequent recovery of the PR interval (**Fig. 4**). Note that the first delay is more than subsequent delays (30 milliseconds vs 10 milliseconds), and this leads to the progressive shortening of the RR intervals before block. The RR interval containing the blocked P wave is shorter than the sum of 2 PP intervals. When the QRS is normal, AV block is almost always in the AV node, with the relatively rare occurrence of intra-Hisian block.[1]

Wenckebach phenomenon can occur at any level of the conduction system outside of the AV node. In **Fig. 5**, Wenckebach block occurs below the His bundle recording with the same findings of grouped beating. Note that the patient has a

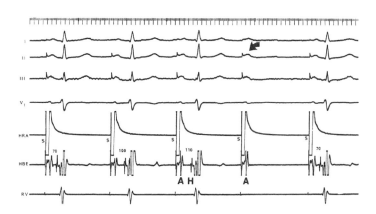

Fig. 4. Second degree type 1 (Wenckebach) AV nodal block. Arrow points to a nonconducted P wave. (*From* Prystowsky EN, Klein GJ, Daubert JP. Cardiac Arrhythmias: Interpretation, Diagnosis, and Treatment, 2nd edition. New York: McGraw Hill; 2020; with permission.)

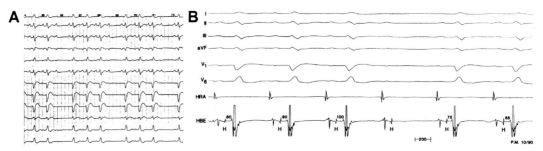

Fig. 5. (*A*) Minimal PR prolongation leading up to AV block in the setting of left bundle branch block suggests infra-His block. (*B*) Infra-His Wenckebach shown with progressive HV prolongation prior to AV block. The patient in this example was taking both propafenone and amiodarone to suppress VT in the era before ICDs. (**Fig. 1**; ICD, implantable cardiac defibrillator).

left bundle branch block, evidence of HPS disease. However, Wenckebach block even in the presence of a wide QRS complex usually occurs in the AV node. There are some clues to block below the AV node in such patients: minimal increase in the PR interval, normal or minimal PR interval prolongation at baseline, and block occurring at faster heart rates. Diseased HPS is more prone to block as the heart rate increases.

Delay in the AV node alone is not life threatening, with Wenckebach being relatively common and without the need for permanent pacemaker placement. However, block below the AV node is concerning and warrants intervention.

Atypical Wenckebach is a phenomenon where the greatest increment in AV conduction time is noted with the last PR interval prior to block. This is likely caused by the presence of dual AVN physiology.

SECOND DEGREE TYPE 2 ATRIOVENTRICULAR BLOCK (MOBITZ II)

As one considers higher levels of AV block it is prudent to recognize the clinical importance of identifying these abnormalities and proceeding with appropriate intervention to avoid increased morbidity and mortality. Second degree type 2 AV block occurs without warning, that is, there is no prolongation of PR interval preceding the blocked P wave, but rather sudden AV block. With rare exception, block occurs within the

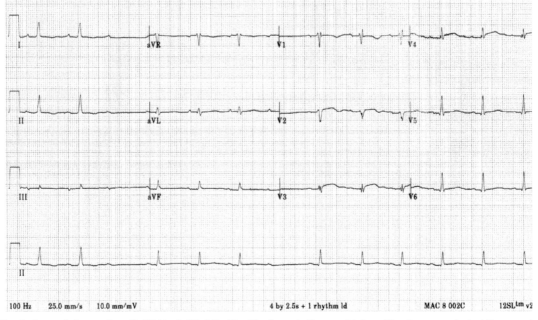

Fig. 6. Second degree type 2 AV block (Mobitz II) with sinus rhythm and intermittent nonconducted P waves in the absence of progressive PR prolongation.

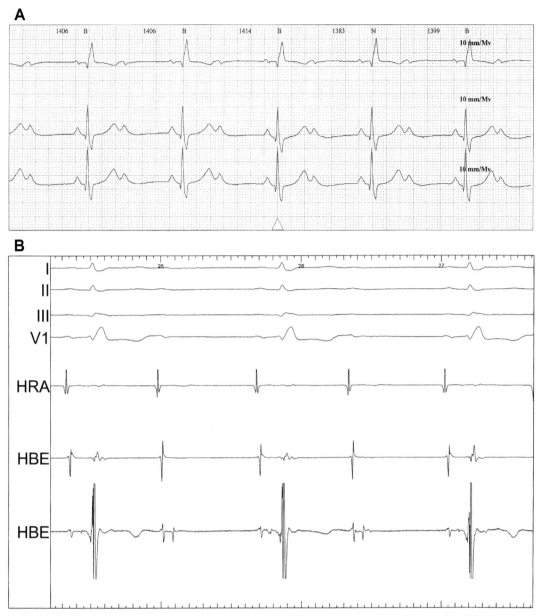

Fig. 7. (*A*) Right bundle branch block with 2:1 conduction. (*B*) Intracardiac tracing showing block below the His recording (see text for details).

HPS, and the QRS complex is wide. Typically, there is 1 nonconducted P wave with recurrence of conduction with the subsequent P wave. This is illustrated in **Fig. 6**.

TWO TO ONE ATRIOVENTRICULAR BLOCK

The phenomenon of 2:1 AV block is its own separate category, for every other beat is blocked, precluding diagnostic information gained from progressive or sudden changes in AV conduction.

In a patient with normal QRS complex and substantial PR prolongation on the conducted beat, block is almost always in the AV node; if the PR interval is normal, one needs to consider block within the His bundle, for in the authors' experience, it is rare to have 2:1 block in the AV node with a normal QRS and PR interval.[1]

Patients with a wide QRS complex and 2:1 AV block present a challenge, for block may be in the AV node or HPS. An important clue to HPS block is a normal or nearly normal PR interval in

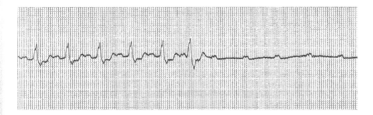

Fig. 8. Sinus rhythm with PR prolongation and bundle branch block followed by complete AV block preceded by a PVC consistent with paroxysmal AV block.

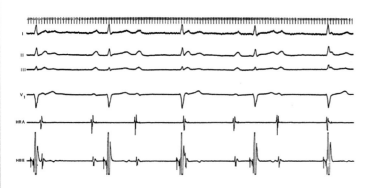

Fig. 9. Complete AV block with sinus rhythm completely dissociated from the junctional escape rhythm. Note a His deflection in front of each QRS complex.

the conducted beat (**Fig. 7**). This observation is based on the fact that in patients with block in the AV node, there is typically a prolonged AH interval (120 milliseconds or more) on nonblocked beats. Thus, one merely needs to do the math; if it takes about 30 to 40 milliseconds for a sinus beat to reach the AVN, and about 35 to 55 milliseconds to go through the HPS, then the shorter the PR interval, the less likely the AH is abnormal. So, if the PR interval is normal, block in the HPS is most likely, and needs to be considered even if the patient is asymptomatic.

PAROXYSMAL ATRIOVENTRICULAR BLOCK

Paroxysmal AV block occurs suddenly following a premature atrial or ventricular complex (**Fig. 8**). In the few cases where there are intracardiac recordings during block, the block has been in the HPS. Block can be prolonged because of the lack of a stable escape rhythm and lead to syncope or even sudden death. The lack of a stable escape rhythm is concerning, and although this phenomenon is rare, it also warrants pacemaker implantation.

COMPLETE HEART BLOCK

In complete heart block (third degree AV block) there is complete AV dissociation, with an atrial rhythm totally independent of an escape rhythm. That escape rhythm can either be junctional (typical of congenital heart block), resulting in conduction with narrow QRS complex, or bundle branch block pattern if the patient had a bundle branch block at baseline, or from a subnodal focus with a wide QRS complex. **Fig. 9** is an example from a patient with congenital heart block and shows a junctional escape rhythm independent of the sinus rhythm and a normal QRS complex.

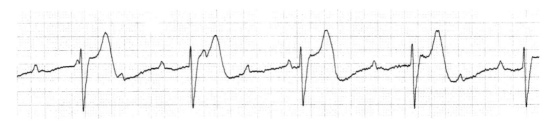

Fig. 10. Complete heart block as evidenced by sinus rhythm completely dissociated from a wide QRS complex escape rhythm.

An escape rhythm from the HPS or ventricle is typical in a patient with acquired complete heart block (**Fig. 10**).

It is important to look for irregularities of the escape rhythm when assessing for the presence of complete AV block. Complete AV dissociation most commonly includes a stable escape rhythm without significant R-R variation. If variation in the R-R interval is identified, then one should determine if there is incomplete AV dissociation with occasional capture beats.

CLINICS CARE POINTS

- When assessing an ECG for second degree type 1 AV block (Wenckebach) look for grouped beating with progressive PR prolongation and progressive shortening of the RR intervals prior to a blocked P wave.

- Block below the AV node may be suggested by a minimal increase in the PR interval, and block occurring at faster heart rates.

- When assessing 2:1 AV block, look for a short PR interval and wide QRS to suggest infranodal disease, whereas a prolonged PR interval is suggestive of AV nodal disease. Both a short PR and narrow QRS suggest intra-His disease.

DISCLOSURE

None.

REFERENCES

1. Prystowsky EN. Cardiac conduction. In: Prystowsky EN, Klein GK,, Daubert JP, editors. Cardiac arrhythmias: interpretation, diagnosis, and treatment. 2nd edition. New York: McGraw Hill; 2020. p. 3–33.

2. Josephson ME. Atrioventricular conduction. In: Josephson ME, editor. Clinical cardiac electrophysiology. 5th edition. Philadelphia: Lippincott Williams & Wilkins; 2016. p. 93–112.

3. Scheinman MM, Peters RW, Modin GU, et al. Prognostic value of infranodal conduction time in patients with chronic bundle branch block. Circulatio 1977;56: 240–344.

4. Cheng S, Keyes MJ, Larson MG, et al. Long-term outcomes in individuals with prolonged PR interval or first-degree atrioventricular block. JAMA 2009; 301(24):2571–7.

5. Aro AL, Anttonen O, Kerola T, et al. Prognostic significance of prolonged PR interval in the general population. Eur Heart J 2014;35(2):123–9.

6. Prystowsky EN. Atrioventricular node reentry: physiology and radiofrequency ablation. Pacing Clin Electrophysiol 1997;20(Pt. II):552–71.

7. Markowitz SM, Lerman BB. A contemporary view of atrioventricular nodal physiology. J Interv Card Electrophysiol 2018;52:271–9.

8. Kertesz NJ, Fogel RI, Prystowsky EN. Mechanism of induction of atrioventricular node reentry by simultaneous anterograde conduction over the fast and slow pathways. J Cardiovasc Electrophysiol 2005; 16(3):251–5.

Physiologic Variants of Cardiac Conduction (Aberration, Gap, Supernormal Conduction)

William M. Miles, MD*, Philip George, MD

KEYWORDS

- Aberration • Bundle branch block • Long-short aberration • Rate-dependent aberration
- Gap phenomenon • Supernormal conduction

KEY POINTS

- Several criteria help distinguish ventricular tachycardia from supraventricular tachycardia with aberrancy, but exceptions occur with all of them.
- Major categories of aberration are long-short aberration and rate-dependent (acceleration- and deceleration-dependent) aberration.
- Long-short aberration can occur in normal His-Purkinje tissue, and once initiated at the onset of tachycardia, commonly persists for a variable duration caused by concealed transseptal conduction.
- Gap phenomenon and supernormal conduction are two potential explanations for unexpected improvement in conduction on shortening of the coupling interval.

INTRODUCTION

In the normal electrocardiogram (ECG), the QRS complex is "narrow," meaning it is less than 120 milliseconds in duration. There are several mechanisms that cause wide (>120 milliseconds) QRS complexes that must be differentiated (**Box 1**). Most importantly, ventricular tachycardia must be distinguished from supraventricular tachycardia with wide QRS complexes. Supraventricular tachycardia may present as a wide QRS complex tachycardia caused by either a fixed bundle branch block or a functional (ie, intermittent) bundle branch block. Functional bundle branch block may occur because of two basic mechanisms[1]:

1. *Long-short aberration* (Ashman phenomenon) occurs when a long RR interval is followed by

a short RR interval that meets refractoriness in one or both of the bundle branches. This phenomenon is usually physiologic and occurs in patients with otherwise normal hearts.

2. *Rate-dependent aberration* comes in two varieties. In the acceleration-dependent (sometimes termed tachycardia-dependent) variety, bundle branch block occurs suddenly on gradual acceleration of the heart rate, and the QRS duration normalizes on deceleration. In the less common deceleration-dependent (bradycardia-dependent) variant, the QRS suddenly widens on critically long RR intervals and disappears with shorter RR intervals. Rate-dependent aberration is usually associated with structural heart disease, although it can occur early in a cardiomyopathy before any other manifestations are apparent.

This article originally appeared in *Cardiac Electrophysiology Clinics*, Volume 13 Issue 4, December 2021.
University of Florida College of Medicine, 1329 S.W. 16th Avenue, PO Box 100288, Gainesville, Florida 32608, USA
* Corresponding author.
E-mail address: william.miles@medicine.ufl.edu

Cardiol Clin 41 (2023) 315–332
https://doi.org/10.1016/j.ccl.2023.03.006

Two other etiologies of wide QRS complexes generated by supraventricular ventricular activation are preexcitation and toxic-metabolic QRS changes. In preexcitation, the ventricle is activated via fusion of anterograde conduction via the atrioventricular (AV) node/His-Purkinje system and an accessory pathway. This can result in minor QRS widening at baseline but prominent QRS widening after an atrial extrasystole that encounters physiologically slowed conduction in the AV node but not in the accessory pathway (**Fig. 1**).

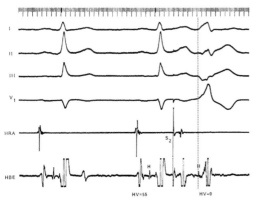

Fig. 1. QRS widening caused by ventricular preexcitation, exposed by an atrial extrastimulus. Sinus rhythm demonstrates a normal His-ventricular (HV) interval and normal QRS duration. Because of the left lateral location of the accessory pathway, AV nodal conduction beats it out during sinus rhythm and there is little to no preexcitation. However, an atrial extrastimulus (S2) exposes the accessory pathway by prolonging the AH interval, allowing the accessory pathway to widen the QRS complex with an initial slur (delta wave) and a resultant HV "interval" of 0. In preexcitation, the HV interval does not represent a true conduction interval, but varies with the degree of AV node/accessory pathway fusion.

Causes of toxic-metabolic widening of the QRS complex include hyperkalemia (**Fig. 2**), acidosis, ischemia, and overdoses of medications that block the fast sodium channel (eg, class IA or IC antiarrhythmic drugs, such as quinidine, propafenone, or flecainide; tricyclic antidepressants; and certain other drugs, such as loperamide[2]). Toxic-metabolic QRS widening resolves quickly once the drug/toxin is removed or metabolic abnormalities reversed.

DIFFERENTIATION OF VENTRICULAR TACHYCARDIA FROM SUPRAVENTRICULAR TACHYCARDIA WITH ABERRANCY

A variety of criteria may be helpful for differentiation of ventricular tachycardia from supraventricular tachycardia with aberrancy using the surface ECG; however, there are exceptions to these general rules (especially in patients with preexcitation), and sometimes the differentiation cannot be established with confidence from the surface ECG and requires intracardiac recordings.

1. AV dissociation and the occurrence of capture and/or fusion beats during tachycardia strongly suggest ventricular tachycardia.
2. If available, the mode of tachycardia initiation may be helpful; if the first wide QRS follows a premature atrial depolarization, supraventricular tachycardia with aberration is favored. If the first beat of tachycardia is a fusion beat, ventricular tachycardia is favored (**Fig. 3**).
3. Regularity versus irregularity may be helpful. A markedly irregular wide QRS rhythm suggests atrial fibrillation with aberration or preexcitation; sustained ventricular tachycardia is commonly but not always regular.
4. QRS duration greater than 140 milliseconds suggests ventricular tachycardia rather than aberration, but preexisting wide QRS complexes and/or drug effects may cause an aberrated QRS to be greater than 140 milliseconds.
5. The more bizarre the QRS axis, the more likely the rhythm is ventricular tachycardia or preexcitation. Precordial QRS complexes that are all concordant and oriented in the same direction suggest ventricular tachycardia rather than aberration.
6. Criteria have been developed for helping differentiate wide QRS tachycardias based on QRS morphology.[3–6] If the QRS has a right bundle branch block–like morphology in lead V1, then a monophasic R wave in V1, a qR in V1, a deep S wave in V6, or R wave taller than the r prime in V1 all suggest ventricular tachycardia rather than aberration. If the wide QRS complex has a left bundle branch block–like morphology in V1, then an R wave in V1 of greater than or

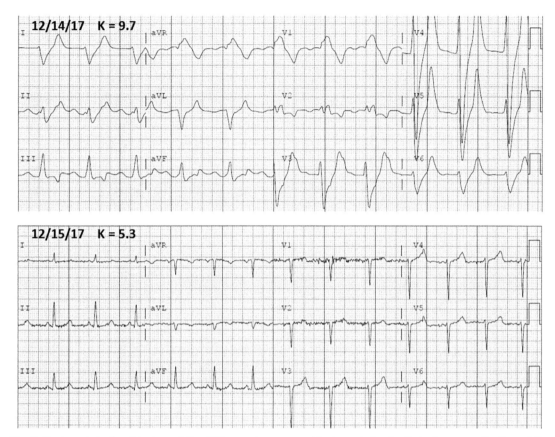

Fig. 2. Toxic-metabolic widening of the QRS complexes caused by hyperkalemia. Note the normalization of the QRS with correction of the hyperkalemia.

equal to 30 milliseconds, a slurred or notched downstroke of the S wave in V1/V2, QRS duration greater than or equal to 70 milliseconds from the onset to the nadir in V1/V2, or any Q waves in V6 suggest ventricular tachycardia rather than aberration. Thus, in general, the more the QRS morphology resembles that of typical right or left bundle branch block, the more likely it represents aberration. If there is a known bundle branch block during sinus rhythm, a wide QRS tachycardia with a similar QRS morphology is likely supraventricular.

7. aVR alone may be a reasonably good discriminator: an initial R wave, an initial r or q wave greater than 40-millisecond duration, notching on the initial downstroke of a predominantly negative QRS, or a ratio of the vertical excursion (in millivolt) recorded during the initial and terminal 40 milliseconds of the QRS less than or equal to 1 suggest VT.[7]

LONG-SHORT ABERRANCY

The term "aberration" was coined by Sir Thomas Lewis and clearly illustrated in an ECG from his 1910 publication.[8] Aberrant conduction of a short-coupled supraventricular impulse following a long RR interval is termed long-short aberrancy (Ashman phenomenon). Typical scenarios where long-short aberrancy commonly occurs include premature atrial contractions, atrial fibrillation, and atrial tachycardia/flutter with variable AV conduction. Long-short aberrancy is a manifestation of normal His-Purkinje physiology,[9] not infrequently seen in young people with normal hearts and robust AV node function, allowing tightly coupled atrial impulses to reach the bundle branches.

Long-short aberrancy occurs because His-Purkinje refractoriness is directly dependent on cycle length; that is, the longer the RR interval, the longer the bundle branch refractory periods.[10] Thus, in contrast to AV nodal tissue, a short-coupled impulse is more likely to block in His-Purkinje tissue if preceded by a long RR interval than a shorter RR interval (**Fig. 4**). Because the right bundle branch refractory period is usually longer than that of the left bundle branch at most physiologic heart rates,[11] right bundle branch block is more common in long-short aberrancy than left bundle branch block. If the refractory

SVT with Aberration

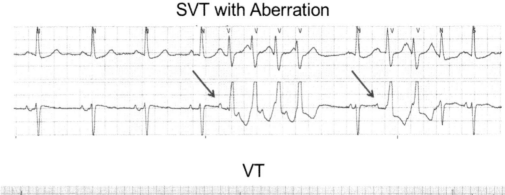

VT

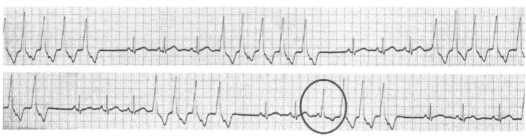

Fig. 3. Short runs of wide QRS tachycardia caused by aberration versus ventricular tachycardia. (*Top*) The clue that this is supraventricular tachycardia with aberration is the identification of the premature P wave preceding the initial long-short aberrated QRS (*arrows*). (*Bottom*) The clue that this represents ventricular tachycardia is that an initial QRS complex (*circle*) demonstrates a short PR and a fusion complex (ie, contributions by the sinus impulse arriving via the His-Purkinje system and the first beat of ventricular tachycardia). SVT, supraventricular tachycardia; VT, ventricular tachycardia.

period of both bundle branches is exceeded by the short-coupled RR interval, no AV conduction occurs because of bilateral bundle branch block or intra-His block. This may occur at initiation of tachycardia and can persist as 2:1 AV conduction during AV node reentrant or atrial tachycardia (discussed later).

Once aberration is initiated at the onset of tachycardia, functional bundle branch block may continue, resolving either spontaneously after a short period of time or when the tachycardia is perturbed. Perpetuation of aberration beyond the first long-short beat is caused by concealed transseptal conduction (**Fig. 5**). The blocked bundle branch is repetitively activated retrogradely via transseptal conduction arriving late (toward the end of the QRS complex) via the contralateral (conducting) bundle branch. Thus, as tachycardia continues, the blocked bundle branch, having been activated late by the preceding beat, "sees" a shorter bundle-to-bundle interval on the subsequent beat than the actual tachycardia cycle length; the blocked bundle branch thus remains refractory, and the aberration persists. This phenomenon of transseptal conduction can result in alternating forms of aberration (**Fig. 6**).

On initiation of tachycardia, most bundle branch refractory period shortening occurs immediately

following the first beat at the shorter cycle length, but further gradual shortening occurs as tachycardia continues, resulting in a new steady state after several complexes at the new cycle length (accommodation of refractoriness).[12,13] As bundle branch refractoriness gradually shortens, it may allow the aberration to resolve spontaneously, even if there is no change in cycle length (**Fig. 7**). In addition to accommodation of refractoriness, other mechanisms may contribute to resolution of aberration. Some authors have postulated a progressive decrease in the degree of transseptal retrograde penetration into the blocked bundle branch with each beat of tachycardia, eventually allowing resumption of anterograde conduction in the blocked bundle branch. In addition, activation of the sympathetic nervous system by the tachycardia may promote slight shortening of the bundle branch refractory period. Tachycardia cycle length wobble, if present, could also allow recovery of anterograde bundle branch conduction on the longer RR intervals (**Fig. 8**).

FUNCTIONAL 2:1 ATRIOVENTRICULAR BLOCK

In some individuals, especially young, healthy patients and during adrenergic stimulation to accelerate AV nodal conduction, long-short aberration

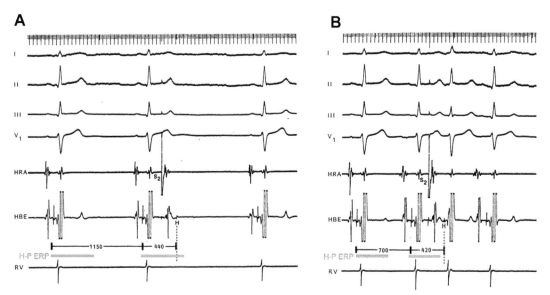

Fig. 4. Long-short refractoriness is directly dependent on the preceding RR interval. (*A*) Sinus rhythm has a cycle length of 1150 ms. An atrial extrastimulus results in an HH interval of 440 ms and functional long-short block below His (block in distal His or both left and right bundle branches). (*B*) An even shorter HH interval following the atrial extrastimulus conducts over both bundle branches and generates a normal QRS complex. This paradox is explained by the much longer RR interval preceding the atrial extrastimulus in *A* compared with *B*. The His-Purkinje effective refractory periods (ERP), represented by the *horizontal bars*, are estimated for each panel; the longer ERP caused by the longer sinus cycle length causes infra-His block of the atrial extrastimulus, and the shorter ERP at the shorter sinus cycle length allows conduction. The refractory period of His-Purkinje tissue (and atrial, ventricular, and accessory pathway tissue, but not AV nodal tissue) is directly related to the cycle length of the preceding RR interval.

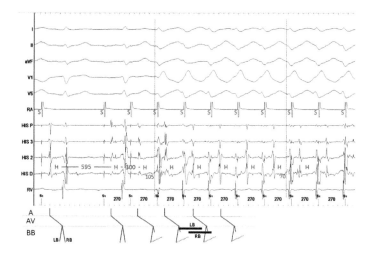

Fig. 5. Intracardiac recordings of initiation and persistence of long-short aberrancy on sudden initiation of rapid atrial pacing. When atrial pacing cycle length is suddenly decreased from 600 to 270 ms (resulting in an HH interval of 595 followed by 300 ms), long-short functional right bundle branch block aberration occurs. Following the first long-short right bundle branch block complex, the aberration persists as atrial pacing continues at a cycle length of 270 ms, despite no further long-short intervals. This persistence of aberration after its initiation by the long-short interval is caused by concealed transseptal conduction; that is, after the right bundle branch blocks anterogradely, the distal right bundle branch is activated retrogradely late in the QRS complex via left-to-right transseptal conduction (*ladder diagram*). Thus, when the subsequent atrial paced impulse arrives at the His bundle, the right bundle branch "sees" a shorter coupling interval than the left bundle branch block (*horizontal bars*), and remains blocked even as the left bundle branch has recovered excitability. This perpetuation of functional aberrancy with continuation of tachycardia is a common phenomenon following long-short aberrancy, despite no further long-short intervals.

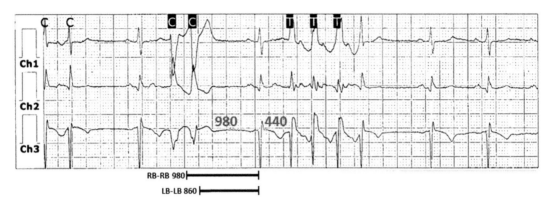

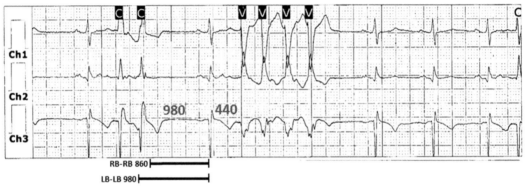

Fig. 6. Alternating aberrancy resulting from differences in bundle branch coupling intervals because of concealed transseptal conduction. Both strips demonstrate sinus rhythm with two- to four-beat bursts of long-short aberrated atrial ectopy. Similar coupling intervals (980, 440 ms) have been selected for display, and channel 3 is similar to a lead V1. (*Top*) The atrial couplet demonstrates left bundle branch block aberration. After the pause, the four-beat run has right bundle branch block aberration. (*Bottom*) Conversely, the atrial couplet has right bundle branch block aberration, and the subsequent four-beat run has left bundle branch block aberration despite the same coupling intervals as the *Top*. The explanation for the alternating aberration is that each bundle branch "sees" a different coupling interval as defined by its concealed transseptal activation. In the *Top* (as demonstrated by the *black horizontal bars*) when functional left bundle branch block occurs, concealed transseptal conduction from the right bundle branch retrogradely invades the left bundle branch late in the QRS, causing the subsequent right-bundle to right-bundle interval to be longer than the left-bundle to left-bundle interval; this discrepancy in bundle-bundle activation favors long-short right bundle branch aberration of the subsequent run of atrial tachycardia, consistent with the rules of long-short aberrancy. The converse is the case for the *Bottom*.

from a premature impulse at the onset of tachycardia can result in either intra-His block or simultaneous left and right bundle branch block, resulting in AV block of the atrial extrasystole. Just as functional bundle branch block can persist during tachycardia after the initial long-short aberration as described previously, functional 2:1 AV block can also persist, giving rise to tachycardias, such as AV node reentry or atrial tachycardia with functional (physiologic) 2:1 AV conduction (**Fig. 9**). The site of functional block is either within both bundle branches simultaneously, or in the proximal or distal His bundle. If the site of block is distal to the His recording site, intracardiac tracings reveal a His potential associated with every QRS complex, even those without conduction to the ventricle; if the site of block is within the His bundle proximal to the His recording site, a His potential may not be recorded before block. However, during 2:1 tachycardia, the ability of ventricular extra-stimuli to "peel back" His-Purkinje refractoriness and allow resumption of 1:1 AV conduction during tachycardia illustrates that the site of block is in His-Purkinje rather than AV nodal tissue.[14]

After the long-short initiation of infra-His block, the functional persistence of 2:1 AV conduction is explained by a repetitive long-short pattern effecting the bundle branches during tachycardia (**Fig. 10**). The His bundle "sees" the actual tachycardia cycle length, but the bundle branches

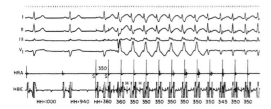

Fig. 7. Initiation, persistence, and resolution of functional aberrancy. There is onset of long-short right bundle branch block aberrancy on initiation of atrial pacing at a cycle length of 350 ms. There is persistence of right bundle branch block for seven complexes (via concealed transseptal conduction, as discussed previously). The aberrancy then resolves spontaneously despite no change in the pacing cycle length or the HH intervals. Spontaneous resolution of functional bundle branch block commonly occurs after several beats of tachycardia and thought to be related to accommodation of refractoriness. On initiation of tachycardia, most of the eventual decrease in His-Purkinje refractoriness occurs after the first beat of tachycardia; however, there is some gradual further shortening of bundle branch refractoriness to the new steady state as the increased rate persists, and if shortening is sufficient, aberrancy resolves. (*From* Miles WM, Prystowsky EN. Alteration of human right bundle branch refractoriness by changes in duration of the atrial drive train. Circulation 1986;73:244-8; with permission)

"see" a much longer interval, setting up a repetitive long-short infra-His block pattern until perturbation by ventricular ectopy, ventricular extrastimuli, slight alterations in the tachycardia cycle length or sympathetic output that allow recovery of bundle branch refractoriness. This postulated mechanism suggests the site of block is proximal in the His-Purkinje system, possibly within the His bundle itself.

Long-short block below His is usually physiologic and not an indication for a pacemaker. If there is doubt about its pathologic significance, one should see if infra-His block occurs while pacing the atria at gradually shorter cycle lengths; if this occurs, significant conduction system disease is present (one unusual exception is infra-His block at fast rates in a young patient with particularly robust AV node conduction).

ACCELERATION-DEPENDENT AND DECELERATION-DEPENDENT ABERRANCY

Acceleration-dependent aberrancy occurs when a gradual increase in the patient's heart rate (ie, decrease in cycle length) results in sudden development of a bundle branch block.[15] Acceleration-dependent aberrancy is not dependent on a sudden long-short sequence, and there may be several beats at the same cycle length before the acceleration-dependent aberrancy manifests (**Fig. 11**). In contrast to long-short aberrancy, left bundle branch block aberrancy is more common than right bundle branch block. Acceleration-dependent aberrancy does not represent normal physiology (except if it occurs only at extremely rapid rates), and it usually occurs in patients with underlying cardiac disease.

The cycle length at which bundle branch block occurs on acceleration is shorter than the cycle length at which bundle branch block disappears on deceleration ("hysteresis") (see **Fig. 11**). This is thought to be caused by concealed transseptal conduction: at the onset of acceleration-dependent bundle branch block, the bundle branch that was blocked anterogradely is now activated retrogradely late in the QRS complex via concealed transseptal conduction. On deceleration of the rate, this bundle branch does not "see" the dominant heart rate, but rather "sees" the interval between its retrograde transseptal invasion and the next anterograde impulse, which is shorter than the true cycle length. Therefore, for the blocked bundle branch to recover anterograde conduction, the heart rate must be slower on deceleration than it was on acceleration by approximately the duration of transseptal conduction.

The mechanism of rate-dependent aberrancy is not totally clear; the concepts of "phase 3 block" and "phase 4 block" have been used to explain acceleration-dependent and deceleration-dependent block, respectively, but these concepts probably do not adequately explain the phenomena. In contrast to long-short aberrancy, acceleration-dependent aberrancy is "time dependent" rather than "voltage dependent." The aberrancy commonly occurs at long cycle lengths, much longer than the bundle branch action potential duration. Therefore, its mechanism is not related to membrane voltage, but may be related to a phenomenon called "source-sink mismatch."[16,17] In this model, the ability of an impulse to conduct across a diseased region of Purkinje tissue depends on a balance of the intensity of input current proximally (current supply, "source") versus the passive and active membrane properties responsible for excitability and action potential propagation distal to the diseased region (current requirement, "sink").

Deceleration-dependent aberrancy is manifest by widening of the QRS on slowing of the dominant rhythm, with subsequent narrowing of the QRS on acceleration.[18] It is less common than acceleration-ependent aberration, but is also usually indicative of cardiac pathology. The source-sink mismatch model described previously may

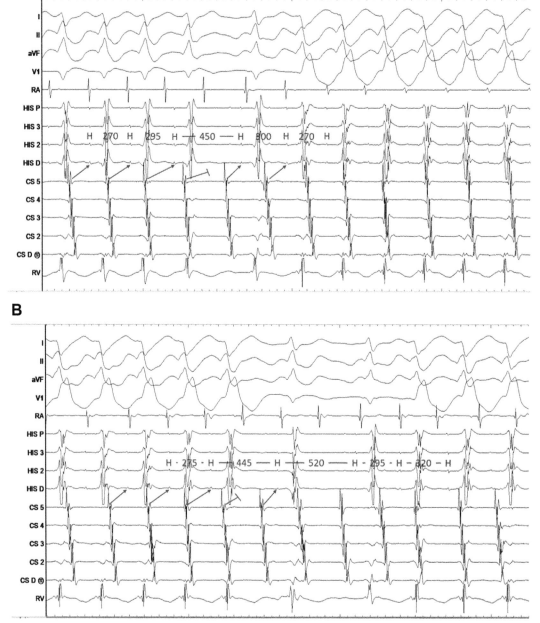

Fig. 8. Long-short aberrancy caused by Wenckebach AV conduction during atrial tachycardia. (*A*) Atrial tachycardia with narrow QRS complexes and gradual prolongation of the AH interval in a Wenckebach pattern. The nonconducted beat of the atrial tachycardia sets up a long-short RR interval (HH 450 to HH 270) that results in functional right bundle branch block aberration. Once initiated, the right bundle branch block persists because of concealed transseptal conduction, as discussed previously. (*B*) Wenckebach AV node conduction during the atrial tachycardia prolongs the HH interval, allowing transient normalization of the aberration; however, a subsequent long-short HH interval on resumption of 1:1 AV conduction (HH 520 to HH 295) reinitiates aberration. The arrows represent conduction from atria to His.

also apply to the mechanism of deceleration-dependent aberrancy (and supernormal conduction, as discussed later). In addition, "phase 4 aberrancy" could play some role in deceleration-

dependent aberrancy; that is, at longer cycle lengths the resting membrane potential gradually becomes less negative, and depolarization from a less negative resting potential results in a slower

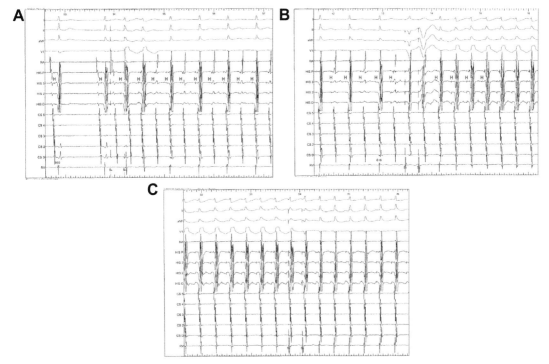

Fig. 9. Functional 2:1 infra-His AV block during AV nodal reentrant tachycardia. (*A*) Two atrial extrastimuli introduced during sinus rhythm result in two QRS complexes with functional right bundle branch block and then sustained AV nodal reentrant tachycardia with 2:1 AV block below the His recording. (*B*) During AV node reentry with 2:1 infra-His block, two ventricular extrastimuli retrogradely invade the bundle branches early, allowing 1:1 AV conduction via the left bundle branch to recover (continued right bundle branch block). (*C*) Two ventricular extrastimuli are introduced during AV node reentry with right bundle branch block aberrancy. They retrogradely invade the right bundle branch, activating it early enough to subsequently restore 1:1 anterograde conduction over the right bundle branch as tachycardia continues with narrow QRS complexes.

phase 0 upstroke and delay in conduction, resulting in a deceleration-dependent bundle branch block.

Another phenomenon, overdrive suppression of conduction, may occur in diseased His-Purkinje tissue (see **Fig 11**).[19] In this phenomenon, overdrive ventricular pacing or the occurrence of ventricular tachycardia transiently suppresses His-Purkinje conduction, resulting in a period of delayed AV conduction or AV block that eventually resolves over time.

MECHANISTIC IMPLICATIONS OF ABERRATION: BUNDLE BRANCH BLOCK DURING SUPRAVENTRICULAR TACHYCARDIA

Aberrant conduction during supraventricular tachycardia is used for diagnostic purposes during supraventricular tachycardia. An example is functional aberration in patients with AV reentry using an accessory pathway. If functional bundle branch block occurs during AV reentry ipsilateral to (on the same side as) the accessory pathway, the ventriculoatrial (VA) interval (measured from the onset

of the QRS in any lead to the A in the lead of interest) during tachycardia prolongs, and usually (but not always, depending on the AV nodal response) the tachycardia cycle length prolongs (**Fig. 12**). This can provide an important clue on surface ECG and intracardiac tracings as to the presence of the accessory pathway and its participation in the tachycardia.

MECHANISTIC IMPLICATIONS OF ABERRATION: CONCEALED HIS EXTRASYSTOLES

A rare cause of intermittent, sudden, unexpected PR prolongation or AV block is concealed His extrasystoles (**Fig. 13**).[20,21] Extrasystoles arising from the His bundle commonly do not conduct retrogradely through the AV node to the atria, but they can intermittently conduct to the ventricles with aberration. Electrocardiographically, they appear as junctional extrasystoles with/without aberration. However, if one or more His extrasystoles encounter functional block simultaneously in both bundle branches, the surface ECG may

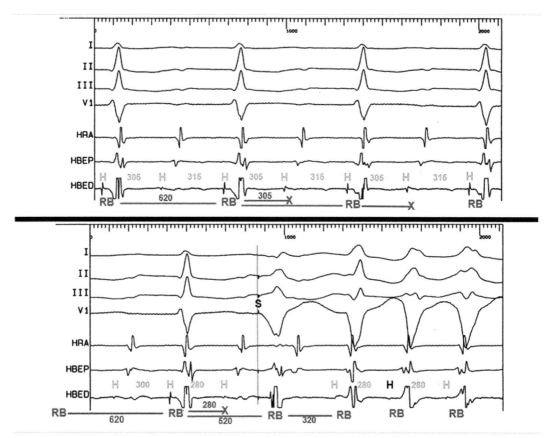

Fig. 10. Mechanism of persistence of 2:1 infra-His conduction once initiated. (*Top*) Tachycardia with 2:1 infra-His block in a patient with no conduction system disease. The HH intervals vary slightly from 305 to 315 ms. However, the right bundle branch below the site of block "sees" alternating intervals of 620 and 305 ms, setting up a repetitive long-short pattern that perpetuates the functional infra-His 2:1 AV block. (*Bottom*) A ventricular extrastimulus introduced during 2:1 infra-His block prematurely activates the right bundle branch (approximately 520 rather than 620 ms), prolonging the subsequent right bundle right bundle interval and allowing recovery of anterograde 1:1 conduction in the right bundle branch (functional left bundle branch block persists).

demonstrate either intermittent unexpected PR prolongation or type 1 or 2 second-degree AV block, despite the patient having a normal AV conduction system. The tip-off that His extrasystoles and not intrinsic conduction system disease are causing the AV block is the observation of coexisting junctional extrasystoles, often aberrantly conducted, scattered throughout the tracings.

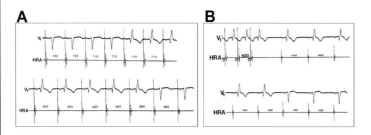

A   **B**

Fig. 11. Acceleration dependent bundle branch block with its typical "hysteresis." (*A*) The cycle length at which bundle branch block occurs on acceleration of the rate is shorter than the cycle length allowing normalization of conduction on deceleration of the rate. This phenomenon is caused by late activation of the blocked bundle branch (in this case the right bundle branch, although less common than the left in acceleration-dependent aberrancy) via concealed transseptal conduction. This late delayed activation creates an RB-RB interval shorter than the actual pacing cycle length and thus explains the slower rate required for resolution of the bundle branch block. (*B*) Overdrive suppression of conduction in the same patient as *A*. After rapid atrial pacing, right bundle branch conduction has been depressed even further than in *A*, and block occurs at even longer cycle lengths.

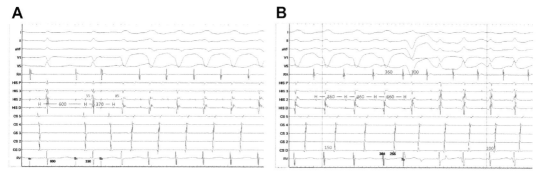

Fig. 12. Functional bundle branch block during AV reentrant tachycardia. (*A*) Induction of AV reentrant tachycardia with an atrial extrastimulus. The long-short interval results in a functional left bundle branch block during tachycardia. The reentrant tachycardia circuit incorporates anterograde conduction via the AV node/right bundle branch and retrograde conduction via a left free wall accessory pathway. (*B*) Normalization of the functional left bundle branch block by a single ventricular extrastimulus (atrial preexcitation when His is refractory proves the existence of a retrogradely conducting accessory pathway). The VA interval during tachycardia (measured from the onset of ventricular activation in any lead to an atrial electrogram) shortens on resolution of the functional left bundle branch block. During AV reentrant tachycardia, functional bundle branch block ipsilateral to (on the same side as) an accessory pathway increases the VA interval by the transseptal conduction time, because the impulse must travel anterogradely over the contralateral bundle branch and traverse the septum to reach the ventricular insertion of the accessory pathway. Conversely, the VA interval shortens on resolution of the ipsilateral bundle branch block.

GAP PHENOMENON

The gap phenomenon refers to an apparent paradoxic improvement in AV (or VA) conduction on shortening of the coupling interval of an atrial (or ventricular) extrastimulus. Differential diagnosis includes paradoxic improvement in conduction because of equal delay within the two bundle branches, or unexpected improvement in conduction because of supernormal conduction (discussed later). The gap phenomenon occurs because of differences in conduction properties between a proximal and distal portion of the

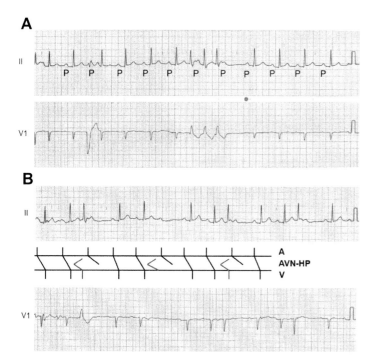

Fig. 13. Aberration provides a clue for the diagnosis of concealed His extrasystoles as a cause of "pseudo-AV block." Both panels display simultaneously recorded strips from an ambulatory monitor. (*A*) Sinus rhythm with multiple supraventricular ectopics not preceded by P waves. Sinus rhythm is not interrupted by the extrasystoles, implying that the extrasystoles do not conduct retrogradely to the atria. The extrasystoles intermittently conduct with either functional left bundle branch block (fourth complex) or right bundle branch block (ninth to eleventh QRS complexes). (*B*) An unexplained nonconducted P wave. Inferring from the fact that the His extrasystoles have demonstrated functional left and right bundle branch aberrancy, the nonconducted P wave is likely related to a concealed His extrasystole (*ladder diagram*); that is, one that blocks simultaneously in both bundle branches but manifests itself by leaving a wake of AV nodal refractoriness that causes the AV block.

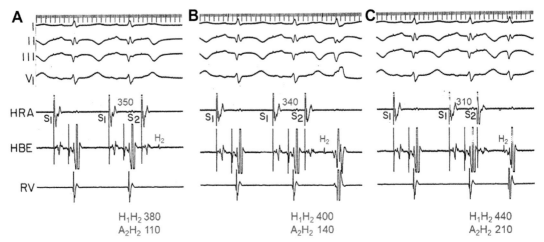

Fig. 14. Anterograde gap caused by prolongation of AV nodal conduction allowing recovery of His-Purkinje conduction. In the three panels, atrial extrastimuli are introduced progressively earlier. (*A*) The atrial extrastimulus reaches the His but fails to activate the ventricle because the H1-H2 interval of 380 ms is shorter than the refractory period of the His-Purkinje system. (*B*) AV nodal conduction and the H1-H2 interval prolong with the more tightly coupled extrastimulus, and the left bundle branch (but not right bundle branch) recovers. (*C*) The more tightly coupled atrial extrastimulus results in even more AH delay and sufficient prolongation of the H1-H2 interval to allow recovery of both bundle branches with normalization of the QRS.

conduction system. For example, when the effective refractory period of a more distal component of the conduction system is longer than the functional refractory period (shortest obtainable coupling interval) of a proximal component, a moderately premature extrastimulus may block in the distal component of the conduction system if there is little slowing in the proximal component; however, an even more premature extrastimulus may effect sufficient delay proximally to allow recovery of the more distal component, manifested by resumption of conduction. The gap may be manifest by either resolution of AV block or resolution of a bundle branch block following the earlier atrial extrastimulus.

The gap phenomenon is observed in either anterograde[22–24] or retrograde cardiac conduction.[25] The most common variety of anterograde

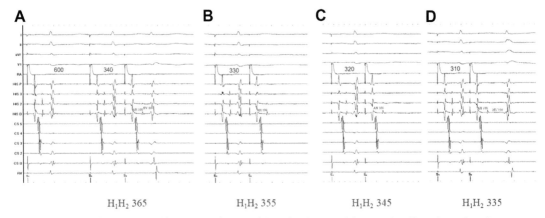

Fig. 15. Anterograde gap caused by proximal His-Purkinje slowing. Atrial extrastimuli are introduced at progressively shorter cycle lengths. (*A*) The resultant H1-H2 interval of 365 ms results in right bundle branch block aberrancy. (*B*) Shortening of the H1-H2 to 355 ms results in functional block below His. (*C*) The H1-H2 interval shortens to 345 ms and there is still block below His. (*D*) The H1-H2 interval shortens even further, but His-Purkinje conduction resumes, albeit with an extremely prolonged HV interval. This is presumably because of substantial slowing of conduction in the more proximal His-Purkinje system caused by the more tightly coupled H1-H2, allowing recovery of the more distal His-Purkinje system with resultant conduction to the ventricle. Note that delay must occur in some portion of the conduction system in order for a gap phenomenon to occur.

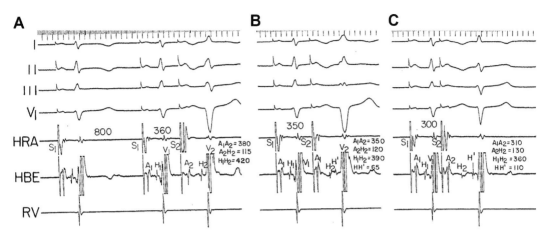

Fig. 16. Normalization left bundle branch block caused by intra-His gap with a split His potential. Atrial extrastimuli are introduced at progressively shorter coupling intervals. (*A, B*) Left bundle branch block aberrancy. Note that in each successive panel, the H1-H2 becomes progressively shorter, but as the His potential splits, the interval between H1 and the split second His component becomes longer because of intra-His delay. (*C*) This delay becomes long enough to allow normalization of conduction with a narrow QRS.

gap involves the AV node as the proximal component and the His-Purkinje system as the distal component (**Fig. 14**). Because an atrial extrastimulus is introduced at progressively earlier coupling intervals, infra-His block occurs when the His-His interval is shorter than the effective refractory period of the more distal His-Purkinje system. However, as the atrial extrastimulus is introduced even earlier, AV nodal conduction delays physiologically, the His-His interval may prolong progressively until it is longer than the His-Purkinje refractory period, and infra-His conduction may return ("type 1 gap"). In the second variety of anterograde gap, the proximal and distal sites of delay are in the His-Purkinje system (**Fig. 15**). Gaps may be suspected from electrocardiographic tracings but are best characterized with intracardiac recordings. The presence of a gap phenomenon necessarily requires prolongation of conduction somewhere along the system; clues to localize a gap phenomenon within the His-Purkinje system include prolongation of the His-ventricular interval and, on rare occasions, split His potentials (**Fig. 16**).

A form of anterograde gap may also occur because of "latency" at the atrial pacing site (**Fig. 17**). In this instance, premature atrial extrastimuli (S-S) may result in delay of the resultant A-A interval because of delay in recruiting local atrial tissue activation as a short S-S coupling interval approaches the effective refractory period of the atria. Thus, as the A-A interval delays despite shortening of the S-S coupling interval, the A-A interval may become long enough to allow resumption of AV node and His-Purkinje conduction.

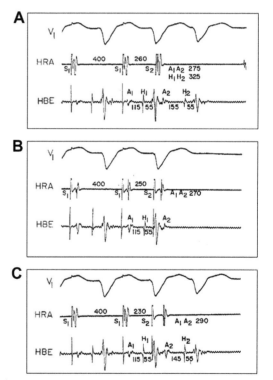

Fig. 17. (*A–C*) Anterograde AV nodal gap caused by atrial latency. Atrial extrastimuli are introduced at progressively shorter coupling intervals (S1-S2), but the resultant A1-A2 intervals do not shorten to the same extent because of local latency (ie, decreasing ability to recruit sufficient tissue to propagate an action potential as one encroaches on the atrial effective refractory period). The slight shortening of A1-A2 in *B* is sufficient to block in the AV node, but the prolongation of A1-A2 in *C* is sufficient to allow recovery of the AV node and conduction to the ventricles.

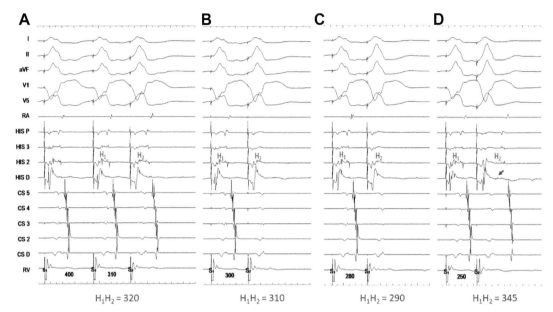

Fig. 18. Retrograde gap phenomenon. (*A–D*) From left-to-right, progressively more premature ventricular extra-stimuli are introduced. Retrograde His activation is labeled as H1 during the drive train and H2 after the extra-stimulus. With progressively tighter ventricular extrastimuli, the retrograde H1-H2 shortens, resulting in retrograde AV nodal block in *B* and *C*. However, with the more tightly coupled ventricular extrastimulus in *D*, there is marked delay in the retrograde His potential (*arrow*), likely caused by retrograde block in the right bundle branch and activation of the left bundle branch via transseptal conduction. This provides sufficient His-Purkinje delay to allow recovery of retrograde AV node conduction to the atria.

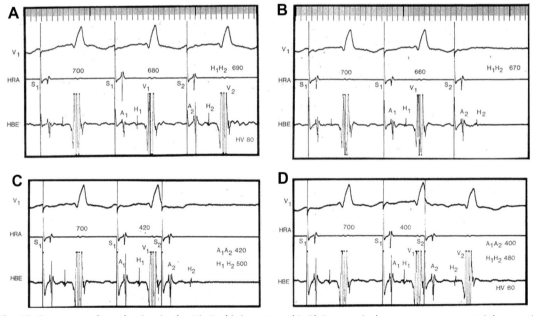

Fig. 19. Supernormal conduction in the His-Purkinje system. (*A–D*) Progressively more premature atrial extrasti-muli are introduced. A fixed right bundle branch block is present. Note that the coupling intervals are long. The H1-H2 interval progressively decreases as the atrial coupling interval decreases. The refractory period of the left bundle branch is exceeded in *B* and *C*, as documented by the block below His. However, in *D*, despite the continued shortening of the H1-H2 interval, His-Purkinje conduction resumes with a right bundle branch block. In distinction to the required delay that must occur in the phenomena of gap or equal bundle branch delay, here the HV interval even shortens slightly.

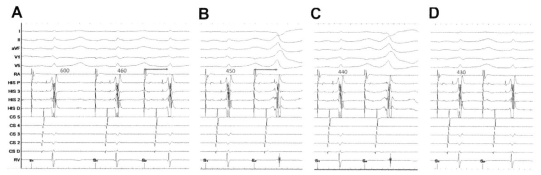

Fig. 20. Supernormal conduction in an accessory pathway. (*A–D*) Atrial extrastimuli introduced at progressively shorter coupling intervals. Note that the coupling intervals are long. (*A*) The atrial extrastimulus conducts with the physiologic AH prolongation, normal HV interval, and a narrow QRS complex. With the shorter A-A intervals in *B* and *C*, there is marked shortening of the AV interval with preexcitation (as demonstrated by the *horizontal arrows*) because of sudden unexpected anterograde conduction via a left free wall accessory pathway. The shortened AV interval proves that preexcitation is not manifest simply because of AV nodal delay. (*D*) The accessory pathway blocks, the AV interval prolongs, and normal conduction resumes. This illustrates a "supernormal" window of atrial coupling intervals in which accessory pathway conduction occurs, whereas either shorter or longer A-A coupling intervals result in accessory pathway block. Only accessory pathways with poor conduction properties demonstrate this phenomenon.

Likewise, a retrograde gap phenomenon is demonstrated during introduction of ventricular extrastimuli (**Fig. 18**). In this situation, the retrograde His-Purkinje system may provide the "proximal" site of delay and the AV node the "distal" site of block, manifesting retrograde block at intermediate ventricular coupling intervals but recovery of retrograde conduction on introduction of more tightly coupled ventricular extrastimuli.

EQUAL BUNDLE BRANCH DELAY

In some patients with abnormal His-Purkinje function, the bundle branch block pattern on ECG may be caused by conduction slowing rather than complete block in one of the bundle branches compared with the other. In these patients, certain atrial coupling intervals may result in equal conduction delay in the two bundle branches and unexpected normalization of the QRS duration.

SUPERNORMAL CONDUCTION

One can make a distinction between supernormal excitability and supernormal conduction. Supernormal excitability refers to transient hyperpolarization of the transmembrane action potential at the end of repolarization; for this short window of time, the transient dip in resting voltage decreases the action potential stimulation threshold just after completion of repolarization.[26,27] Supernormal excitability may explain certain clinical phenomena, such as transient lower pacemaker capture thresholds just after repolarization.[27]

Supernormal conduction has been most commonly thought to manifest in His-Purkinje tissue and accessory pathways. Supernormal conduction, like rate-dependent aberrancy, can manifest at long coupling intervals. Its mechanism may be related to source-sink mismatch as described previously for rate-dependent aberrancy. A supernormal window of improvement in His-Purkinje (**Fig. 19**)[28] or accessory pathway conduction (**Figs. 20 and 21**)[29,30] with more tightly coupled extrastimuli is presumably related to this balance between the current supply of the proximal source and the current requirements of the distal sink in abnormal conduction tissue at various coupling intervals.

The common feature of supernormal conduction in either His-Purkinje tissue or accessory pathways is the existence of a window of conduction at intermediate atrial coupling intervals, with conduction block at atrial coupling intervals either longer or shorter than those that demonstrate conduction. In contrast to the gap and equal delay phenomena, there is no overall delay in the PR interval or elsewhere in the conduction system associated with normalization of conduction; in fact, one may even detect a slight improvement in the conduction intervals. The existence of supernormal conduction has been controversial, and alternative explanations need to be excluded.[31,32]

Wellens[33] published an example of atrial fibrillation with rate-dependent bundle branch block and also unexpected normalization of the QRS after short RR intervals; without intracardiac tracings,

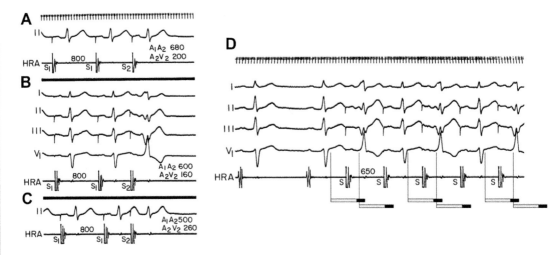

Fig. 21. 2:1 accessory pathway conduction as a manifestation of supernormal conduction. (*A–C*) Illustration of progressively more premature atrial extrastimuli, with a window of accessory pathway supernormal conduction demonstrated in *B*. (*D*) 2:1 accessory pathway conduction on initiation of atrial pacing, with the first short-coupled premature resulting in shortening of the AV interval because of accessory pathway conduction that was not present during sinus rhythm. The subsequent 2:1 accessory pathway conduction may be explained by alternation in the timing of the supernormal period (represented by the *terminal black portion of the horizontal bars*). When there is preexcitation, the accessory pathway is activated at the onset of the QRS, but when there is no preexcitation, the accessory pathway is activated retrogradely, late in the QRS complex. This alternation in activation timing allows the accessory pathway to fall in or out of the supernormal period on every other beat. If there were no supernormal period, once the accessory pathway blocked it would likely remain blocked because of repetitive concealed retrograde conduction into the accessory pathway. (*Adapted from* Chang MS, Miles WM, Prystowsky EN. Supernormal conduction in accessory atrioventricular connections. Am J Cardiol 1987;59:852-6; with permission)

supernormal conduction versus gap-like phenomena or equal bundle branch delay as the mechanism could not be distinguished. We obtained intracardiac tracings from a similar patient, demonstrating slight shortening of the His-ventricular interval in the short-coupled normalized QRS (**Fig. 22**),[34] thus excluding gap or equal delay as the mechanism for normalization of the QRS duration; the latter two mechanisms require prolongation of conduction somewhere in the system.

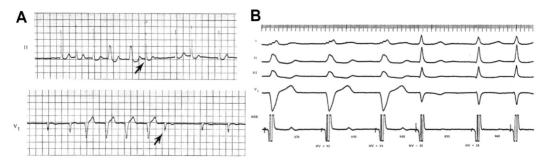

Fig. 22. Surface ECG and intracardiac tracing in a patient with atrial fibrillation, acceleration-dependent bundle branch block, and supernormal bundle branch conduction. (*A*) Electrocardiographic strips reveal atrial fibrillation with acceleration-dependent bundle branch block. However, the *arrows* point to unexpected QRS normalization at particularly short RR coupling intervals. This could be explained by either equal bundle branch delay or gap versus supernormal bundle branch conduction. (*B*) The His bundle recording reveals that the HV interval of the short-coupled normalized QRS complexes is slightly shorter than the others during normal conduction or left bundle branch block. Because there is no delay in conduction, equal bundle branch delay and gap are excluded and supernormal conduction is presumably the mechanism. (*From* Miles WM, Prystowsky EN, Heger JJ, Zipes DP. Evaluation of the patient with wide QRS tachycardia. Med Clin North Am 1984;68:1015-38; with permission).

SUMMARY

Wide QRS complexes during supraventricular rhythms are caused by fixed bundle branch block, functional (intermittent) bundle branch block, pre-excitation, or transient QRS widening from toxic/metabolic causes. Functional bundle branch block is caused by long-short aberrancy (usually physiologic), or acceleration/deceleration dependent aberrancy (usually pathologic). ECG criteria have been proposed to help differentiate aberration from ventricular tachycardia; they are helpful but not always accurate.

The gap phenomenon can occur in the AV conduction system during anterograde or retrograde conduction. The principle of the gap phenomenon "paradox" is that with increasingly premature extrastimuli, progressive proximal delay in the conduction system allows time for distal recovery of excitability. Although not well characterized, the phenomenon of supernormal conduction can explain unusual conduction phenomena in patients with abnormal His-Purkinje function or poorly conducting accessory pathways.

DISCLOSURE

The authors have nothing to disclose.

CLINICS CARE POINTS

- ECG criteria can be very helpful for distinguishing SVT with aberrancy from VT, but sometimes an electrophysiology study is necessary for confirmation.
- Once functional bundle branch block occurs during SVT, the bundle branch block tends to perpetuate and may mimic VT.
- Bundle branch block or block below His due to functional long-short aberrancy represents normal His-Purkinje physiology and is not an indication for a pacemaker; in contrast, block below His occurring during gradual decremental pacing is usually pathologic.
- 2:1 AV block during SVT does not exclude AV node reentry.
- In acceleration-dependent bundle branch block, either narrow-QRS or wide-QRS complexes may be seen within a defined intermediate range of heart rates, depending on whether the rate has been accelerating or decelerating ("hysteresis").

REFERENCES

1. Fisch C. Aberration: seventy five years after Sir Thomas Lewis. Br Heart J 1983;50:297–302.
2. Wu PE, Juurlink DN. Clinical review: loperamide toxicity. Ann Emerg Med 2017;70:245–52.
3. Wellens HJ, Bar FW, Lie KI. The value of the electrocardiogram in the differential diagnosis of a tachycardia with a widened QRS complex. Am J Med 1978;64:27–33.
4. Brugada P, Brugada J, Mont L, et al. A new approach to the differential diagnosis of a regular tachycardia with a wide QRS complex. Circulation 1991;83:1649–59.
5. Kindwall KE, Brown J, Josephson ME. Electrocardiographic criteria for ventricular tachycardia in wide complex left bundle branch block morphology tachycardias. Am J Cardiol 1988;61:1279–83.
6. Wellens HJ. Ventricular tachycardia: diagnosis of broad QRS complex tachycardia. Heart 2001;86:579–85.
7. Vereckei A, Duray G, Szenasi G, et al. New algorithm using only lead aVR for differential diagnosis of wide QRS complex tachycardia. Heart Rhythm 2008;5:89–98.
8. Lewis T. Paroxysmal tachycardia, the result of ectopic impulse formation. Heart 1910;1:262–82.
9. Myerburg RJ, Steward JW, Hoffman BF. Electrophysiological properties of the canine peripheral A-V conducting system. Circ Res 1970;26:361–78.
10. Denes P, Wu D, Dhingra R, et al. The effects of cycle length on cardiac refractory periods in man. Circulation 1974;49:32–41.
11. Chilson DA, Zipes DP, Heger JJ, et al. Functional bundle branch block: discordant response of right and left bundle branches to changes in heart rate. Am J Cardiol 1984;54:313–6.
12. Janse MJ, van der Steen ABM, van Dam RT, et al. Refractory period of the dog's ventricular myocardium following sudden changes in frequency. Circ Res 1969;24:251–62.
13. Miles WM, Prystowsky EN. Alteration of human right bundle branch refractoriness by changes in duration of the atrial drive train. Circulation 1986;73:244–8.
14. Man KC, Brinkman K, Bogun F, et al. 2:1 atrioventricular block during atrioventricular node reentrant tachycardia. J Am Coll Cardiol 1996;28:1770–4.
15. Fisch C, Zipes DP, McHenry P. Rate dependent aberrancy. Circulation 1973;48:714–24.
16. Jalife J, Antzelevitch C, Lamanna V, et al. Rate-dependent changes in excitability of depressed cardiac Purkinje fibers as a mechanism of intermittent bundle branch block. Circulation 1983;67:912–22.
17. Davidenko JM, Antzelevitch C. Electrophysiological mechanisms underlying rate-dependent changes of refractoriness in normal and segmentally depressed canine Purkinje fibers. Circ Res 1986;58:257–68.

18. Fisch C, Miles WM. Deceleration-dependent left bundle branch block: a spectrum of bundle branch conduction delay. Circulation 1982;65:1029–32.

19. Chiale PA, Sanchez RA, Franco DA, et al. Overdrive prolongation of refractoriness and fatigue in the early stages of human bundle branch disease. J Am Coll Cardiol 1994;23:724–32.

20. Rosen KM, Rahimtoola SH, Gunnar RM. Pseudo A-V block secondary to premature nonpropagated His bundle depolarizations. Circulation 1970;42:367–73.

21. Fisch C, Zipes DP, McHenry PL. Electrocardiographic manifestations of concealed junctional ectopic impulses. Circulation 1976;53:217–23.

22. Gallagher JJ, Damato AN, Caracta AR, et al. Gap in A-V conduction in man: types I and II. Am Heart J 1973;85:78–82.

23. Agha AS, Castellanos A, Wells D, et al. Type I, type II, and type III gaps in bundle-branch conduction. Circulation 1973;47:325–30.

24. Wu D, Denes P, Dhingra R, et al. Nature of the gap phenomenon in man. Circ Res 1974;34:682–92.

25. Akhtar M, Damato AN, Caracta AR, et al. The gap phenomena during retrograde conduction in man. Circulation 1974;49:811–7.

26. Spear JF, Moore EN. Supernormal excitability and conduction in His-Purkinje system of the dog. Circ Res 1974;35:782–92.

27. Moore EN, Spear JF, Fisch C. "Supernormal" conduction and excitability. J Cardiovasc Electrophysiol 1993;4:320–37.

28. Elizari MV, Schmidberg J, Atienza A, et al. Clinical and experimental evidence of supernormal excitability and conduction. Curr Cardiol Rev 2014;10:202–21.

29. Przybylski J, Chiale PA, Sanchez RA, et al. Supernormal conduction in the accessory pathway of patients with overt or concealed ventricular pre-excitation. J Am Coll Cardiol 1987;9:1269–78.

30. Chang MS, Miles WM, Prystowsky EN. Supernormal conduction in accessory atrioventricular connections. Am J Cardiol 1987;59:852–6.

31. Moe GK, Childers RW, Merideth J. An appraisal of "supernormal" A-V conduction. Circulation 1968;38:5–28.

32. Gallagher JJ, Damato AN, Varghese PJ, et al. Alternative mechanisms of apparent supernormal atrioventricular conduction. Am J Cardiol 1973;31:362–71.

33. Wellens H. Unusual occurrence of nonaberrant conduction in patients with atrial fibrillation and aberrant conduction. Am Heart J 1969;77:158–66.

34. Miles WM, Prystowsky EN, Heger JJ, et al. Evaluation of the patient with wide QRS tachycardia. Med Clin North Am 1984;68:1015–38.

Genetic Abnormalities of the Sinoatrial Node and Atrioventricular Conduction

Andreu Porta-Sánchez, MD, PhD[a,b,c], Silvia Giuliana Priori, MD, PhD[a,d,e],*

KEYWORDS

- Inherited arrhythmias • Atrioventricular node • Electrophysiology • Sinoatrial node dysfunction
- Arrhythmia

KEY POINTS

- Inherited sinoatrial node dysfunction (SAND) should be suspected in individuals with significant bradycardia at young age and a positive family history when reversible causes have been ruled out.
- Inherited cardiac conduction system disorders (CCSDs) may have a significant degree of overlap with SAND and may also be the first manifestation of an underlying inherited cardiomyopathy.
- Storage diseases such as amyloidosis, Anderson-Fabry, Danon disease, and PRKAG2 syndrome usually present with progressive nonobstructive cardiomyopathy phenotypes and CCSD.
- Neuromuscular disorders such as Myotonic Dystrophy 1, Emery-Dreifuss, and desminopathies present often with CCSD.
- Specific treatment for storage diseases includes enzyme replacement therapy, and small molecule therapeutic drugs, including substrate reduction and chaperone therapies. Management of CCSD may include permanent pacing based on the diagnosis, clinical, electrophysiological, and arrhythmic burden observed in the patient.

INTRODUCTION

The uniqueness of the physiology of the sinoatrial node (SAN) and the specialized cardiac conduction system (CCS) that allows a steady life-long rhythmic and synchronous activation of the heart has fascinated scientists for decades. The dysfunction of the SAN and the CCS is seen in congenital heart defects or linked to the aging heart but in some instances, those diseases may present at an early age and may have an underlying genetic cause. The incidence of inherited arrhythmia syndromes linked to SAN dysfunction (SAND) and CCS disease (CCSD) is estimated to be low. In a recent report from systematic screening with a Health Questionnaire and ECG in 26,900 individuals aged between 14 and 35 years, ECG abnormalities suggesting SAND were found in 10 patients (0.04%) and CCSD were found in 197 patients (0.73%), including nonspecific intraventricular conduction delay in 117 cases, ventricular preexcitation in 42 cases, right bundle branch block (RBBB) in 34 cases, left bundle branch block (LBBB) in 3 cases, and 1 patient with complete heart block.[1] Although rare, the implications for patients and families suffering from such diseases are extremely important because recent reports have raised concerns about the possibility of an underlying cardiomyopathy in a substantial proportion of young patients

This article originally appeared in *Cardiac Electrophysiology Clinics*, Volume 13 Issue 4, December 2021.
[a] Cardiología Molecular, Fundación Centro Nacional de Investigaciones Cardiovasculares Carlos III (CNIC) Madrid, Spain; [b] Departamento de Cardiología, Unidad de Arritmias, Hospital Universitario Quironsalud Madrid, Spain; [c] Departamento de Medicina, Universidad Europea de Madrid, Spain; [d] Molecular Medicine Department, University of Pavia, Italy; [e] Istituti Clinici Scientifici Maugeri, IRCCS, Pavia, Italy
* Corresponding author. Molecular Cardiology, Istituti Clinici Scientifici Maugeri, IRCCS, Via Salvatore Maugeri 10, Pavia 27100, Italy.
E-mail address: silvia.priori@icsmaugeri.it

Cardiol Clin 41 (2023) 333–347
https://doi.org/10.1016/j.ccl.2023.03.014

needing pacemakers due to complete heart block.[2] This hypothesis could be behind the finding of increased long-term mortality of this population compared with healthy controls despite pacemaker implantation. In other instances, mutations in genes causing overt channelopathies such as Brugada syndrome (BrS) may manifest as CCSD highlighting the importance of genetic testing to identify the underlying defect and prompt the appropriate treatment and risk stratification. In this review, we will describe the most frequent clinical phenotypes of the genetic mutations that cause inherited SAND and/or CCSD. The most common clinical presentations are in the form of channelopathies or cardiomyopathies (mainly dilated cardiomyopathy [DCM] or hypertrophic cardiomyopathy [HCM]) associated with CCSD). **Fig. 1** shows a schematic representation of the cellular function/location of each of the genes described.

ION CHANNELS
SCN5A and SCN1B Subunit Mutations

The SCN5A gene encodes for Nav1.5, the alpha-subunit of the sodium channel located in the sarcolemma of cardiac myocytes. The normal function of the Nav1.5 is of paramount importance to ensure the proper propagation of the cardiac impulse both in the atria and ventricle and is the key component of the phase 0 of the action potential. The variety and severity of cardiac clinical manifestations linked to the dysfunction (both gain of function [GOF] or loss of function [LOF]) of the cardiac sodium channel Nav1.5 are very heterogeneous. The 2 most common cardiac manifestations of SCN5A mutations are BrS and Long QT syndrome type 3 (LQT3) caused, respectively, by LOF and GOF mutations. Interestingly, mutations that have at the same time an LOF (such as

a reduction of the peak INa current and a GOF such as a slower recovery from fast inactivation of the INa) may present different phenotypes among family members with the same mutation.[3] With regards to SAND and CCSD, several mutations have been linked to familial phenotypes that include progressive and nonprogressive heart block and sick sinus syndrome.[4–7] Interestingly, the coexistence of CCSD and BrS has been linked to adverse prognosis in some series.[8] In mechanistic terms, LOF mutations have been shown in animal models to underlie the lack of lateralization of gap junctions[9] and decrease the conduction velocity of the myocardium, making it prone to ventricular fibrillation inducibility.[10] With regards to the pathophysiology of SAND, despite the fact that the impulse generation in the central SAN cells is mainly driven by the *If* current, the effect of LOF mutations in the peripheral SAN cells (known to have Nav1.5 expression) has been hypothesized to lead to SAN exit block or arrest because of slowing of impulse generation and conduction to the surrounding atrial tissue[11,12].

With regards to SCN1B, which encodes for the beta-regulatory subunit of Nav1.5, mutations in this gene have been associated with familial atrial fibrillation[13] and with BrS with cardiac conduction defects.[14]

Key findings and clinical recommendations

- Presentation:
  - Clinically, patients carrying LOF SCN5A mutations usually present with sinus bradycardia, prolonged PR interval, and wide QRS with a left-axis deviation and/or RBBB. BrS can coexist with CCSD.
  - Syncope at rest or during fever episodes can be an initial presentation of an SCN5A mutation.

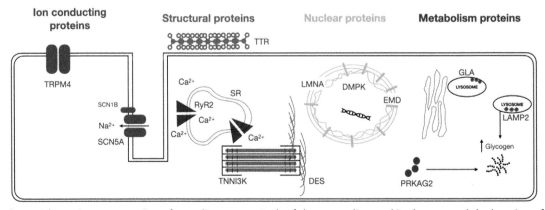

Fig. 1. Schematic representation of a cardiomyocyte. Each of the genes discussed in the text and the location of the encoded proteins is illustrated. Color coding for the proteins as in the text: ion channels in gray, structural proteins in blue, nuclear proteins in yellow, and metabolism proteins in red.

- Genetics:
  - Truncating mutations in SCN5A have been linked to severe forms of conduction disease.[15]
  - SCN5A mutations can also present with familial DCM and CCSD.[16]
  - SCN1B mutations are linked to familial atrial fibrillation or BrS with progressive CCSD.
- Management:
  - Targeted genetic testing to SCN5A is recommended in patients with DCM and CCSD.[17]
  - In families with CCSD, genetic study for SCN5A mutations may reveal the presence of an LOF mutation suggestive of a concealed BrS. Carriers of an SCN5A pathogenic LOF mutation with CCSD and no spontaneous type I BrS pattern may undergo an ajmaline or flecainide test to unmask the Brugada pattern.[18]
  - Avoidance of drugs known to block the Na$^+$ channel (https://www.brugadadrugs.org/) and prompt reduction of body temperature during fever is recommended for patients with a pathogenic LOF mutation in SCN5A.
  - If progressive CCSD is present in a patient who also needs an Implantable Cardioverter Defibrillator (ICD), an endovascular device should be considered rather than a subcutaneous ICD to allow for pacing during follow-up.
  - Patients with CCSD due to SCN1B mutations may present with RBBB or LBBB although the penetrance is very variable and family members with the same mutation may not show any signs of CCSD.[14]

TRPM4

The TRPM4 gene encodes a nonselective cation channel belonging to the transient receptor potential melastatin family of ion channels. TRPMs are calcium-activated nonselective channels showing an equal permeability to Na+ and K+ ions, and they are activated via an increase of the intracellular calcium concentration and membrane depolarization.[19] In the heart, TRPM4 channels are expressed in atrial and ventricular cardiomyocytes, SAN, conductive tissue, and atrial and ventricular fibroblasts.[20]

Brink and coworkers were the first to identify in an Afrikaner kindred with progressive heart block mapping to chromosome 19q13.3 (PFHB1B; 604559), a heterozygous missense mutation (E7K) in the TRPM4 gene.[21,22] The mutation segregated with the disease in the kindred. To identify

the mechanism of the mutation studied the mutant channels *in vitro* showing that the E7K mutation impairs the dynein-based TRPM4 channel endocytosis leading to an augmented amount of the protein expression.[22] They also went on to study post-translational modifications and hypothesized and demonstrated that SUMOylation of the channel is impaired in the presence of the mutation leading to disruption of endocytosis and elevated TRPM4 channel density at the cell surface.[22]

It is interesting to observe that pathogenic variants of the TRPM4 gene have also been identified in patients with different forms of cardiac disorders such as BrS and long QT syndrome. These variants have been characterized *in vitro* and they induce either GOF or LOF of TRPM4 channels.[23]

Subsequently, functional studies have shown that TRPM4 plays a role in the repolarization of the atrial action potential, and atrioventricular block at different levels has been shown in a mice model of the disease.[24] Reports in French and Lebanese families with of other TRPM4 mutations leading to CCSD were reported by Liu and colleagues[25] and further cases in patients with early-onset atrioventricular heart block leading to the discovery of other TRPM4 variants by Syam and colleagues[26] and Bianchi and colleagues.[27] Interestingly, only few of the newly identified mutations confirmed that the pathogenetic mechanism is associated with the increase in the expression of the channel in the membrane due to attenuated endocytosis[25] with increased susceptibility to arrhythmia.[28] More recently, also LOF TRPM4 mutations have been associated with CCSD and the underpinning mechanism of these mutations is still debated. A BrS phenotype due to TRPM4 variants has also been described in patients with[29] and without coexisting SCN5A mutations. In those with only TRPM4 variants, 11 mutations were identified and 9 were new mutations. Functional studies of 4 of those mutations showed that 2 led to an increase in TRPM4 expression and 2 led to a decrease in expression.[23]

Key findings and clinical recommendations

- Presentation:
  - Familial early-onset bundle branch block (mostly RBBB) or progressive atrioventricular block initially presenting as RBBB is the most common presentation of TRPM4 mutations (progressive familial heart block type 1). Characterization of the level of block (Atrioventricular Node (AVN) or His-Purkinje system) has not been systematically analyzed in cohorts of patients with mutations.

○ In kindreds with several affected members, genetic screening on TRPM4 gene may be reasonable to identify in a presymptomatic stage affected family members to keep them under medical control and monitor aggravation of clinical manifestations.

○ TRPM4 has been proposed to account for a fraction of cases of BrS[23] and LQTS[30]; however, the causative effect of TRPM4 mutations for BrS and LQT remains elusive.

- Genetics:
  ○ Mutations in TRPM4 (both GOF and LOF) could lead to Nav1.5 disfunction because of a change in the availability of Nav1.5 via hyperpolarization (LOF) or depolarization (GOF) of the membrane potential leading to CCSD and proarrhythmia.

- Management:
  ○ In cases where CCSD is diagnosed because of a TRPM4 mutation, a provocative pharmacologic test with flecainide or ajmaline may be performed in a setting suitable for managing worsening of CCSD and inducibility of ventricular fibrillation.
  ○ Na+ channel blocking drugs should not be prescribed to patients with a BrS phenotype.
  ○ Pacemaker implantation is needed if CCSD progresses to advanced atrioventricular block and patients become symptomatic for syncope.[31]

STRUCTURAL PROTEINS
TTR

Transthyretin amyloidosis (ATTR) is a cause of progressive cardiomyopathy due to the deposition of misfolded transthyretin. An acquired form of the disease occurs as a consequence of aging, whereas the genetic form is caused by mutations in the TTR gene encoding for the protein transthyretin that is a protein that is found in serum and cerebrospinal fluid. The function of TTR is to transport retinol (vitamin A) through the holo-retinol-binding protein (RBP) and thyroxin (T4). Both mutant and wild-type amyloid cause the disease (ATTR) that is caused by the deposition of misfolded amyloid aggregates in organs such as heart, liver, pancreas, and retinal pigment.

The cardiac manifestations of full-blown amyloidosis are hypertrophic or restrictive cardiomyopathy often accompanied by neurologic symptoms and carpal tunnel syndrome. Patients with the hereditary form of amyloidosis may present with mild signs of CCSD at their first cardiac evaluation and echocardiography may show mild cardiac hypertrophy without electrocardiographic evidence of left ventricular hypertrophy.[32] Often,

CCSD may occur several years ahead of the onset of heart failure symptoms. Electrophysiological studies of patients diagnosed with cardiac amyloidosis have shown impaired atrioventricular conduction with prolongation of the HV interval with or without QRS widening.[33] In a recent cohort reported by Rehorn and collaborators, patients with cardiac amyloid of different etiology showed that pacemaker or ICD implantation often preceded the diagnosis of amyloidosis, which became clinically evident 4 to 5 years later. In their population, the cause of device implantation was SAND in 27% of patients, high-degree AV block in 64%, and tachy-brady syndrome in 9%. Over time, a typical finding in patients who have received a pacemaker is the increase in the percentage of pacing indicating the progressive nature of this disease.[34] Atrial arrhythmias are also quite common in amyloidosis and they carry a very high risk of stroke. New therapies have recently shown promising results for the treatment of ATTR such as *patisiran, inotersen,* and *tafamidis. Tafamidis* was able to show an all-cause mortality benefit versus placebo in a trial involving 441 patients with amyloid cardiomyopathy and 24% of them having hereditary ATTR cardiomyopathy.[35] Solomon and colleagues showed that in a prespecified subgroup of patients with hereditary ATTR *patisiran* treatment was associated with a decrease in LV wall mass and an increase in cardiac output compared with placebo.[36] Nonetheless, whether *tefamidis* treatment is also able to slow the progression of CCSD is still unknown.

Key findings and clinical recommendations

- Presentation:
  ○ The appearance of CCSD (most commonly prolonged PR with RBBB[34]) with unexplained polyneuropathy should raise the suspicion of hereditary amyloidosis even with minor degrees of LV hypertrophy with disproportionate increase in NT-proBNP levels.[37]
  ○ Diagnosis of the hereditary form of amyloidotic cardiomyopathy is based on the combination of increase in LV mass mimicking nonobstructive HCM or restrictive cardiomyopathy and compatible imaging in scintigraphy and often an ECG with relatively low voltages discrepant with the degree of increase in LV mass.
  ○ As both wild-type amyloid and mutant amyloid can cause cardiac amyloidosis, a negative genetic screening for TTR in a patient with CCSD suspected of having amyloidosis should not rule out the diagnosis.

- Genetics:
  - Many distinct phenotypical manifestations of amyloidosis have been observed among carriers of different point mutations scattered along the 127 amino acids of the TTR protein. The pattern of inheritance of the disease is predominantly autosomal dominant while selected mutations are inherited as homozygous mutations such as the V30M and the V122I mutations.
- Management:
  - Conduction disturbances in hATTR-CM are very common and the most frequent reasons for pacing include SAND, atrioventricular block, and atrial fibrillation with slow ventricular response.[34]
  - In patients with second-degree Mobitz II AV block or high-grade AV block or third-degree AV block permanent pacing should be considered independently from symptoms.[31]
  - Resynchronization therapy could be considered in patients fulfilling guideline criteria for CRT implantation and could be associated with better outcomes than conventional pacing (observational retrospective data).[38]
  - There are currently no clear indications for ICD on primary prevention as some studies have shown no impact on the prognosis of patients who received one.[39]
  - ICD implantation should be considered in patients who have survived a cardiac arrest and those exhibiting a high burden of nonsustained ventricular tachycardia (NSVT) or syncope of likely cardiogenic cause or those patients listed for heart transplantation.[31,40]

DES

The DES gene encodes for desmin, one of the proteins of the intermediate filament of the cytoskeleton of cardiomyocytes and skeletal muscle cells. Mutations in the DES gene may transmit the diseases either as a dominant or as a recessive condition. Desmin protein forms a scaffold around the Z-disk of the sarcomere and connects the Z-disk to the subsarcolemmal cytoskeleton. Desmin also connects the sarcomere to organelles such as the nucleus and the mitochondria. These connections are important to preserve the architecture and the contractile apparatus of cardiomyocytes. The diseases associated with mutations in the DES gene may manifest as a combined cardiac and skeletal muscle disease or as an isolated cardiac phenotype that may include besides the development of a DCM also CCSD and risk of sudden cardiac death.[41]

Key findings and clinical recommendations

- Presentation:
  - The clinical manifestations of mutations in DES are very broad: most mutations are linked to muscular dystrophy with or without overt cardiomyopathy.[42] Selected mutations may cause an early-onset cardiomyopathy and advanced CCSD (mostly RBBB[43]) needing pacemaker implantation during infancy without accompanying signs of neuromuscular involvement.[44]
- Genetics:
  - Most common DES mutations lead to myopathy due to disruption of desmin filament assembly.[42]
  - Other DES mutations such as p.Glu401Asp lead to severe forms of arrhythmogenic cardiomyopathy with no significant CCSD but a very high arrhythmic burden without extracardiac involvement.[45]
- Management:
  - Extensive neurologic evaluation is important to rule out muscular weakness that is a sign of skeletal muscle myopathy.
  - The progressive nature of the DCM phenotype leads to early heart failure and premature death.[41,43,46,47]

TNNI3K

This gene encodes for troponin I interacting kinase that belongs to the MAPKKK family of protein kinases expressed only in cardiomyocytes.[48] Theis and colleagues described a family with recurrent supraventricular tachycardia, CCSD and DCM with different degrees of systolic dysfunction.[49] Later reports by other groups have shown similar findings caused by different mutations but a clear pathogenic mechanism for the TNNI3K variants is not yet conclusively defined although increased autophosphorylation and aggregation defect has been proposed as a mechanism based on *in vitro* data.[50,51]

Key findings and clinical recommendations

- Presentation:
  - A familial history of recurrent supraventricular tachycardia during childhood/early adulthood (junctional tachycardia, atrioventricular nodal reentrant tachycardia, or atrial tachycardia) with sinus arrhythmia and mild degrees of atrioventricular conduction impairment (prolonged PR interval, variable degrees of RBBB, and left anterior hemiblock[51]) is the most common presentation of TNNI3K mutations.[50]

- Genetics:
  - Heterozygous missense mutations and mutations that disrupt the splice sites have been identified in families with the disease.
- Management:
  - In most of the patients ($\approx$75%), CCSD is diagnosed during invasive electrophysiological testing (HV prolongation, infrahisian or intra-hisian block).
  - DCM pattern or heart failure symptoms are present in $\approx$25% of patients.[49–51]

NUCLEAR PROTEINS
LMNA

The LMNA gene encodes for lamin A/C, an intermediate filament protein of the nuclear membrane involved in nuclear stability, chromatin structure, and gene expression. Mutations in LMNA are linked to a broad spectrum of phenotypes presenting cardiac and extracardiac manifestations (laminopathies: Charcot-Marie-Tooth disease, type 2B; Emery-Dreifuss muscular dystrophy 2; Emery-Dreifuss muscular dystrophy 3; Heart-hand syndrome, Slovenian type; Hutchinson-Gilford progeria; Lipodystrophy, familial, partial type 2; Malouf syndrome; Mandibuloacral dysplasia; Muscular dystrophy, congenital; and Restrictive dermopathy, lethal). Several LMNA mutations are linked to a severe form of DCM without muscular involvement which frequently presents initially as an isolated CCSD at young ages that may be present years before other clinical signs or imaging findings of cardiomyopathy arise.[52] Compared to sporadic forms of DCM, LMNA mutation carriers have younger age at disease onset, are more commonly females, and are more likely to present with CCSD, which in a published series was present in 43% of patients at diagnosis and in 19% of patients was in the form of complete heart block.[53] Patients with LMNA-related cardiomyopathy experience severe ventricular arrhythmias at early stages of the disease and often independently from the degree of cardiac systolic function.[54] The risk of sudden cardiac death is so high that ICD implantation in primary prevention is often advocated. As a consequence, the need for pacing should lead the treating physician to consider ICD implantation as a first choice.[55,56] Nonmissense mutations have been linked to worse prognosis, similarly the documentation of NSVT at Holter monitoring is considered a marker of high risk of sudden death. Although male sex was previously linked to higher mortality, recent series have not confirmed this association.[57,58]

Key findings and clinical recommendations

- Presentation:
  - Sinus dysfunction with brady-tachycardia syndrome, prolonged PR, bundle branch block (mostly LBBB[57]), or progressive heart block at young ages (2nd or 3rd decade of life) or advanced degrees of AV block with initially normal left ventricular function are common presentations of LMNA-related DCM. Ventricular arrhythmias often accompany the initial presentation.
  - In one study of 64 mutation carriers, the time between the initial ECG abnormality and the onset of LV dysfunction was 7 years.[59]
  - The arrhythmic burden of the disease is independent of the left ventricular ejection fraction (LVEF) and should be assessed periodically.
- Genetics:
  - Mutations in the LMNA gene is a well-established cause of inherited DCM.[60]
  - Subjects with truncating mutations have earlier onset of the disease and lower LVEF than those with missense mutations.[61]
- Management:
  - Targeted genetic testing to LMNA is recommended in patients with DCM and CCSD and it is useful for risk-stratification.[17,56]
  - As per current guidelines,[62] in patients with DCM due to LMNA mutation who have 2 or more risk factors (NSVT, LVEF <45%, non-missense mutation, male sex), an ICD can be beneficial if life expectancy is >1 year.
  - In patients with CCSD linked to LMNA mutations needing cardiac pacing, a consideration of ICD implantation should be made even if only mildly depressed LVEF is present.[31,56]
  - If cardiac resynchronization is needed, physiologic conduction system pacing could be a reasonable approach to maintain intraventricular synchrony (His or left bundle branch pacing) as well as conventional cardiac resynchronization therapy.[63]
  - Management of patients suffering from ventricular tachycardia due to LMNA cardiomyopathy is difficult and catheter ablation outcomes are poor.[64]

EMD

EMD encodes for Emerin, which is a protein located in the nuclear membrane that mediates membrane anchorage to the cytoskeleton. Mutations in EMD are responsible for the Emery-

Dreifuss muscular dystrophy type 1, autosomal recessive. They can also manifest in a nonsyndromic fashion and cause X-linked SAND and atrial fibrillation.[65] In syndromic forms of Emerin mutations, the overt phenotype includes both CCSD with DCM and progressive muscular dystrophy and early contractures of the elbows and Achilles tendons.[66] Recently, new mutations in EMD have been linked to the development of severe early-onset atrial arrhythmia progressing to atrial standstill and left ventricular noncompaction without extracardiac manifestations.[67] A recent report of a cohort with 11 years of median follow-up by Marchel and collaborators has shown that patients with EMD mutations experience frequently atrial arrhythmia (flutter or fibrillation in 50%) and that the presenting rhythm was atrial standstill in 50% of cases reflecting severe SAND. With regards to CCSD, advanced degrees of atrioventricular block were also common with second degree in 20% of patients and third degree in 27% at presentation.[68]

Key findings and clinical recommendations

- Presentation:
  - Patients with the disease will present usually with limb muscle wasting and weakness and joint contractures of the neck and elbows during the 1st and 2nd decade of life. Cardiac involvement may not be apparent at the onset of muscular symptoms and appears after muscular involvement is diagnosed.[68]
  - Patients will present most frequently with atrial standstill or sinoatrial block (SAND) or CCSD with second-degree or third-degree atrioventricular block with junctional escape.[68,69]
  - The most common echocardiographic imaging findings are the presence of left ventricular dilatation with mildly reduced LVEF and biatrial dilatation.[70]
- Genetics:
  - Emerin is involved in a large number of biological processes such as regulation of transcription factors, intracellular signaling, nucleocytoskeletal mechanotransduction, nuclear structure, and chromatin condensation among others. Mutated Emerin leads to a dysfunctional protein that has weaker interactions with the nuclear lamina components causing structural abnormalities in the cardiomyocyte and skeletal muscle cells.[71,72]
- Management:
  - Permanent pacing is indicated if a PR interval of greater than 240 ms and LBBB are present or high-grade AV block occurs irrespective of symptoms.[31] This often occurs before the age of 30 years.
  - Stroke risk may remain high because of atrial standstill and atrial fibrillation and thus patients may need chronic anticoagulation.[73]

DMPK

Myotonic dystrophy 1 (DM1) is an autosomal dominant, inherited neuromuscular disorder caused by the expansion of a CTG repeat in the 3′-untranslated region of the gene encoding DMPK (myotonic dystrophy protein kinase). Cardiac involvement is one of the leading causes of death in patients affected by the disease. The cardiac phenotype is characterized by HCM and CCSD.[74] Recently, a large retrospective series of patients has shown that ECG markers such as prolonged PR interval greater than 200 ms and a QRS complex of greater than 120 ms were independent predictors of prolonged HV interval of greater than 70 ms at the invasive EP testing, thus needing pacemaker implantation.[75] Periodic cardiac follow-up of those patients is advised.[73,76]

Key findings and clinical recommendations

- Presentation:
  - Clinical presentation of Myotonic Dystrophy 1 disease is usually in the 2nd to 4th decade of life with skeletal myotonia and progressive muscle weakness and wasting.
  - The most common CCSD-related ECG findings at presentation are: prolonged PR interval (28%), LBBB 6%, RBBB 5%, and QRS greater than 120 ms in 20% of patients indicating that other forms of intraventricular conduction delay are present[77]
- Genetics:
  - The CTG repeat in the gene DMPK is linked to an increase in mutant RNA repeats, which exert a toxic effect and interfere with RNA-binding proteins leading to changes in CUGBP/Elav-like family member 1 (CELF1) and Muscle blind-like (MBNL) proteins. The RNA expansions fold and accumulate in the nucleus and reduce the function of the MBNL protein and interfere in the splicing in multiple other genes such as BIN1, skeletal muscle chloride channel, the insulin receptor, Troponin T, and NKX2-5, which could explain the CCSD defects of DM1 patients.[78–80]
- Management:
  - In the study by Brembilla and colleagues that included 129 patients, multivariate predictors of pacemaker implantation were as

follows: age and the presence of left anterior hemiblock or any bundle branch block at the baseline ECG. Those were also multivariate predictors of mortality[81]

○ The presence of second-degree AV block or third-degree AV block or HV interval of greater than 70 ms or PR interval greater than 240 ms or QRS duration greater than 120 ms, regardless of symptoms, needs to prompt permanent pacing.[31]

○ ICD implantation should be considered if there are concomitant ventricular arrhythmias or left ventricular dysfunction.[62]

○ Patients with a PR interval greater than 200 ms or a QRS greater than 100 ms were shown to experience a survival benefit in an observational trial with an invasive strategy including EP study and pacemaker implantation if HV was over 70 ms.[30,76]

METABOLISM PROTEINS
PRKAG2

PRKAG2 encodes for a regulatory subunit of adenosine monophosphate-activated protein kinase (AMPK), which plays a key role in regulating cellular energetic metabolism. In normal conditions, when intracellular ATP levels are reduced, AMPK activates other energy-producing pathways and inhibits energy-consuming processes, causing changes in the biosynthesis of fatty acids and cholesterol. PRKAG2 mutations cause a phenotype that combines HCM and ventricular preexcitation (familial Wolff-Parkinson-White (WPW) syndrome) because of accessory pathways that abnormally connect the atrium with the ventricles allowing for reentrant arrhythmias to occur and increasing the risk of atrial fibrillation.[82] The mechanism hypothesized by Arad and colleagues is that accumulation of glycogen in cardiomyocytes causes disruption of the fibrous annulus that separates the atrium from the ventricle based on the findings of a transgenic mice model that recapitulated the clinical human phenotype.[83] The clinical presentation of patients will be with arrhythmic symptoms such as palpitations, presyncope at young age (2nd and 3rd decade of life) with WPW and cardiac hypertrophy. Patients often have multiple accessory pathways and SAND and CCSD is responsible for a high rate of pacemaker implantation.[84] The clinical course of the disease is aggressive with 13% mortality and 4% heart transplantation after 6 years of clinical follow-up.[85]

Key findings and clinical recommendations

• Presentation:

○ The combination of an ECG with high voltages, ventricular preexcitation and HCM on echocardiography is the most common finding in patients with PRKAG2 mutations. Diagnosis is usually established during the 4th decade of life.

○ The CCSD is progressive and may lead to pacemaker implantation at young ages (3rd or 4th decade of life). Atrial fibrillation is a common complication during the course of the disease.[85]

○ Mutations in PRKAG2 can also be linked to CCSD and WPW in children in the absence of hypertrophy.[82]

• Genetics:

○ PRKAG2 mutations are linked to glycogen accumulation in the cardiomyocytes.

○ Although the most frequent mutations do not have extracardiac manifestations, rare mutations can be associated also with the development of skeletal myopathy with elevation in creatinine phosphokinase.[86]

• Management:

○ In patients manifesting signs and/or symptoms of WPW an electrophysiological testing is recommended to study the pathway characteristics and ablation can be performed during the same procedure. Often these patients have multiple accessory pathways. Noninvasive markers of low-risk accessory pathways such as intermittent preexcitation or disappearance of the delta wave during stress testing have been recently questioned as good markers of low-risk pathways so an invasive testing will always be the most reliable diagnostic and therapeutic strategy.[87]

○ Sudden cardiac death can occur (mean age 33.4 years) in a significant proportion of patients (8.7%) both due to complete heart block or rapid unstable tachyarrhythmia.[88] ICD implantation should be individualized.

○ Cardiac transplantation may be required in cases of advanced heart failure. In a cohort with a median follow-up of 6 years, heart transplantation was needed in 4% of patients.[89]

LAMP2

Mutations in LAMP2 are responsible for Danon's disease. The gene LAMP2 encodes for a protein that is part of the family of membrane glycoproteins (lysosome-associated membrane protein 2), which plays an important role in chaperone-mediated autophagy, a process that mediates lysosomal degradation of proteins in response to various stresses and part of the normal turnover of proteins with a long biological half-live. Mutations in LAMP2 impair the fusion of the autophagosome and lysosome leading to inefficient lysosome maturation and impairment of the metabolism of glycogen that subsequently accumulates in the heart and other organs causing a neuromuscular disease and intellectual disability. The histopathological study of these patients shows clusters of vacuolated myocytes and cardiomyopathy features such as myocyte disarray, myocardial fibrosis, and small vessel hypertrophy.[90] Male patients show signs of the disease earlier in life.[91,92] Extracardiac manifestations such as myopathy or cognitive dysfunction and visual alterations are very common.[85,93]

The cardiac manifestations are severe degrees of concentric hypertrophy and in some instances left ventricular systolic dysfunction and dilatation. Most of the time, the cardiomyopathy coexists with CCSD, which is present in most of the patients. CCSD phenotype includes WPW syndrome (present in 49% of patients in recent cohorts) and third-degree heart block in 33% of patients.[85]

Key findings and clinical recommendations

- Presentation:
  - The most common triad at presentation are as follows: nonobstructive HCM, skeletal myopathy, and cognitive impairment.
  - LAMP2 mutations are responsible for approximately 5% of pediatric cases of HCM. The disease shows an X-linked inheritance pattern and is often accompanied by skeletal myopathy. The prognosis is poor with a mean age at the time of death of 23 years.[94]
  - Males exhibit a more severe phenotype at earlier ages (2nd or 3rd decade of life). Neurologic involvement with cognitive impairment is common.[85]
  - Patients frequently exhibit ventricular pre-excitation[93] followed frequently by CCSD with complete heart block over time.[95]
- Genetics:
  - LAMP2 mutations result in total or partial loss of the enzyme leading to glycogen accumulation.[95]
  - Most mutations are nonsense or frameshift predicted to truncate the LAMP2 protein, resulting in absence of the transmembrane and cytoplasmic domains and disabling the function as a lysosomal membrane protein[95,96]
- Management:
  - In cases when permanent pacing is needed, ICD implantation should be considered

based on the degree of hypertrophy and other possible factors related to the risk of sudden death.
  - The severity of the cardiac phenotype leads to heart failure at early ages and is the leading cause of death.[93]
  - Cardiac transplantation or LVAD implantation may be needed in a high proportion of patients (27% in a European registry after a median follow-up of 6 years).[85,93]

GLA

The gene GLA encodes for the protein alpha-galactosidase (AGAL-A), which is responsible for the hydrolyzation of glycolipids and glycoproteins. Mutations in GLA cause Anderson-Fabry disease (AFD) and have an X-linked pattern of inheritance causing the accumulation of glycosphingolipids in multiple organs. Cardiac involvement presents myocardial hypertrophy and commonly chronotropic incompetence, severe CCSD, and proarrhythmia.[97] Most prevalence studies are based on the screening of patients with unexplained HCM: 1% to 12% in those highly selected populations.[98,99] Neonatal screening studies have suggested an incidence of disease-causing variants between 1:1250 and 1:7800.[100] Specific treatments for the disease with a pharmacologic chaperone and enzyme replacement therapy exist but the effect on CCSD is unknown.[101]

Key clinical findings and clinical recommendations

- Presentation:
  - Age at presentation is often in the 4th decade of life and recent data have suggested that AFD patients present more often with a shorter PR interval, RBBB pattern, and ST-segment depression compared with non-Fabry HCM patients.[102]
  - Extracardiac involvement includes cutaneous lesions (angiokeratoma), hypohidrosis, peripheral neuropathy (acral pain and painful febrile crisis), stroke, and renal insufficiency with proteinuria.
- Genetics:
  - The diagnosis is based on both the absence or severe reduction of the activity of AGAL-A enzyme (<1% of normal in males) and GLA sequencing in females.
- Management:
  - Patients with AFD are at risk of AV block and atrial or ventricular arrhythmias. In adult patients with AFD, the incidence of pacing or defibrillator implantation ranges between 1% and 2% per year.[102,103]

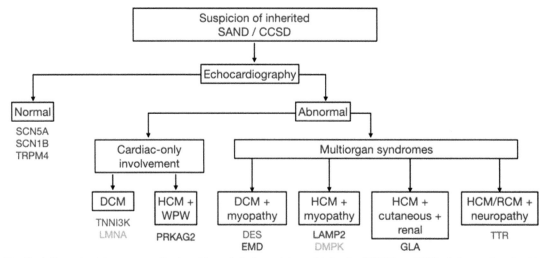

Fig. 2. A flow chart to assess patients with a clinical suspicion of inherited SAND or CCSD. Color coding for the gene names as in **Fig. 1**: ion channels in gray, structural proteins in blue, nuclear proteins in yellow, and metabolism proteins in red. RCM, restrictive cardiomyopathy.

- Current guidelines recommend pacemaker implantation if a patient with Fabry disease has a QRS of greater than 110 ms.[31]
- Implantation of pacemaker should also be done if advanced AV block occurs or if symptomatic proven chronotropic incompetence is diagnosed. Consideration for cardiac resynchronization therapy should be done if the baseline LVEF is less than 50% and the percentage of ventricular pacing is expected to be very high.[104]
- Implantation of primary prevention ICD should be individualized and performed in those patients with ventricular arrhythmia.[31,104]
- Enzyme replacement therapy for confirmed cases of AFD is available and it has shown beneficial cardiovascular effects when initiated early in the course of the disease. Despite the treatment, some patients experience severe complications due to progression of the disease.[101,105]
- Specific treatment with the pharmacologic chaperone *migalastat* is available for some GLA mutations to increase the trafficking of the enzyme into lysosomes.[106]

Fig. 2 shows a simplified flow chart to assess the most common phenotype-genotype correlation.

SUMMARY

The inherited forms of SAND and CCSD are complex and heterogeneous disorders. Genetic defects at different levels translate into dysfunctional proteins causing a wide range of clinical manifestations ranging from asymptomatic sinus bradycardia to life-threatening cardiomyopathies with multiorgan damage and poor outcomes. The familial pattern and the mutation identification are key to risk stratification and to select the most appropriate therapy and follow-up for each clinical presentation. Genetic screening of the conditions described in this review could provide valuable information and in some instances risk stratification for patients with a familial or with early-onset sporadic CCSD presentation. Overall, patients with familial forms of cardiac conduction diseases with or without additional cardiac or extracardiac phenotypes should be screened for mutations in the following genes:

SCN5A (OMIM#60016)
LMNA (OMIM#150330)
TRPM4 (OMIM#606936)
DESMIN (OMIM #125660)
PRKAG2 (OMIM#602743)
TNNI3K (OMIM #613932)
SCN1B (OMIM#612838)
NKX2.5 (OMIM#600584)
TBX5 (OMIM#601620)

The OMIM number refers to the classification of inherited diseases reported in the Online Mendelian Inheritance in Man Web site https://www.omim.org/ that is *"a comprehensive, authoritative compendium of human genes and genetic phenotypes that is freely available and updated daily."* For readers interested to expand their knowledge on the topic discussed in this review, the OMIM Web site is the best starting point.

CLINICS CARE POINTS

- The appropriate diagnosis of an inherited form of SAND/CCSD is critical for the most precise and personalized management of patients and their families.
- In some inherited diseases, SAND or CCSD can be the initial manifestation of an underlying cardiomyopathy such as LMNA-related cardiomyopathy.
- Inherited storage diseases such as inherited amyloidosis, Anderson-Fabry, Danon Disease, and PRKAG2 syndrome usually manifest with increased left ventricular mass. They are progressive diseases and may have a very severe clinical presentation.
- Clinical management with pacemaker implantation may be the only treatment for most of the inherited forms of SAND or CCSD. In cases of channelopathies or mutations manifesting as dilated cardiomyopathy or hypertrophic cardiomyopathy, the risk of sudden arrhythmic death needs to be assessed. Consideration for ICD implantation should be made based on the severity of arrhythmias present in the patient or on the prospective risk of developing life-threatening ventricular arrhythmias.

DISCLOSURE

No disclosures.

REFERENCES

1. Dhutia H, Malhotra A, Finnochiaro G, et al. Diagnostic yield and financial implications of a nationwide electrocardiographic screening programme to detect cardiac disease in the young. Europace 2021. https://doi.org/10.1093/europace/euab021.
2. Dideriksen JR, Christiansen MK, Johansen JB, et al. Long-term outcomes in young patients with atrioventricular block of unknown aetiology. Eur Heart J 2021;42(21):2060–8.
3. Sasaki T, Ikeda K, Nakajima T, et al. Multiple arrhythmic and cardiomyopathic phenotypes associated with an SCN5A A735E mutation. J Electrocardiol 2021;65:122–7.
4. Benson DW, Wang DW, Dyment M, et al. Congenital sick sinus syndrome caused by recessive mutations in the cardiac sodium channel gene (SCN5A). J Clin Invest 2003;112(7):1019–28.
5. Schott J-J, Alshinawi C, Kyndt F, et al. Cardiac conduction defects associate with mutations in SCN5A. Nat Genet 1999;23(1):20–1.
6. Probst V, Kyndt F, Potet F, et al. Haploinsufficiency in combination with aging causes SCN5A-linked hereditary Lenegre disease. J Am Coll Cardiol 2003;41(4):643–52.
7. Tan HL, Bink-Boelkens MT, Bezzina CR, et al. A sodium-channel mutation causes isolated cardiac conduction disease. Nature 2001;409(6823):1043–7.
8. Maury P, Rollin A, Sacher F, et al. Prevalence and prognostic role of various conduction disturbances in patients with the Brugada Syndrome. Am J Cardiol 2013;112(9):1384–9.
9. Mohler PJ, Rivolta I, Napolitano C, et al. Nav1. 5 E1053K mutation causing Brugada syndrome blocks binding to ankyrin-G and expression of Nav1. 5 on the surface of cardiomyocytes. Proc Natl Acad Sci 2004;101(50):17533–8.
10. Park DS, Cerrone M, Morley G, et al. Genetically engineered SCN5A mutant pig hearts exhibit conduction defects and arrhythmias. J Clin Invest 2015;125(1):403–12.
11. Butters TD, Aslanidi OV, Inada S, et al. Mechanistic Links between Na+ channel (SCN5A) mutations and impaired cardiac pacemaking in sick sinus syndrome. Circ Res 2010;107(1):126–37.
12. Asseman P, Berzin B, Desry D, et al. Persistent sinus nodal electrograms during abnormally prolonged postpacing atrial pauses in sick sinus syndrome in humans: sinoatrial block vs overdrive suppression. Circulation 1983;68(1):33–41.
13. Watanabe H, Darbar D, Kaiser DW, et al. Mutations in sodium channel β1-and β2-subunits associated with atrial fibrillation. Circ Arrhythmia Electrophysiol 2009;2(3):268–75.
14. Watanabe H, Koopmann TT, Le Scouarnec S, et al. Sodium channel beta1 subunit mutations associated with Brugada syndrome and cardiac conduction disease in humans. J Clin Invest 2008;118(6):2260–8.
15. Ziyadeh-Isleem A, Clatot J, Duchatelet S, et al. A truncating SCN5A mutation combined with genetic variability causes sick sinus syndrome and early atrial fibrillation. Heart Rhythm 2014;11(6):1015–23.
16. McNair WP, Ku L, Taylor MRG, et al. SCN5A mutation associated with dilated cardiomyopathy, conduction disorder, and arrhythmia. Circulation 2004;110(15):2163–7.
17. Ackerman MJ, Priori SG, Willems S, et al. HRS/EHRA expert consensus statement on the state of genetic testing for the channelopathies and cardiomyopathies this document was developed as a partnership between the Heart Rhythm Society (HRS) and the European Heart Rhythm Association (EHRA). Heart Rhythm 2011;8(8):1308–39.
18. Hong K, Brugada J, Oliva A, et al. Value of electrocardiographic parameters and ajmaline test in the

diagnosis of Brugada syndrome caused by SCN5A mutations. Circulation 2004;110(19):3023–7.

19. Launay P, Fleig A, Perraud AL, et al. TRPM4 is a Ca2+-activated nonselective cation channel mediating cell membrane depolarization. Cell 2002; 109(3):397–407.

20. Amarouch MY, El Hilaly J. Inherited cardiac arrhythmia syndromes: focus on molecular mechanisms underlying TRPM4 channelopathies. Cardiovasc Ther 2020;2020:6615038.

21. Brink AJ, Torrington M. Progressive familial heart block–two types. South Afr Med J 1977;52(2):53–9.

22. Kruse M, Schulze-Bahr E, Corfield V, et al. Impaired endocytosis of the ion channel TRPM4 is associated with human progressive familial heart block type I. J Clin Invest 2009;119(9):2737–44.

23. Liu H, Chatel S, Simard C, et al. Molecular genetics and functional Anomalies in a series of 248 Brugada cases with 11 mutations in the TRPM4 channel. PloS one 2013;8(1):e54131.

24. Demion M, Thireau J, Gueffier M, et al. Trpm4 gene invalidation leads to cardiac hypertrophy and electrophysiological alterations. PloS one 2014;9(12): e115256.

25. Liu H, El Zein L, Kruse M, et al. Gain-of-Function mutations in TRPM4 cause autosomal dominant isolated cardiac conduction disease. Circ-Cardiovasc Gene. 2010;3(4). 374-U326.

26. Syam N, Chatel S, Ozhathil LC, et al. Variants of transient receptor potential melastatin member 4 in childhood atrioventricular block. J Am Heart Assoc 2016;5(5):e001625.

27. Bianchi B, Ozhathil LC, Medeiros-Domingo A, et al. Four TRPM4 cation channel mutations found in cardiac conduction diseases lead to altered protein stability. Front Physiol 2018;9:177.

28. Pironet A, Syam N, Vandewiele F, et al. AAV9-mediated overexpression of TRPM4 increases the incidence of stress-induced ventricular arrhythmias in mice. Front Physiol 2019;10:802.

29. Gualandi F, Zaraket F, Malagù M, et al. Mutation Load of multiple ion channel gene mutations in Brugada syndrome. Cardiology 2017;137(4):256–60.

30. Hof T, Liu H, Sallé L, et al. TRPM4 non-selective cation channel variants in long QT syndrome. BMC Med Genet 2017;18(1):31.

31. Kusumoto FM, Schoenfeld MH, Barrett C, et al. 2018 ACC/AHA/HRS guideline on the evaluation and management of patients with bradycardia and cardiac conduction delay: a report of the American College of cardiology/American heart association Task Force on clinical practice guidelines and the heart rhythm Society. J Am Coll Cardiol 2019;74(7):e51–156.

32. Rapezzi C, Quarta CC, Obici L, et al. Disease profile and differential diagnosis of hereditary transthyretin-related amyloidosis with exclusively cardiac phenotype: an Italian perspective. Eur Heart J 2012;34(7):520–8.

33. Barbhaiya CR, Kumar S, Baldinger SH, et al. Electrophysiologic assessment of conduction abnormalities and atrial arrhythmias associated with amyloid cardiomyopathy. Heart Rhythm 2016; 13(2):383–90.

34. Rehorn MR, Loungani RS, Black-Maier E, et al. Cardiac implantable electronic devices: a window into the evolution of conduction disease in cardiac amyloidosis. JACC: Clin Electrophysiol 2020;6(9): 1144–54.

35. Maurer MS, Schwartz JH, Gundapaneni B, et al. Tafamidis treatment for patients with transthyretin amyloid cardiomyopathy. N Engl J Med 2018;379(11): 1007–16.

36. Solomon SD, Adams D, Kristen A, et al. Effects of patisiran, an RNA interference therapeutic, on cardiac parameters in patients with hereditary transthyretin-mediated amyloidosis: analysis of the APOLLO study. Circulation 2019;139(4): 431–43.

37. Garcia-Pavia P, Rapezzi C, Adler Y, et al. Diagnosis and treatment of cardiac amyloidosis: a position statement of the ESC working group on myocardial and Pericardial diseases. Eur Heart J 2021;42(16): 1554–68.

38. Donnellan E, Wazni OM, Hanna M, et al. Cardiac resynchronization therapy for transthyretin cardiac amyloidosis. J Am Heart Assoc 2020;9(14): e017335.

39. Kim E-J, Holmes BB, Huang S, et al. Outcomes in patients with cardiac amyloidosis and implantable cardioverter-defibrillator. Europace 2020;22(8): 1216–23.

40. Varr BC, Zarafshar S, Coakley T, et al. Implantable cardioverter-defibrillator placement in patients with cardiac amyloidosis. Heart Rhythm 2014;11(1): 158–62.

41. Fischer B, Dittmann S, Brodehl A, et al. Functional characterization of novel alpha-helical rod domain desmin (DES) pathogenic variants associated with dilated cardiomyopathy, atrioventricular block and a risk for sudden cardiac death. Int J Cardiol 2021;329:167–74.

42. Taylor MRG, Slavov D, Ku L, et al. Prevalence of desmin mutations in dilated cardiomyopathy. Circulation 2007;115(10):1244–51.

43. van Spaendonck-Zwarts KY, van Hessem L, Jongbloed JD, et al. Desmin-related myopathy. Clin Genet 2011;80(4):354–66.

44. Otten E, Asimaki A, Maass A, et al. Desmin mutations as a cause of right ventricular heart failure affect the intercalated disks. Heart Rhythm 2010; 7(8):1058–64.

45. Bermúdez-Jiménez FJ, Carriel V, Brodehl A, et al. Novel desmin mutation p. Glu401Asp impairs

filament formation, disrupts cell membrane integrity, and causes severe arrhythmogenic left ventricular cardiomyopathy/dysplasia. Circulation 2018; 137(15):1595–610.

46. Goldfarb LG, Park K-Y, Cervenáková L, et al. Missense mutations in desmin associated with familial cardiac and skeletal myopathy. Nat Genet 1998;19(4):402–3.

47. Dalakas MC, Park K-Y, Semino-Mora C, et al. Desmin myopathy, a skeletal myopathy with cardiomyopathy caused by mutations in the desmin gene. N Engl J Med 2000;342(11):770–80.

48. Zhao Y, Meng X-M, Wei Y-J, et al. Cloning and characterization of a novel cardiac-specific kinase that interacts specifically with cardiac troponin I. J Mol Med 2003;81(5):297–304.

49. Theis JL, Zimmermann MT, Larsen BT, et al. TNNI3K mutation in familial syndrome of conduction system disease, atrial tachyarrhythmia and dilated cardiomyopathy. Hum Mol Genet 2014; 23(21):5793–804.

50. Podliesna S, Delanne J, Miller L, et al. Supraventricular tachycardias, conduction disease, and cardiomyopathy in 3 families with the same rare variant in TNNI3K (p.Glu768Lys). Heart Rhythm 2019;16(1):98–105.

51. Xi Y, Honeywell C, Zhang D, et al. Whole exome sequencing identifies the TNNI3K gene as a cause of familial conduction system disease and congenital junctional ectopic tachycardia. Int J Cardiol 2015;185:114–6.

52. Fatkin D, MacRae C, Sasaki T, et al. Missense mutations in the rod domain of the lamin A/C gene as causes of dilated cardiomyopathy and conduction-system disease. N Engl J Med 1999;341(23): 1715–24.

53. Taylor MRG, Fain PR, Sinagra G, et al. Natural history of dilated cardiomyopathy due to lamin A/C gene mutations. J Am Coll Cardiol 2003;41(5):771–80.

54. Gigli M, Merlo M, Graw SL, et al. Genetic risk of arrhythmic phenotypes in patients with dilated cardiomyopathy. J Am Coll Cardiol 2019;74(11): 1480–90.

55. Kumar S, Baldinger SH, Gandjbakhch E, et al. Long-term arrhythmic and Nonarrhythmic outcomes of lamin A/C mutation carriers. J Am Coll Cardiol 2016;68(21):2299–307.

56. Priori SG, Blomström-Lundqvist C, Mazzanti A, et al. 2015 ESC guidelines for the management of patients with ventricular arrhythmias and the prevention of sudden cardiac death: the Task Force for the management of patients with ventricular arrhythmias and the prevention of sudden cardiac death of the European Society of cardiology (ESC) Endorsed by: association for European Paediatric and congenital cardiology (AEPC). Europace 2015;17(11):1601–87.

57. Barriales-Villa R, Ochoa JP, Larrañaga-Moreira JM, et al. Risk predictors in a Spanish cohort with cardiac laminopathies. The REDLAMINA registry. Rev Esp Cardiol (Engl Ed) 2020;74(3):216–24.

58. Van Rijsingen IA, Arbustini E, Elliott PM, et al. Risk factors for malignant ventricular arrhythmias in lamin A/C mutation carriers: a European cohort study. J Am Coll Cardiol 2012;59(5):493–500.

59. Brodt C, Siegfried JD, Hofmeyer M, et al. Temporal relationship of conduction system disease and ventricular dysfunction in LMNA cardiomyopathy. J Card Fail 2013;19(4):233–9.

60. Parks SB, Kushner JD, Nauman D, et al. Lamin A/C mutation analysis in a cohort of 324 unrelated patients with idiopathic or familial dilated cardiomyopathy. Am Heart J 2008;156(1):161–9.

61. Nishiuchi S, Makiyama T, Aiba T, et al. Gene-based risk stratification for cardiac disorders in LMNA mutation carriers. Circ-Cardiovasc Gene. 2017;10(6): e001603.

62. Al-Khatib SM, Stevenson WG, Ackerman MJ, et al. 2017 AHA/ACC/HRS guideline for management of patients with ventricular arrhythmias and the prevention of sudden cardiac death: a report of the American College of cardiology/American heart association Task Force on clinical practice guidelines and the heart rhythm Society. J Am Coll Cardiol 2018;72(14):e91–220.

63. Huang WJ, Su L, Wu SJ, et al. A novel pacing strategy with low and stable output: pacing the left bundle branch immediately beyond the conduction block. Can J Cardiol 2017;33(12):1736.e1-3.

64. Kumar S, Androulakis AFA, Sellal J-M, et al. Multicenter experience with catheter ablation for ventricular tachycardia in lamin A/C cardiomyopathy. Circulation Arrhythmia Electrophysiol 2016;9(8): e004357.

65. Karst ML, Herron KJ, Olson TM. X-linked nonsyndromic sinus node dysfunction and atrial fibrillation caused by emerin mutation. J Cardiovasc Electrophysiol 2008;19(5):510–5.

66. Bonne G, Di Barletta MR, Varnous S, et al. Mutations in the gene encoding lamin A/C cause autosomal dominant Emery-Dreifuss muscular dystrophy. Nat Genet 1999;21(3):285–8.

67. Ishikawa T, Mishima H, Barc J, et al. Cardiac emerinopathy: a nonsyndromic nuclear Envelopathy with increased risk of Thromboembolic stroke due to progressive atrial standstill and left ventricular Noncompaction. Circ Arrhythmia Electrophysiol 2020;13(10):e008712.

68. Marchel M, Madej-Pilarczyk A, Tyminska A, et al. Cardiac arrhythmias in muscular dystrophies associated with emerinopathy and laminopathy: a cohort study. J Clin Med 2021;10(4):732.

69. Boriani G, Gallina M, Merlini L, et al. Clinical relevance of atrial fibrillation/flutter, stroke, pacemaker

implant, and heart failure in emery-dreifuss muscular dystrophy. Stroke 2003;34(4):901–8.

70. Marchel M, Madej-Pilarczyk A, Tyminska A, et al. Echocardiographic features of cardiomyopathy in emery-dreifuss muscular dystrophy. Cardiol Res Pract 2021;2021:8812044.

71. Ellis JA, Yates JRW, Kendrick-Jones J, et al. Changes at P183 of emerin weaken its protein-protein interactions resulting in X-linked Emery-Dreifuss muscular dystrophy. Hum Genet 1999; 104(3):262–8.

72. Sakata K, Shimizu M, Ino H, et al. High incidence of sudden cardiac death with conduction disturbances and atrial cardiomyopathy caused by a nonsense mutation in the STA gene. Circulation 2005;111(25):3352–8.

73. Brignole M, Auricchio A, Baron-Esquivias G, et al. 2013 ESC Guidelines on cardiac pacing and cardiac resynchronization therapy. Eur Heart J 2013; 34(29):2281–329.

74. de Die-Smulders CE, Höweler CJ, Thijs C, et al. Age and causes of death in adult-onset myotonic dystrophy. Brain 1998;121(8):1557–63.

75. Joosten IBT, van Lohuizen R, den Uijl DW, et al. Electrocardiographic predictors of infrahissian conduction disturbances in myotonic dystrophy type 1. Europace 2020;23(2):298–304.

76. Wahbi K, Meune C, Porcher R, et al. Electrophysiological study with prophylactic pacing and survival in adults with myotonic dystrophy and conduction system disease. JAMA 2012;307(12): 1292–301.

77. Petri H, Vissing J, Witting N, et al. Cardiac manifestations of myotonic dystrophy type 1. Int J Cardiol 2012;160(2):82–8.

78. Ebralidze A, Wang Y, Petkova V, et al. RNA Leaching of transcription factors disrupts transcription in myotonic dystrophy. Science 2004;303(5656):383–7.

79. Udd B, Krahe R. The myotonic dystrophies: molecular, clinical, and therapeutic challenges. Lancet Neurol 2012;11(10):891–905.

80. Yadava RS, Frenzel-McCardell CD, Yu Q, et al. RNA toxicity in myotonic muscular dystrophy induces NKX2-5 expression. Nat Genet 2008;40(1): 61–8.

81. Brembilla-Perrot B, Luporsi JD, Louis S, et al. Long-term follow-up of patients with myotonic dystrophy: an electrocardiogram every year is not necessary. Europace 2011;13(2):251–7.

82. Gollob MH, Seger JJ, Gollob TN, et al. Novel PRKAG2 mutation responsible for the genetic syndrome of ventricular preexcitation and conduction system disease with childhood onset and absence of cardiac hypertrophy. Circulation 2001;104(25): 3030–3.

83. Arad M, Moskowitz IP, Patel VV, et al. Transgenic mice overexpressing mutant PRKAG2 define the cause of Wolff-Parkinson-White syndrome in glycogen storage cardiomyopathy. Circulation 2003;107(22):2850–6.

84. Gollob MH, Green MS, Tang AS-L, et al. Identification of a gene responsible for familial Wolff–Parkinson–white syndrome. N Engl J Med 2001;344(24): 1823–31.

85. Lopez-Sainz A, Salazar-Mendiguchia J, Garcia-Alvarez A, et al. Clinical findings and prognosis of Danon disease. An analysis of the Spanish multicenter Danon registry. Rev Esp Cardiol (Engl Ed) 2019;72(6):479–86.

86. Laforêt P, Richard P, Said MA, et al. A new mutation in PRKAG2 gene causing hypertrophic cardiomyopathy with conduction system disease and muscular glycogenosis. Neuromuscul Disord 2006;16(3):178–82.

87. Escudero CA, Ceresnak SR, Collins KK, et al. Loss of ventricular preexcitation during noninvasive testing does not exclude high-risk accessory pathways: a multicenter study of WPW in children. Heart Rhythm 2020;17(10):1729–37.

88. Porto AG, Brun F, Severini GM, et al. Clinical spectrum of PRKAG2 syndrome. Circulation Arrhythmia Electrophysiol 2016;9(1):e003121.

89. Dominguez F, Lopez-Sainz A, Rocha-Lopes L, et al. Clinical characteristics and natural history of PRKAG2 syndrome. Eur Heart J 2020; 41(Supplement_2). p. 2086.

90. Maron BJ, Roberts WC, Arad M, et al. Clinical outcome and phenotypic expression in LAMP2 cardiomyopathy. JAMA 2009;301(12):1253–9.

91. Arad M, Maron BJ, Gorham JM, et al. Glycogen storage diseases presenting as hypertrophic cardiomyopathy. N Engl J Med 2005;352(4):362–72.

92. Sugie K, Komaki H, Eura N, et al. A nationwide survey on Danon disease in Japan. Int J Mol Sci 2018; 19(11):3507.

93. Lotan D, Salazar-Mendiguchia J, Mogensen J, et al. Clinical profile of cardiac involvement in Danon disease A multicenter European registry. Circulation Genomic Precision Med 2020;13(6): 660–70.

94. Cenacchi G, Papa V, Pegoraro V, et al. Review: Danon disease: review of natural history and recent advances. Neuropathol Appl Neurobiol 2020; 46(4):303–22.

95. D'souza RS, Levandowski C, Slavov D, et al. Danon disease. Circ Heart Fail 2014;7(5):843–9.

96. Nishino I, Fu J, Tanji K, et al. Primary LAMP-2 deficiency causes X-linked vacuolar cardiomyopathy and myopathy (Danon disease). Nature 2000; 406(6798):906–10.

97. Hagege A, Reant P, Habib G, et al. Fabry disease in cardiology practice: Literature review and expert point of view. Arch Cardiovasc Dis 2019;112(4): 278–87.

98. Monserrat L, Gimeno-Blanes JR, Marín F, et al. Prevalence of Fabry disease in a cohort of 508 unrelated patients with hypertrophic cardiomyopathy. J Am Coll Cardiol 2007;50(25):2399–403.

99. Chimenti C, Pieroni M, Morgante E, et al. Prevalence of Fabry disease in female patients with late-onset hypertrophic cardiomyopathy. Circulation 2004;110(9):1047–53.

100. Spada M, Pagliardini S, Yasuda M, et al. High incidence of later-onset Fabry disease revealed by newborn screening. Am J Hum Genet 2006;79(1):31–40.

101. Dutra-Clarke M, Tapia D, Curtin E, et al. Variable clinical features of patients with Fabry disease and outcome of enzyme replacement therapy. Mol Genet Metab Rep 2021;26:100700.

102. Vitale G, Ditaranto R, Graziani F, et al. Standard ECG for differential diagnosis between Anderson-Fabry disease and hypertrophic cardiomyopathy. Heart 2021. https://doi.org/10.1136/heartjnl-2020-318271.

103. Sene T, Lidove O, Sebbah J, et al. Cardiac device implantation in Fabry disease: a retrospective monocentric study. Medicine 2016;95(40):e4996.

104. Linhart A, Germain DP, Olivotto I, et al. An expert consensus document on the management of cardiovascular manifestations of Fabry disease. Eur J Heart Fail 2020;22(7):1076–96.

105. Schiffmann R, Kopp JB, Austin HA, et al. Enzyme replacement therapy in Fabry disease - a randomized controlled trial. JAMA 2001;285(21):2743–9.

106. Germain DP, Hughes DA, Nicholls K, et al. Treatment of Fabry's disease with the pharmacologic chaperone migalastat. N Engl J Med 2016;375(6):545–55.

Sinus Node Dysfunction

Neeraj Sathnur, MD[a,b,c], Emanuel Ebin, MD[a,b], David G. Benditt, MD[a,b,*]

KEYWORDS

- Sick sinus syndrome ● Sinus node dysfunction ● Bradycardia ● Bradycardia-tachycardia syndrome

KEY POINTS

- Sinus node dysfunction (SND) is multifaceted disorder most prevalent in older individuals.
- The diagnosis of SND may be suspected based on careful history.
- Both bradycardia and tachycardia may coexist in the same patients.
- Treatment strategy is largely dictated by symptoms and ECG manifestations and may require a pacemaker.
- Anticoagulant therapy to prevent stroke is often needed.

INTRODUCTION

Sinus node dysfunction (SND) encompasses a range of sinus node and/or atrial electrophysiologic/arrhythmic disturbances with clinical consequences ranging from none or minimal to severe disability. On initial assessment, slow heart rates or paroxysmal atrial tachyarrhythmias may not seem to bother some individuals, yet in many instances, more detailed history taking may elicit subtle disturbances that were previously unreported and perhaps even unrecognized by the patient. For instance, gradual cognitive and functional deterioration due to arrhythmic or embolic complications associated with SND, particularly in elderly patients.

Many of the arrhythmias now incorporated within the SND landscape have been known since the development of electrocardiographic (ECG) recordings in the early part of the 20th century, but the concept of SND as a syndrome only began in the mid-1950s to early 1970s[1–7] (**Figs. 1 and 2**). Herein, we provide an overview of the pathophysiology and principal clinical manifestations of SND, as well as current guideline-based treatment recommendations.

Sinus Node Anatomy and Physiology

Activation of each normal cardiac impulse arises from pacemaker cells capable of spontaneously depolarizing; these lie principally within a relatively diffuse "sinus node" anatomic region approximately situated laterally in the epicardial groove of the sulcus terminalis of the right atrium.[8–12] The arterial supply to the node (sinus node artery) is usually derived from the proximal portion of the right coronary artery (55%), with the remainder (45%) arising from the left circumflex coronary artery.[11–14]

Although often inappropriately depicted as a discrete structure, the sinus node region is complex and incorporates considerable redundancy including "principal" pacemaker cells, as well as auxiliary pacemaker cell nests that operate as backup or subsidiary pacemakers[8–12]; these latter cell groups may become the principal pacemaker sites under a variety of physiologic and pathologic conditions (eg, vagal stimulation, sympathetic stimulation, electrolyte disturbances). The result is a shift of the origin of the cardiac impulse within the sinus node region; apart from causing alterations of P-wave morphology, such shifts also complicate electrophysiologic assessment of sinus node function.[8–10,14]

This article originally appeared in *Cardiac Electrophysiology Clinics*, Volume 13 Issue 4, December 2021.

[a] Cardiac Arrhythmia Service, Cardiovascular Division, University of Minnesota Medical School, Minneapolis, MN, USA; [b] Cardiovascular Medicine, University of Minnesota Medical School, Mail Code 508, 420 Delaware St SE, Minneapolis, MN 55455, USA; [c] Cardiac Electrophysiology, Park-Nicollet Medical Center, St Louis Park, Minneapolis, MN, USA

* Corresponding author.

E-mail address: bendi001@umn.edu

cardiology.theclinics.com

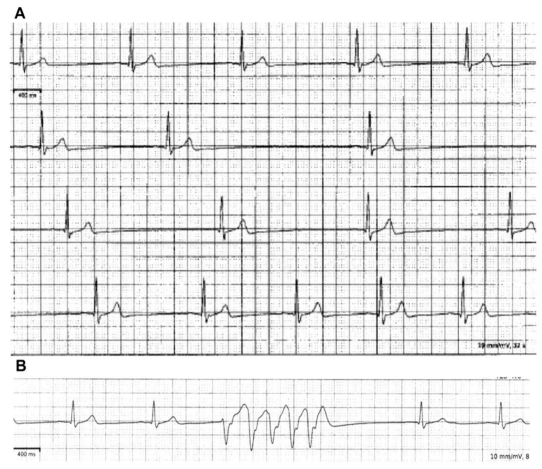

Fig. 1. (*A*) Rhythm strip illustrating onset of seemingly asymptomatic bradycardia in a 68-year-old woman. However, more careful history taking revealed progressive fatigue over the past 6 months. (*B*) Rhythm strip from the same patient revealing nonsustained ventricular tachycardia (VT) may be as a consequence of persistent sinus bradycardia. Pacemaker therapy improved her energy and eliminated VT events during subsequent monitoring.

Impulse conduction within sinus node tissue is relatively slow (2–5 cm/s). Although in health, slow conduction tends to improve safety factor for impulse propagation, it also introduces a greater propensity for intranodal conduction failure due to adverse outside influences. The same slow conduction physiology may also be the substrate for re-entry rhythms, particularly sinoatrial re-entry tachycardia (**Fig. 3**A and B).

Electroanatomic mapping studies not only support the distributed nature of sinus node activation[8–14] but also suggest that there may be multiple preferential conduction routes from pacemaker cells to the atrium.[8–11,15] The conduction routes have importance, as a small group of pacemaker cells must generate an electrical impulse capable of activating a relatively large mass of atrial tissue. This is a "source-sink" problem; in essence, the small electrical source must generate sufficient space constant to activate downstream cells and create an effective depolarizing wavefront.[15–18]

Several anatomic and electrophysiological factors are believed to be helpful in permitting the few sinus node cells to activate the much larger atrial structure. In this regard, fibrous barriers within the sinus node may act to reduce, from the source perspective, the effective "physical size" of the sink. In addition, the inherently slow conduction, perhaps somewhat paradoxically, provides for an increased safety factor for electrical transmission from the pacemaker cell nests to the periphery.[15–17]

SND: Intrinsic and Extrinsic

SND may be the result of "intrinsic" factors that directly alter sinus node and perinodal structure

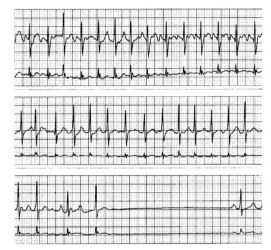

Fig. 2. ECG recording revealing atrial fibrillation with a rapid ventricular response, which terminates abruptly with a prolonged pause before resumption of stable rhythm.

and function or "extrinsic" contributors such as drugs and/or autonomic disturbances that may cause so-called "extrinsic" SND[9,17–19] (**Table 1**).

Intrinsic SND

Intrinsic SND is believed to be a nonreversible condition that progresses over time and exhibits variable manifestations. Most often progressive fibrosis (beyond that normally associated with sinus node anatomy) and cell death (which may be

due to a variety of disease processes) are considered to be the primary causes.[17–29] In addition, genetic abnormalities, remodeling of membrane ion channels, and alterations of intracellular Ca++ cycling have been increasingly implicated.[17,18]

i) Adults

Replacement or displacement of normal SA cells by fibrous tissue with alteration of regional architecture is among the more common pathologic observations of cardiac tissues from SND patients. Potential causes include ischemia, atrial myopathy (stand-alone or in conjunction with cardiomyopathy affecting other cardiac tissues), surgical trauma, and inflammation (eg, pericardial disease, rheumatic heart disease, viral myocarditis, collagen vascular diseases). In some instances, the condition appears to be familial in origin[22–29] and possible genetic contributions have become of increased interest.

Acute disturbances of sinus node function may occur in the setting of acute myocardial infarction, especially of the right coronary artery. In such cases, ischemia may be the primary driver, but neural reflex effects attributed to mechanical or chemoreceptors within the ventricular wall are potential contributors; in any event, the problem tends to be transient.[30–36]

Coronary atherosclerosis is often listed among the more frequent causes of chronic SND,[34] but the relationship may be coincidental, since both tend to occur in older individuals. Shaw and

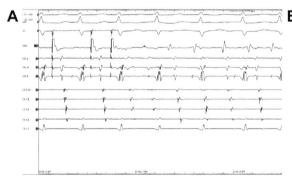
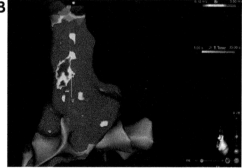

Fig. 3. (A) ECGs and intracardiac electrograms in a patient with an attempted but incompletely successful sinus node modification for IST 4 years earlier. She returned with a paroxysmal supraventricular tachycardia (PSVT) consistent with sinus node reentry tachycardia likely resulting from residual ablation scar. Depicted here are ECG leads I, aVF, and V1, along with an atrial electrogram in the sinus node region (HRA) and His (HBE) bundle and coronary sinus electrograms. The PSVT was readily inducible by premature beats, and terminated with pacing. The activation atrial sequence was similar to that recorded in sinus rhythm and during atrial pacing from the sinus node region, as shown here. The PSVT, consistent with Sinus Node Reentry Tachycardia, exhibited 2:1 AV block. (B) Voltage map depicting the right atrium from a lateral view with SVC at the top in the patient described in panel A. The dark red zone indicates scar and the pink-purple indicates healthy tissue. Entrainment was successful in the green zone just anterior to the most dense scar. The presence of the phrenic nerve nearby complicated the ablation procedure. Nonetheless, ablation centered on the entrainment site eliminated induction of tachycardia, with no spontaneous recurrence during 6 months follow-up.

Table 1
Principal "intrinsic" and "extrinsic" factors that may undermine sinus node and perinodal structure and function and thereby contribute to clinical SND

Intrinsic Sinus Node Dysfunction	Extrinsic Sinus Node Dysfunction
Idiopathic degenerative disease (probably most common) • Including effects of hypertension • Atrial myopathy (primary or secondary associated with other disease state noted below)	Drug effects (see **Box 1**)
Ischemic: • Chronic (may involve sinus node artery) • Acute MI (particularly inferior wall, may be reflex (see "Extrinsic")	Electrolyte disturbances: particularly hyperkalemia
Infiltrative disorders: • Amyloidosis, • Hemochromatosis, • Sarcoid	Endocrine conditions: hypothyroidism, or less commonly hyperthyroidism
Genetic • SCN5A • HCN4 • Ryanodine	Myocardial infarction, acute inferior wall (neural reflex effects)
Inflammatory or postinflammatory: • Pericarditis, myocarditis • Rheumatic fever • Chagas disease • Diphtheria	
Musculoskeletal disorders: • Duchenne's • Myotonic dystrophy • Friedreich's ataxia	Miscellaneous - Intracranial hypertension - Obstructive jaundice
Collagen-vascular disease: Lupus erythematosus, scleroderma	
Postoperative: • Mustard/Senning procedure, • Atrial septal defect repair	
Obstructive sleep apnea	
Consequences of Valvular heart disease	

colleagues[34] investigated sinus node blood supply in 25 SND patients and reported greater than 50% stenosis of the sinus node artery in 7 cases, but in none of 54 heart block patients. Thus, chronic SND in adults may be due to sinus node artery ischemia in about one-third of cases.

ii) Children and young adults

In children and young adults, intrinsic SND is most commonly associated with presumed direct damage to the sinus node region due to previous atrial surgery, especially after Mustard/Senning operations for transposition of the great arteries.[37–42] However, SND has also been observed in patients with unoperated congenital heart disease and even in ostensibly normal children and adolescents.[43–46] Genetic disturbances may be the cause in the latter group. For instance, mutations of the cardiac sodium channel SCN5A and the HCN4 gene have been described. Although the sodium channel gene SCN5A is not crucial in sinus node cells, it may be an important contributor in the sinus node periphery impacting transmission of the electrical impulse to the atrium. The result could be sinus bradycardia or pauses or even atrial inexcitability. Of the HCN gene family, HCN4 is the most important in the atria and encodes the channel responsible for the I_f current. Consequently, an HCN4 mutation may yield sinus bradycardia.[45,46] Multiple HCN4 mutations have been described with diverse outcomes including bradycardia-induced syncope, chronotropic incompetence (CI), and somewhat unexpected torsades. Other mutations, including gap junction connexin proteins, have also been encountered and could be rare causes of SND. Genetic causes should be considered when SND is identified in younger patients (ie, teenage years and early adulthood), and other potentially affected family members should be screened.

Extrinsic SND

Autonomic factors and drugs (sometimes acting in concert) are important common extrinsic influences that can contribute to SND.[8,10,23–25] Parasympathetic and sympathetic neurohumors (ie, acetylcholine, norepinephrine, epinephrine) alter spontaneous depolarization rates of sinus node cells and may also influence the site of the principal pacemaker within the node. Similarly, many drugs may affect sinus node function; while beta-adrenergic blockers are perhaps the most widely known, vagomimetic agents such as the cardiac glycosides and vagolytic drugs (eg, quinidine, disopyramide) also fall into this category. Electrolyte (eg, hyperkalemia) and endocrine (eg, hyperthyroidism) disturbances may also play a role.

i) Drugs

Drug-induced SND is relatively uncommon, but is of particular concern in elderly patients (**Box 1**). Adrenergic blockers are particularly troublesome in older individuals as sinus node function tends to be increasingly dependent on sympathetic tone with aging (see later). However, many other agents may also adversely impact sinus node function including calcium channel blockers and "membrane active" antiarrhythmics.[23,24,48,49] The latter may act directly to impair impulse formation and transmission but also indirectly through their impact on autonomic tone.

ii) Autonomic control

Disturbances of sinus node autonomic control can be responsible for ECG findings suggestive of SND. In health, intrinsic sinus node function tends to decline with age,[47] leading to slower heart rates, while sinoatrial conduction time (SACT) and sinus node recovery time (SNRT) tend to lengthen. However, these aging changes usually have only a minor effect on heart rate in the innervated sinus node as autonomic changes compensate; in essence, sympathetic tone increases, or vagal influence decreases, or both (**Fig. 4**).[47] Unfortunately, these same alterations of autonomic influence with age have a downside: susceptibility to drug-induced SND changes as patients age. For instance, if the aging sinus node increasingly relies on sympathetic tone, as is currently suspected, to maintain heart rate, then adrenergic blockers may have greater potential for inducing symptomatic bradycardia or pauses in the elderly.

Box 1
Commonly Prescribed Drugs Affecting Sinus Node Function

Antiarrhythmic agents

- Amiodarone: may cause de novo SND
- Flecainide, propafenone, sotalol, dronedarone: may exacerbate sinus node dysfunction
- Quinidine, disopyramide, procainamide: lesser concern possibly due to vagolytic properties
- Adenosine*

    * Transient action

Antihypertensives (sympatholytic)

- Alpha-methyldopa*, reserpine*, clonidine
- Amlodipine

    * No longer widely used in developed countries

Beta-adrenergic blocking drugs

- Without ISA*: metoprolol, propranolol, nadolol,
- With ISA*, less severe affects: pindolol, acebutolol, etc.
- Ophthalmic drops: Timolol (and others)

    * ISA = intrinsic sympathomimetic activity

Calcium channel blockers (non-dihydropyridine forms)

- Verapamil
- Diltiazem

Cardiac glycosides

Miscellaneous

- Cimetidine
- Lithium
- Phenytoin
- Phenothiazine
- Ivabradine*

    * I_f channel blocker designed to slow sinus node

In summary, SND may result from factors that directly alter the intrinsic anatomy and function of the pacemaker complex or from extrinsic influences (eg, drugs, autonomic tone). Distinguishing these pathophysiologies has important prognostic and therapeutic implications.

Epidemiology and Natural History

SND occurs most commonly in individuals in the sixth or seventh decade of life, with some studies

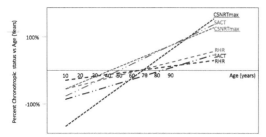

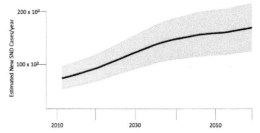

Fig. 4. Graphs illustrating the effect of aging on measures of sinus node function. Shown in blue, after autonomic blockade (atropine plus propranolol), the aging effect on intrinsic sinus node function is evident with progressive increase of resting heart rate (RHR), corrected sinus node recovery time (CSNRT), and SACT. In the absence of autonomic blockade, the advancing age effect is moderated. These observations, adapted from the observations of de Marneffe[47] suggest that a greater sympathetic versus parasympathetic balance plays a role in maintaining sinus node function in the older individual.

Fig. 5. Graph depicting increasing prevalence of SND with advancing age. The blue area depicts the estimated annual incident SND number (95% confidence limits). (*Adapted from* Jensen PN, Gronroos NN, Chen LY, et al. Incidence of and risk factors for sick sinus syndrome in the general population. J Am Coll Cardiol. 2014;64(6):531-538.   doi:10.1016/j.jacc.2014.03.056; with permission)

revealing a bimodal distribution with a small additional peak among individuals in their twenties. The latter, as discussed earlier, may relate to increasingly recognized genetic/familial causes of SND, or the consequences of prior cardiac surgery for congenital heart disease.

Although the prevalence of SND increases with advancing age, establishing an accurate assessment is difficult. Furthermore, SND diagnostic criteria are not consistent among published reports, and distinguishing intrinsic SND from extrinsic causes during the review of individual medical records is impractical, thereby undermining the value of epidemiologic estimates. In an early study, Kulbertus and colleagues[50] estimated that in persons older than 50 years attending a cardiology clinic, the incidence of symptomatic SND is approximately 5 in 3000 (about 0.17%). More recently, using access to much larger study populations (Atherosclerotic Risk in Communities study [ARIC] and Cardiovascular Health Study [CHS]), Jensen and colleagues[51] estimated the development of SND in 20,572 subjects (mean age 59 years) who were deemed free of SND findings at entry. Over a 17-year follow-up, 291 SND patients were identified (0.8/1000 patient-years) with increasing incidence with age (**Fig. 5**).

The course of SND progression[52–57] in terms of 5- to 10-year survival is similar in both SND patients and patients with other forms of conduction system disease. When mortality in SND patients was compared with otherwise well-matched control subjects, the SND exhibited only a 4% to 5% excess annual mortality in the first 5 years of follow-up.[56] However, in those SND patients without other coexisting diseases at the time of initial diagnosis, mortality did not differ significantly from that observed in control subjects. Sutton and Kenny,[55] reporting data from the early 1980s, calculated the following overall survival statistics for SND patients: 1 year, 85% to 92%; 5 years, 62% to 65%; 7 years, 52%.

Among SND patients, bradycardia-tachycardia patients tend to have a worse outcome, possibly due to thromboembolic complications.[58] Whether these outcome differences have changed with the wider application of anticoagulation is unclear. For instance, Bodin and colleagues[59] examined outcomes in a large longitudinal study in France encompassing almost 1.7 million individuals of whom about 100,000 had solitary SND and 27,000 had SND and atrial fibrillation. Findings revealed that SND alone had a risk of ischemic stroke during follow-up that was greater than was observed in patients with other cardiac diseases, but less than in patients with atrial fibrillation. The additional risk associated with atrial fibrillation remained relatively constant until patients had a CHADS-Vasc score of ≥ 7.

Embolic events (primarily cerebrovascular embolism) were previously reported to account for 30% to 50% of deaths in SND patients but, apart from the findings reported by Bodin and colleagues,[59] the impact of embolic events may be diminished given more widespread anticoagulant therapy and greater use of atrial based pacing systems. In the Mode Selection Trial,[60] a 6-year study of pacing in SND, the basis of death switched from embolism concerns to left ventricular ejection fraction (LVEF). As LVEF increased from less than 35% to 36% to 49%, to greater than 50%, both sudden death risk and heart failure death risk decreased. The sudden death rates were similar to those observed in implantable cardioverter defibrillator

(ICD) primary prevention trials. The potential impact of anticoagulation was not studied, but mortality and stroke were greater in patients in whom implanted devices recorded high rate atrial events of 5 minutes or longer.[61] Atrial fibrillation was diminished with atrial-based pacing, but mortality, stroke, and heart failure outcomes were not impacted.[60]

Other outcomes in untreated SND patients were assessed in a small patient population by Menozzi and colleagues.[54] Prospective evaluation of 35 patients with sinus bradycardia or pauses followed over 4 years revealed adverse events in 20 of 35 patients (57%); syncope occurred in 23%, heart failure in 17%, and atrial tachyarrhythmias in 17%. The authors pointed out that symptoms in affected patients often showed spontaneous and unexplained fluctuations. Nonetheless, they suggested that intervention could safely be delayed in younger patients (<65 years) with resting heart rates greater than 40 beats/min and minimum heart rates on ambulatory ECG greater than 35 beats/min. Conversely, a history of syncope and a corrected SNRT greater than 800 ms were indicative of a high likelihood of syncope/collapse recurrence.

In summary, most studies of the natural history of SND are dated and recent epidemiologic reports cannot provide the depth of detail needed (eg, intrinsic vs extrinsic SND, whether "isolated" SND does in fact have undiagnosed atrial fibrillation). In addition, our current understanding has been undermined by the evolution of treatment strategies, including more "physiologic" pacing systems (including benefits of algorithms that minimize ventricular pacing) and more aggressive anticoagulation.

Clinical Recognition

Clinical manifestations of SND vary from seemingly asymptomatic ECG findings to very disabling complaints including manifestations of inadequate cerebral blood flow (eg, syncope, concentration difficulties, lightheadedness), exertional intolerance (eg, CI), and palpitations. However, substantiating a causal relationship between symptoms such as personality changes, memory loss, and diminished exertional tolerance and abnormal ECG findings may be difficult. Finally, apart from overt stroke, multiple smaller embolic phenomena may be the cause of progressive mental status deterioration, or dysfunction of other organ systems.

ECG manifestations of SND range from persistent or intermittent sinus bradycardia and/or sinus pauses, to episodic sinus or atrial tachycardias.

Often, both bradycardia and tachycardia occur episodically, resulting in a subset of SND that is often termed "bradycardia-tachycardia syndrome" (B-T-S) (**Fig. 2**). The arrhythmic landscape includes:

1. Sinus arrhythmia, sinus tachycardia, and inappropriate sinus tachycardia

Sinus arrhythmia, a heart rate variation most often associated with respiratory cycles (rate increases with inspiration and decreases with expiration), is commonly present in healthy individuals, and is not of clinical concern apart from being a useful marker of autonomic tone. Given their cyclic nature, even extreme degrees of sinus arrhythmia can usually be differentiated from more worrisome sinus pauses.

Sinus tachycardia is usually a physiologic phenomenon indicating an appropriate response to demands arising from exercise, fever, anemia, and so forth. As a rule of thumb, the approximate upper limit for sinus rate can be estimated as 220—age in years. Furthermore, sinus tachycardia occurs in response to an appropriate stimulus. Occasionally, however, it may be difficult to differentiate physiologic sinus tachycardia from pathologic rhythm disturbances[62] such as atrial tachycardia, postural orthostatic tachycardia syndrome (POTS), or sinus node reentry tachycardia. In particular, the syndrome of intractable nonphysiological sinus tachycardia, often termed "inappropriate sinus tachycardia" (IST) is an infrequent but clinically troublesome problem[63]; in some patients, IST may be difficult to distinguish from POTS.[64,65]

The basis for IST is unknown. There may be abnormally enhanced automaticity within the sinus node or nearby atrial regions, possibly contributed to by diminished parasympathetic control. Ivabradine and/or beta-blockade therapy may help, but often do not provide complete relief. On occasion, but only in the most severely affected individuals, refractory IST may lead to attempted transcatheter ablation/modification of the sinoatrial region. The long-term results of these interventions have to date not been very effective.[63,66]

2. Sinus bradyarrhythmias and pauses

Sinus bradycardia, typically defined as a persistent sinus rate less than 50 beats/min during waking hours, is the most common bradyarrhythmia in SND (**Fig. 6**). However, in some individuals, heart rates as low as 35 to 40 beats/min may be perfectly acceptable. Such rates are often present in young athletic individuals at rest and in many adults during sleep. As a rule, such individuals are without symptoms attributable to slow heart

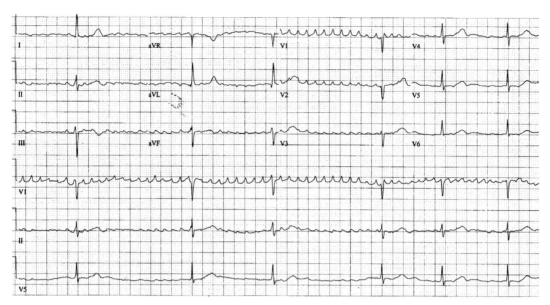

Fig. 6. ECG tracing in a 78-year-old male with progressive exertional fatigue. ECG findings revealed permanent atrial fibrillation with a slow ventricular rate and poor chronotropic response with exercise.

rates and they exhibit normal heart rate responses during physical exertion (ie, normal chronotropic competence). On the contrary, the presence of symptoms or the identification of coexisting CI implies that the sinus bradycardia may be an indicator of SND.

Sinus rates in the 50 to 70 range are generally accepted as within the normal range. However, under special conditions, these rates may be inadequate. For example, after heart transplantation or in some patients with chronic heart failure, higher heart rates are desired. In such circumstances, treatment intervention may be warranted, although in the heart transplant patient, the problem is usually self-limited and permanent pacing is only infrequently needed.[67,68]

With regard to heart transplant patients, the overall trend for pacemaker implantation has declined over the years. Mallidi and Bates report a 2% incidence after the bicaval approach and 9% with the biatrial technique.[68] Two-thirds of devices were placed within the first 30 days postoperatively. In our institution, permanent pacemakers are implanted in fewer than 5% of transplant patients, especially with use of bicaval operative procedures.

Sinus pauses may be due to sinus "arrest" or sinoatrial exit block (**Fig. 7**). The term "sinus pause" implies failure of an expected atrial activation of sinus node origin, and may be due to either failure of the sinus node to depolarize (sinus arrest) or failure of the impulse to exit into the atrium (exit block). Asymptomatic pauses of ≤3 seconds in duration are relatively common and are usually without adverse implications. On the other hand, pauses greater than 3 seconds are much less common during ambulatory monitoring (0.8% of patients). These longer pauses, especially when occurring during waking hours, may reflect underlying SND and warrant further assessment for correlating symptoms.

Sinoatrial exit block is usually classified in a manner analogous to AV block, and it occurs when there is either delay or failure of a sinus impulse to exit the sinus nodal region. First-degree sinus node exit block (ie, slowed conduction out of the node) cannot be readily identified by ECG inspection alone. In a second-degree sinoatrial exit block, there is periodic failure of a sinus impulse to exit the node and generate a P wave. The latter may occur in a form analogous to type I AV block, in which case Wenckebach periodicity may be suspected by recognition of progressive P-P interval shortening preceding a pause in the atrial rhythm (a "dropped" P wave). In more severe grades of second-degree sinoatrial exit block, several sinus impulses may fail to exit the node, the distinctive ECG feature being a pause duration equal to a whole number multiple (or approximately so) of the immediately preceding P-P interval. The need for treatment is based on the severity of clinical implications associated with the pause in the cardiac rhythm. Assuming associated symptoms are present, and in the absence of a reversible cause (eg, adverse drug effect), a cardiac pacemaker is generally recommended.

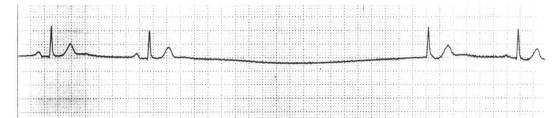

Fig. 7. Sinus bradycardia in an elderly male interrupted by a sinus pause of approx. 4.5 sec duration with a junctional escape. This patient complained of worsening fatigue and occasional lightheaded spells. Correlation of symptoms with slow rates proved to be difficult, but ultimately cardiac pacing substantially diminished symptoms.

In patients with suspected SND, the recent 2018 guidelines indicate that there are no established minimums of heart rate, or maximums of cardiac pauses, that automatically warrant proceeding with cardiac pacing.[67] The guideline implies that symptom–arrhythmia correlation is necessary. However, this recommendation sidesteps the common problem of severe bradycardia in a patient who may not have sufficient insight to recognize progressive physical or cognitive limitations. In such cases, physicians must use clinical judgment and are prudent to provide solid documentation of the rationale to proceed to permanent pacing. In particular, before resorting to pacemaker implantation, caregivers should have a frank discussion with the patient and family that symptoms of fatigue may not vanish completely.

3. Chronotropic incompetence
The term "chronotropic incompetence" (CI) implies inability of the heart to adjust its rate appropriately in response to metabolic demand.[69] Technically, inadequate heart rate responses, as well as 'IST', could be incorporated within CI. Currently, however, IST is usually considered as a separate condition as noted earlier.

There are no universally accepted diagnostic criteria for CI. Exercise testing is often considered as a means to help identify such patients. The Chronotropic Assessment Exercise Protocol (CAEP) is the most thoroughly evaluated,[70] but other low-level exertion protocols such as Naughton or MPREP may be used. However, such testing has important limitations if only high heart rate targets are used as endpoints because CI patients may achieve high target rates when they are being encouraged to persist with the exercise (see later). However, at home, in the absence of such encouragement, these individuals may not reach adequate rates and consequently stop because of fatigue. Other manifestations of CI may include either failure or delay in achieving heart rate targets during exertion, inadequate submaximal

heart rate during activities of daily living, rate instability during sustained exercise, or abrupt heart rate slowing after exercise is completed.[69–73] The utility of pacing depends on the specific arrhythmia-symptom correlation. Ambulatory ECG monitoring may be useful to develop the arrhythmia-symptom correlation; however, to be optimally effective, such a step requires that the patient have sufficient insight to use the device and provide effective feedback.

4. Bradycardia-tachycardia syndrome
B-T-S consists of the coexistence in the same patient of periods of bradyarrhythmia interspersed with bouts of atrial tachyarrhythmias (usually atrial fibrillation, but occasionally atrial flutter or other paroxysmal atrial tachycardias; see **Figs. 2** and **8**). Symptoms may result from either the rapid heartbeat or the bradycardic component (which is often at its most severe immediately after spontaneous tachyarrhythmia termination), or both. As noted earlier, the prognosis in B-T-S is more severe than observed in sinus bradycardia alone. Systemic embolism is a particular concern in B-T-S patients, with current guidelines providing direction for effective anticoagulation. Nonetheless, there remains concern that recurrent episodes of atrial fibrillation also have an adverse direct effect on the heart. Atrial fibrillation itself has an undesirable impact on atrial electrophysiology, and both atrial and ventricular function. In terms of the latter, the most important of the several factors that may adversely impact left ventricular function are the impact of sustained, inappropriately high heart rates on the ventricle (the concept of so-called "tachycardia-mediated cardiomyopathy"),[74–76] and the potential for repetitive coronary artery embolism.

5. Intra-atrial conduction disease and atrial fibrillation with slow ventricular rates
Abnormal intra-atrial conduction (eg, prolonged and/or complex appearing P wave), and, in some cases, disturbances of AV conduction (eg, atrial

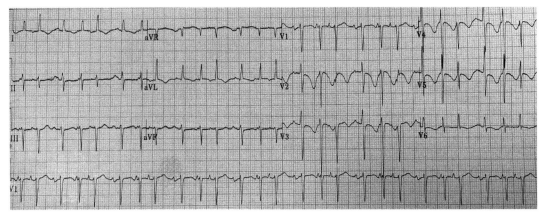

Fig. 8. ECG recording in a patient with SND and chronic pulmonary disease. Findings are those of an atrial tachy-cardia with at least 3 different P-wave morphologies. Technically, this could be considered a multifocal atrial tachycardia.

fibrillation with a slow ventricular response not due to drug therapy) fall within the SND landscape. In the case of slow ventricular rates (see **Fig. 6**), concomitant AV conduction system disease is presumed to be present; however, the development of clinically relevant AV block is uncommon. In fact, some SND patients manifest surprisingly rapid ventricular responses during atrial tachyarrhythmias (**Fig. 9**). Furthermore, the stability of AV conduction over time in SND patients has been illustrated in the DANPACE study.[77,78] Findings revealed the utility of atrial pacing over an approximate 5-year follow-up with a low risk of progression to AV block.

6. Pauses following cardioversion

Prolonged asystolic pauses or sustained periods of junctional or idioventricular escape rhythms following cardioversion of atrial fibrillation are another subset of SND. Failure of appropriate physiologic pacemaker function following termination or cardioversion of an episode of tachycardia, including delay or absence of restoration of a stable sinus rhythm following overdrive pacing or cardioversion of atrial tachyarrhythmias, may be the basis for lightheaded spells or syncope (see **Fig. 2**). Although not often needed for diagnostic purposes, measurement of SNRT and corrected SNRT in the electrophysiology laboratory is

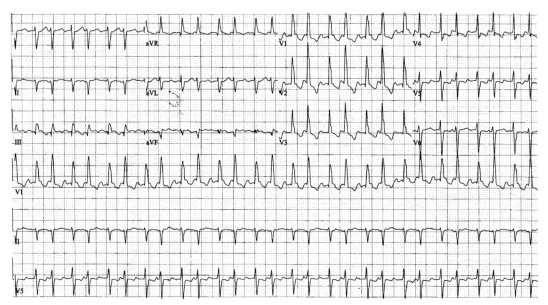

Fig. 9. ECG recording in a 40-year-old male patient with SND in whom paroxysmal atrial fibrillation resulted in rapid ventricular response and symptoms of lightheadedness.

occasionally undertaken to assess sinus node function and quantify susceptibility to prolonged pauses after a period of rapid atrial rate.

7. Sinus node reentrant tachycardia

Slow conduction properties within the sinus node region offer a substrate for reentrant rhythms (so-called "sinus node reentry" tachycardia, SRT). SRT is an infrequent cause for symptoms in SND patients, but can be targeted for ablation if necessary (see **Fig. 3**). The diagnosis of SRT requires that the arrhythmia have a P-wave morphology and an intra-atrial activation sequence very similar to that observed during sinus rhythm in that patient, and the arrhythmia can be initiated and terminated by atrial extra stimuli. Vagal maneuvers, verapamil, or adenosine will also usually terminate SRT abruptly.

Diagnostic Methods

A careful medical history, in conjunction with the application of experienced clinical suspicion, provides the best tool for identifying SND patients. Thereafter, careful use of selected noninvasive diagnostic tools will usually be adequate to substantiate the diagnosis and focus therapy. Invasive electrophysiologic tests are only rarely indicated and have largely been disappointing in terms of clinical utility. The optimum outcome of the diagnostic evaluation is to obtain a symptom-arrhythmia correlation; however, this is often not achieved.

1. Noninvasive diagnostic testing

Ambulatory ECG (AECG) recordings, exercise testing, and to a much lesser extent, pharmacologic assessment of sinus node autonomic control have been used to diagnose SND. However, only AECG recordings (including insertable cardiac monitors [ICMs]) offer insight into the relation between symptoms and arrhythmia. If symptom-arrhythmia correlation is obtained during a recording, the basis for symptoms is then clear, and for the most part, the treatment direction is immediately established.

In most SND patients, symptoms are brief and relatively infrequent. As a result, long-term recording devices (ie, "event" recorders, MCOT systems, and ICMs) may be more helpful than conventional 24- or 48-h Holter-type recordings. However, if it is deemed that the older patient is likely incapable of reacting sufficiently rapidly to use conventional "event recorders" effectively, then MCOT devices and ICMs with remote download features are preferred.

As a rule, exercise testing has limited utility in SND, but if undertaken using specialized protocols (eg,.CAEP), it may be helpful for supporting a suspected diagnosis of CI. As mentioned earlier, maximum heart rate alone is not an adequate end-point. Many SND patients, when subjected to forced treadmill exercise, can achieve heart rates comparable to that of control subjects (**Fig. 10**), although the time taken to achieve such rates may be longer, and feel more exhausting.

Heart rate response to pharmacologic interventions is infrequently warranted in clinical practice. However, if there is concern regarding intrinsic versus extrinsic SND, the assessment of intrinsic heart rate (IHR) may be helpful. In this case, sinus node rate is determined when neural control has been largely eliminated by pharmacologic autonomic blockade (usually propranolol 0.2 mg/kg I.V., followed by atropine 0.04 mg/kg i.v.). For practical purposes, normal values for IHR can be approximately predicted (IHRp) from the linear regression: IHRp = 118.1 - (0.57 × age).[18,21,47,79] The precision of the calculation may be debated, but this method has been used to ascertain the effect of aging on sinus node rate, and to show the importance of increased sympathetic tone for maintaining heart rate with increasing age[47] (see **Fig. 4**).

2. Invasive electrophysiologic testing

Invasive diagnostic testing is rarely needed in SND diagnosis and is only used if it is necessary to assess a clinical suspicion when ECG studies are nondiagnostic.[21] The latter issue is becoming increasingly rare as ambulatory monitoring tools have dramatically improved and ICMs are readily available if very long-term monitoring is needed.[80]

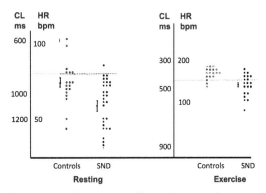

Fig. 10. Data illustrating effect of exercise in control subjects and SND patients based on findings presented by Vallin and Edhag.[72] Note that maximum heart rates are similar in both groups. Thus, maximum exercise rates may not be a useful diagnostic measure for identifying SND. However, although not evaluated in this study, the time taken to achieve maximum rate may help differentiate the groups and be a better indicator of sinus node function.

In general, electrophysiologic testing lacks sensitivity although when used together they exhibit a specificity of 70% to 90%.

Equal in importance to detecting SND is determining whether it is the cause of the patient's symptoms and whether pacing intervention is warranted. Unfortunately, electrophysiologic testing has not proved very effective in this regard. Long-term ambulatory monitoring is a much more powerful tool.

i) Sinus node recovery time SNRT is the most straightforward invasive electrophysiologic test of sinus node function, and takes advantage of a physiologic characteristic of native cardiac pacemaker tissue, namely "overdrive suppression."[21] Specifically in this case, the time taken for sinus node activity to return following termination of a period of rapid atrial stimulation (ie, the SNRT) is used to identify underlying SND.[18,19,21] However, the SNRT measurement is dependent on multiple factors such as autonomic tone, sinoatrial conduction properties, the patient's sinus cycle length at the time of study, and the magnitude of sinus arrhythmia present. The SNRT is usually corrected for baseline sinus cycle length (ie, Corrected SNRT, or CSNRT). Most commonly, this correction is obtained by subtracting the baseline sinus cycle length from the SNRT: CSNRT = SNRT - sinus cycle length. The usual normal value in adults is in the 500 to 550 ms range (most commonly < 525 ms) but is shorter in young children (approx. 275 ms). In adolescents, the CSNRT has been reported to range from 186 to 440 ms (mean value approx. 320 ms).[81]

ii) Sinoatrial conduction time The measurement of SACT teaches important principles of sinus node physiology,[10,20–22] but is otherwise hardly ever used in current practice.[9,19,21] SACT can be determined by both indirect and direct techniques. The classic indirect method described by Strauss and colleagues[22] uses timed premature atrial extra stimuli (A2) introduced at a high lateral right atrial pacing site during sinus rhythm (A1-A1). With insertion of A2, the sequence of sinoatrial activation is reversed for one cycle. Assuming that intrinsic sinus node automaticity is unperturbed by A2, the return cycle (A2-A3) should be equal to A1-A1 plus an interval equal to both the time required for A2 to enter the node and the time taken for the next sinus impulse to exit the node. By repeating this maneuver multiple times, an estimate of the total conduction time into and out of the node (SACT by definition) may be estimated. Although the reported upper limit of normal SACT value varies somewhat in the literature, 205 msec is commonly used. The Narula

('new') method provides an alternative indirect assessment of total SACT; the return cycle is measured following a period of atrial pacing at a rate slightly faster than the sinus rate.[24] If the pacing is not too fast, retrograde atrial capture can be assumed, and then the duration of the pause after pacing termination is then the sum of the basic sinus cycle length and total SACT. Again, multiple measures are made and an average SACT value is determined.

Techniques for direct recording of sinus node electrograms, and thereby obtaining direct estimate of SACT are feasible in the clinical electrophysiology laboratory but are difficult and have limited clinical utility.[24] A value of 112 ms (one direction) is typical for an adult, whereas 15 to 91 ms has been reported in children.

In summary, electrophysiologic techniques have been developed in an attempt to diagnose SND, but have not proved very effective in the clinical setting.

Treatment

In SND when symptoms do occur, they may be due to either bradyarrhythmia or tachyarrhythmia, or both. Therefore, pacemaker therapy (usually atrial-based pacing) may be needed in some cases, arrhythmia suppression by drugs or ablation in others, and various combinations of all of these in some cases.

Pharmacologic Treatment

Apart from anticoagulants, drug therapy has little role to play in terms of the bradycardias associated with SND, but is widely used in an attempt to diminish susceptibility to tachycardias. Antiarrhythmic agents used to suppress tachycardias may aggravate bradyarrhythmias in some patients; alternatively, elimination of certain drugs may be instrumental for eliminating symptoms.

SND patients are often exposed to a wide range of drugs that may exacerbate or unmask underlying susceptibility to bradycardia. For example, cardiac glycosides, beta-adrenergic blockers, calcium channel blockers, and membrane-active antiarrhythmic agents (especially sotalol and amiodarone) are used to treat coexisting paroxysmal atrial tachyarrhythmias. Some of these drugs, and many other bradycardia-promoting sympatholytic agents, are used to treat hypertension, a common problem in the generally older SND population. In addition, certain less commonly used agents such as radiographic contrast materials, lithium carbonate, cimetidine, and adenosine have been associated with depression of sinus node function.

Atrial fibrillation and atrial flutter are common manifestations of SND, and in patients with these arrhythmias, anticoagulation is often a critical treatment component depending on risk score assessment. Long-term anticoagulation after radiofrequency ablation of atrial fibrillation remains the subject of debate. Recent guideline recommendations support the continuation of anticoagulants for at least 2 months after the procedure.[82] Thereafter, the consensus states that continuing should be based on clinical risk assessment, which would reasonably consist of balancing CHADS-VAsc score vs bleeding/falls risk.

The 2018 guidelines[67] provide recommendations for the use of certain agents in the setting of acute bradycardia episodes. Most importantly, atropine is recommended for emergent use when temporary pacing is not immediately available. In addition, theophylline or aminophylline may be helpful in certain specific but limited circumstances.

Pacemaker Therapy

i) Conventional cardiac pacing

Guidelines for the implantation of cardiac pacemakers are periodically reviewed and updated[67] (**Tables 2 and 3**). In general, cardiac pacemaker therapy is indicated and has proved highly effective in SND when bradyarrhythmia has been demonstrated to account for symptoms.[67,83] The Task Force defined "symptomatic bradycardia" as encompassing those "clinical manifestations that are directly attributable to the slow heart rate; transient dizziness, light-headedness, near syncope or frank syncope as manifestations of transient cerebral ischemia, and more generalized symptoms such as marked exercise intolerance or frank congestive heart failure." However, symptomatic bradycardia due to "nonessential" drug therapy is excluded.

Although uncertainty remains, two of the largest studies, MOST and CTOPP, tended to favor the view that pacing techniques that endeavor to maintain a normal atrioventricular (AV) relationship appear to diminish heart failure hospital admission rates, and offer the additional benefit of reducing atrial fibrillation risk, and thereby diminishing the risk of thromboembolism.[83] However, as CI often coexists in SND patients, cardiac pacemakers programmed to an atrial-tracking mode (eg, VDD, DDD modes) may not provide optimal physiologic heart rate response. In this circumstance, sensors in current generation pacing systems (eg, piezoelectric accelerometers, respiratory sensors, and others), although not perfectly

Table 2 Guideline-directed recommendations for acute bradycardia in SND[68]	
Class (all LOE = C)[b]	Recommendations
I	Patients in whom symptoms are attributable to SND, evaluation and removal of reversible causes if possible
IIA	In symptomatic or hemodynamically compromised patients with SND**atropine is reasonable
IIB	In symptomatic or hemodynamically compromised patients with SND** and low probability of cardiac ischemia, isoproterenol, epinephrine, dobutamine or dopamine may be considered
III	Atropine should not be used in patients with prior heart transplantation but no evidence of reinnervation as it may yield paroxysmal AVB or rarely sinus arrest
IIA	In patients, after heart transplant, theophylline or aminophylline may be used to try and increase heart rate if needed.

[a]The guideline does not state "bradycardia with SND" but that is implied.
[b] LOE = level of evidence is sufficiently low that shared decision making is warranted.

physiologic, offer valuable backup to better support heart rate. In addition, there has been a growing appreciation that optimum benefit is obtained if atrial pacing is favored and ventricular stimulation is minimized as much as possible. Reducing ventricular stimulation diminishes adverse effects of ventricular pacing on overall cardiac mechanical function and susceptibility to heart failure.[84–93]

In the MOST study,[60] 2010 SND patients were randomized to either ventricular pacing (n = 996) or dual-chamber pacing (n = 1014), and followed for a median of 33 months. Ignoring the crossover issue, the primary endpoint (all-cause mortality or stroke) did not differ in the 2 groups. The CTOPP (Canadian Trial of Physiologic Pacing)[86] randomized patients undergoing first pacemaker implants (for SND or AV conduction system disease) to ventricular-based single-chamber devices (n = 1474), or more

Table 3
Guideline-directed permanent pacing recommendations (mainly atrial-based) for chronic SND[68]

Class (all LOE = C)[b]	Recommendations
I	Patients in whom symptoms are directly attributable to SND, permanent pacing is indicated[a]
I	Patients who develop symptomatic bradycardia in the course of guideline-directed for which there is no alternative
IIA	Patients with B-T-S attributable to bradycardia[c]
IIA	Patients with symptomatic chronotropic incompetence
IIB	In patients with suspected symptomatic bradycardia atrial of theophylline may be considered before pacing

[a] The guideline does not state "bradycardia with SND" but that is implied.
[b] LOE = level of evidence is sufficiently low that shared decision making is warranted.
[c] The assumption is that the bradycardia triggered tachycardia may be ventricular in some instances.

physiologic AAI or DDD pacing systems (n = 1094). Among these individuals, total mortality tended to be lower in physiologic paced patients (not statistically significant), but cardiovascular death did not differ in the 2 groups. On the contrary, the annual rate of atrial fibrillation was significantly less in the physiologic pacing group (5.3% vs 6.6%, annual relative risk reduction, 18%, $P = .05$). The atrial fibrillation benefit became increasingly apparent with longer follow-up. In terms of the specific context of assessing cardiac pacing in SND, the CTOPP trial data are difficult to assess because only about 40% of patients carried some element of that diagnosis. Furthermore, many of the patients may have required pacing only for brief periods, making it difficult to evaluate the impact of the pacing intervention. In this regard, a substudy analysis of CTOPP results was undertaken, looking at findings in individuals with slower versus faster resting heart rates at entry. The presumption was that patients with lower heart rates would pace more often, and thus more clearly demonstrate differences among pacing modes. In this analysis, Tang and colleagues[87] found that slower unpaced heart rates were accompanied by an increasing annual cardiovascular death or stroke rate. Physiologic paced patients did not evidence

this increase. Thus, to the extent that unpaced slow heart rates are a marker (albeit not very strong) of SND, these individuals were probably benefited by selection of physiologic pacing systems. The benefit in terms of atrial fibrillation suppression is probably of the greatest practical importance.

The ongoing Danish prospective trials also provide evidence favoring the benefits of atrial-based pacing in SND (ie, single-chamber atrial [AAI], or atrioventricular paced) over single-chamber ventricular pacing (VVI).[77,78,94–96] In the initial report, 225 SND patients were randomized to AAI or VVI pacing. At 5.5 years follow-up, AAI paced patients were clearly showing lower incidence of atrial fibrillation, thromboembolism, heart failure, and stroke. Furthermore, all-cause mortality was less in AAI paced patients, although when various preimplant variables were accounted for, it was cardiovascular death rather than total mortality, which was statistically significantly reduced.

The Danish study also compared AAIR pacing with DDDR mode. Findings revealed the utility of atrial pacing over an approximate 5-year follow-up with a low risk of progression to AV block.[77,78] Mortality did not differ in the 2 groups. However, although there was a higher frequency of atrial fibrillation in atrial paced patients in the initial report,[77] this disappeared with longer follow-up (8.9 years). In addition, there was significant mortality, heart failure, or stroke difference between DDDR and AAIR pacing.

In conclusion, when possible, atrial-based pacing is preferred in symptomatic SND. In the setting of intact AV conduction, the use of atrial-single-chambered pacing (AAI, AAIR) can be readily defended, and it is cost-effective. Maintenance of 1:1 conduction to atrial rates of 130/min is easily tested and if stable at that rate, the subsequent risk of abrupt onset heart block is low.

ii) Specialized pacing techniques

Several specialized pacing methods have been proposed that may have utility in SND patients but additional study is needed. These include dual-site atrial pacing,[97,98] pacing the region of Bachman's bundle pacing as a means to diminish intra-atrial conduction delays,[99,100] cardiac resynchronization pacing, and more recently His bundle, and left-bundle branch pacing that offer more physiologic pacing techniques that may reduce valvular regurgitation and intra-atrial pressures. Potentially, these could be assistance in SND patients, but adequate studies have not yet been undertaken.

Ablation

Percutaneous cardiac ablative techniques have had only limited use for the treatment of SND but with the development of cardioneural ablation, the environment may be changing.

i) Conventional ablation methods

Transcatheter radiofrequency ablation of the His bundle with placement of a cardiac pacemaker remains useful in many patients (usually elderly individuals) with refractory primary atrial tachyarrhythmias, including those in whom drug therapy is associated with intolerable side effects. There has been considerable clinical experience gained over the years with the so-called "ablate and pace" technique.[100,101] Quality of life is improved in most patients both by achieving better heart rate control and reducing hospitalization frequency. However, the patient becomes "pacemaker dependent," necessitating careful device monitoring.

Ablation of foci of atrial arrhythmogenesis has increasingly become part of the treatment options in bradycardia tachycardia syndrome. Outcomes are best in patients with minimal structural atrial disease.

ii) Cardioneural ablation

Recently, there has been increasing interest in modulation of the intrinsic cardiac autonomic neural system to treat a variety of arrhythmias,[102–109] including SND with bradycardia and vasovagal or reflex syncope. Although our understanding of the anatomy and physiology of the intrinsic cardiac autonomic neural system is incomplete, the common epicardial locations of several prominent ganglionic plexi (GP) have been identified. Observation of sudden heart rate changes and vagal activity during ablation around these GPs, such as often occur during atrial fibrillation ablation procedures, prompted studies of deliberate autonomic modulation via endocardial catheter ablation at these GP sites, hypothesizing diminished parasympathetic influence on heart rate.

The published literature on cardioneural ablation for SND comprises several nonrandomized observational studies, which all showed improvement in symptomatic bradycardia but, notably, varied considerably with respect to several key factors:

1. The manner of identifying the GP location for ablation, which included some permutation of simply ablating at the common anatomic location of GPs, identifying GPs by observing the response to high-frequency stimulation (HFS) at common locations, spectral mapping for GPs via Fast-Fourier Transforms of endocardial signals, and/or selecting sites of fractionated signals near common locations of GPs.

2. The extent of ablation with respect to the number and location of GP sites.

3. The chosen endpoints of ablation; a combination of persistent increase in sinus rate and AV block cycle length, blunted response to HFS postablation, elimination of local electrograms, and/or changes in the P-P interval.

Further study of both the appropriate endpoints and the most effective method of targeting GPs is required, as well as randomized trials looking at clinical endpoints.

There are published reports of autonomic modulation for IST via stellate ganglion block or surgical denervation, although trial data are lacking to support their use. Moreover, IST may result, at least in some cases, from abnormalities within the intrinsic cardiac autonomic nervous system, as suggested by a case of IST in a transplanted heart with complete surgical denervation. One open-label nonrandomized trial of radiofrequency catheter ablation of the sympathetic input to the sinus node in patient with IST is underway and is estimated to be completed in 2022 (ClinicalTrials. gov Identifier: NCT00584649).

SUMMARY

SND is a common and multifaceted disorder that is most prevalent in older individuals, but may also occur at an earlier age on a genetic basis, or as a complication of cardiac surgery or cardiac inflammation (eg, pericarditis or myocarditis). Often the cause of SND is not readily identified in individual patients, and in fact the trigger may have occurred many years before clinical findings become manifest. The diagnosis of SND may be suspected based on careful history taking in at-risk individuals, particularly elderly individuals, or those who underwent congenital heart disease surgical intervention during childhood. In most cases, the diagnosis is established by documenting its ECG manifestations. Electrophysiologic testing (EPS) has limited utility and while offering many teaching opportunities, EPS is only rarely a crucial tool in clinical practice.

Treatment strategy in SND patients is largely dictated by symptoms and ECG manifestations. Not infrequently both bradycardia and tachycardia coexist in the same patients, along with other diseases common in the elderly (eg, hypertension, coronary artery disease), thereby complicating treatment strategy. Prevention of the adverse consequences of both bradyarrhythmia and tachyarrhythmia is important to reduce susceptibility to syncope, falls, and thromboembolic complications.

CLINICS CARE POINTS

- SND is not a single condition but comprises a range of arrhythmic disorders that vary from patient-to-patient
- SND may be due to intrinsic structural sino-atrial disease, but often extrinsic functional disturbances are the cause (eg, drugs, autonomic disturbances)
- A careful medical history may lead to suspecting SND, but in most cases, long-term ambulatory ECG monitoring provides the most important diagnostic insight.
- Electrophysiologic testing is rarely useful for diagnosis or assessment of SND
- Atrial fibrillation is a common feature of SND, and consequently many of these patients require anticoagulation.
- Bradycardia in SND, if not reversible by adjusting concomitant medical therapy, often leads to the need for pacemaker therapy.

DISCLOSURE STATEMENT

Dr Benditt reports equity interest and consulting fees from Medtronic Inc and St Jude Medical Inc. Dr Benditt was supported in part by a philanthropic grant from the Dr Earl E Bakken family in support of heart-brain research.

Dr Sathnur and Dr Ebin have no conflicts of interest pertinent to the subject of this work.

REFERENCES

1. Short DS. The syndrome of alternating bradycardia and tachycardia. Br Heart J 1954;16:208–14.
2. Lown B. Electrical reversion of cardiac arrhythmias. Br Heart J 1967;29:469–89.
3. Ferrer MI. The sick sinus syndrome in atrial disease. J Am Med Assoc 1968;206:645–6.
4. Ferrer MI. The sick sinus syndrome. Circulation 1973;47:635–41.
5. Rubenstein JJ, Schulman CL, Yurchak PM, et al. Clinical spectrum of the sick sinus syndrome. Circulation 1972;46:5–13.
6. Kaplan BM, Langendorf R, Lev M, et al. Tachycardia-bradycardia syndrome (so-called sick sinus syndrome): pathology, mechanisms and treatment. Am J Cardiol 1973;31:497–508.
7. Bigger JT Jr, Reiffel JA. Sick sinus syndrome. Annu Rev Med 1979;30:91–118.
8. Bonke FIM, Kirchhoff CJHJ, Allessie MA, et al. Impulse propagation from the S-A node to the ventricles. Experientia 1987;43:1044–9.
9. Boineau JP, Canavan TE, Schuessler RB, et al. Demonstration of a widely distributed atrial pacemaker complex in the human heart. Circulation 1988;77:1221–37.
10. Strauss HC, Prystowsky EN, Scheinman MM. Sinoatrial and atrial electrogenesis. Prog Cardiovasc Dis 1977;19:385–404.
11. Bollmann A, Hilbert S, John S, et al. Insights from preclinical high-density electroanatomical sinus node mapping. Europace 2015;17:489–94.
12. James TN. Structure and function of the sinus node, AV node and His bundle of the human heart: part I-structure. Prog Cardiovasc Dis 2002;45:235–67.
13. Berdajs D, Patonay L, Turina MI. The clinical anatomy of the sinus node artery. Ann Thorac Surg 2003;76:732–6.
14. Anderson KR, Ho SY, Anderson RH. Location and vascular supply of sinus node in human heart. Br Heart J 1979;41:28–32.
15. Schuessler RB, Boineau JP, Bromberg BI. Origin of the sinus impulse. J Cardiovasc Electrophysiol 1996;7:263–74.
16. Unudurthi SD, Wolf RM, Hund TJ. Role of sinoatrial node architecture in maintaining a balanced source-sink relationship and synchronous cardiac pacemaking. Front Physiol 2014;5:1–7.
17. Joyner RW, Van Capelle FJ. Propagation through electrically coupled cells. How a small SA node drives a large atrium. Biophys J 1986;50:1157–64.
18. Dobrzynski H, Boyett MR, Anderson RH. New insights into pacemaker activity: promoting understanding of sick sinus syndrome. Circulation 2007;115:1921–32.
19. Jordan JL, Yamaguchi I, Mandel WJ. Studies on the mechanism of sinus node dysfunction in the sick sinus syndrome. Circulation 1978;57:217–23.
20. Langendorf R, Lesser ME, Plotkin P, et al. Atrial parasystole with interpolation. Observations on prolonged sinoatrial conduction. Am Heart J 1962;63:649–58.
21. Pick A, Langendorf R, Katz LN. Depression of cardiac pacemakers by premature impulses. Am Heart J 1951;41:49–57.
22. Strauss HC, Bigger JT Jr, Saroff AL, et al. Electrophysiologic evaluation of sinus node function in patients with sinus node dysfunction. Circulation 1976;53:763–76.
23. Scheinman MM, Strauss HC, Evans GT, et al. Adverse effects of sympatholytic agents in patients with hypertension and sinus node dysfunction. Am J Med 1978;64:1013–20.
24. Benditt DG, Sakaguchi S, Goldstein MA, et al. Sinus node dysfunction: pathophysiology, clinical features, evaluation and treatment. In: Zipes DP, Jalife J, editors. Cardiac electrophysiology: from cell to Bedside. 2nd ed. Philadelphia, Pa: WB Saunders Co; 1995. p. 1215–47.

25. Benson DW, Wang DW, Dyment M, et al. Congenital sick sinus syndrome caused by recessive mutations in the cardiac sodium channel gene (SCN5A). J Clin Invest 2003;112:1019–28.

26. Barak M, Herschkowitz S, Shapiro I, et al. Familial combined sinus node and atrioventricular conduction dysfunctions. Int J Cardiol 1987;15:231–9.

27. Surawicz B, Hariman RJ. Follow-up of the family with congenital absence of sinus rhythm. Am J Cardiol 1988;61:467–9.

28. Tomita T, Kinoshita O, Hanaoka T, et al. Familial sick sinus syndrome complicated by extensive cardiac conduction disturbance. Int J Cardiol 2004;94:343–5.

29. Isobe M, Oka T, Takenaka H, et al. Familial sick sinus syndrome with atrioventricular conduction disturbance. Jpn Circ J 1998;62:788–90.

30. Davies MJ, Pomerance A. Quantitative study of ageing changes in the human sinoatrial node and internodal tract. Br Heart J 1972;34:150–2.

31. Evans R, Shaw DB. Pathological studies in sinoatrial disorder (sick sinus syndrome). Br Heart J 1977;39:778–86.

32. Demoulin J-C, Kubertus HE. Pathological correlates of atrial arrhythmias. In: Kulbertus HE, editor. Reentrant arrhythmias. Mechanisms and treatment. Lancaster: MTP Press; 1977. p. 99–113.

33. Demoulin J-C, Kulbertus HE. Histopathological correlates of sinoatrial disease. Br Heart J 1978;40:1384–9.

34. Shaw DB, Linker NJ, Heaver PA, et al. Chronic sinoatrial disorder (sick sinus syndrome): a possible result of cardiac ischemia. Br Heart J 1987;58:598–607.

35. Alboni C, Baggioni GF, Scarfo F, et al. Role of sinus node artery disease in sick sinus syndrome in inferior wall myocardial infarction. Am J Cardiol 1991;67:1180–4.

36. Morris GM, Kalman JM. Fibrosis, electrics and genetics. Perspectives in sinoatrial disease. Circ J 2014;78:1272–82.

37. Mackintosh AF. Sinuatrial disease in young people. Br Heart J 1981;45:62–6.

38. Sasaki R, Theilen EO, January LE, et al. Cardiac arrhythmias associated with the repair of atrial and ventricular septal defects. Circulation 1958;18:909–15.

39. Young D. Later results of closure of secundum atrial septal defect in children. Am J Cardiol 1973;31:14–22.

40. Greenwood RD, Rosenthal A, Sloss LJ, et al. Sick sinus syndrome after surgery for congenital heart disease. Circulation 1975;52:208–13.

41. Beder SD, Gillette PC, Garson A Jr, Porter CB, et al. Symptomatic sick sinus syndrome in children and adolescents as the only manifestation of cardiac abnormality or associated with unoperated congenital heart disease. Am J Cardiol 1983;51:1133–6.

42. Tuinenburg AE, Van Gelder IC, Van Den Berg MP, et al. Sinus node function after cardiac surgery: is impairment specific for the maze procedure? Int J Cardiol 2004;95:101–8.

43. Yabek SM, Dillion T, Berman W, et al. Symptomatic sinus node dysfunction in children without structural heart disease. Pediatrics 1982;69:590–3.

44. Kardelen F, Celiker A, Ozer S, et al. Sinus node function in children and adolescents: treatment by implantation of a permanent pacemaker in 26 patients. Turk J Pediatr 2002;44:312–6.

45. Verker AO, Wilders R. Pacemaker activity of the human sinoatrial node: an update on the effects of mutations in HCN4on the hyperpolarization activated current. Int J Mol Sci 2015;16:3071–94.

46. Choudhury M, Boyett MR, Morris GM. Biology of the sinus node and its disease. Arrhyth Electrophysiol Rev 2015;4:28–34.

47. de Marneffe M, Jacobs P, Haardt R, et al. Variations of normal sinus node function in relation to age: role of autonomic influence. Eur Heart J 1986;7:662–72.

48. Benditt DG, Benson DW Jr, Dunnigan A, et al. Drug therapy in sinus node dysfunction. In: Rapaport E, editor. Cardiology update. New York: Elsevier; 1984. p. 79–102.

49. Linker NJ, Camm AJ. Drug effects on the sinus node a clinical perspective. Cardiovasc Drugs Ther 1988;2:165–70.

50. Kulbertus HE, de Leval-Rutten F, Demoulin JC. Sino-atrial disease: a report on 13 cases. J Electrocardiol 1973;6:303–12.

51. Jensen PN, Gronroos NN, Chen LY, et al. Incidence of and risk factors for sick sinus syndrome in the general population. J Am Coll Cardiol 2014;64:531–8.

52. Rasmussen K. Chronic sinus node disease: natural course and indications for pacing. Eur Heart J 1981;2:455–9.

53. Shaw DB, Holman RR, Gowers JI. Survival in sinoatrial disorder (sick-sinus syndrome). Br Med J 1980;280:139–41.

54. Menozzi C, Brignole M, Alboni P, et al. The natural course of untreated sick sinus syndrome and identification of the variables predictive of unfavorable outcome. Am J Cardiol 1998;82:1205–9.

55. Sutton R, Kenny RA. The natural history of sick sinus syndrome. PACE 1986;9:1110–4.

56. Skagen K, Hansen JF. The long-term prognosis for patients with sinoatrial block treated with permanent pacemaker. Acta Med Scand 1975;199:13–5.

57. McComb JM, Gribbin GM. Effect of pacing mode on morbidity and mortality: update of clinical pacing trials. Am J Cardiol 1999;835B:211–3.

58. Fairfax AJ, Lambert CD, Leatham A. Systemic embolism in chronic sinoatrial disorder. N Engl J Med 1976;295:190–2.

59. Bodin A, Bisson A, Gaborit C, et al. Ischemic stroke in patients with sinus node disease, atrial fibrillation and other cardiac conditions. Stroke 2020;51:1674–81.

60. Lamas G, Lee KL, Sweeney MO, et al. Mode Selection Trial in Sinus-Node Dysfunction. Ventricular pacing or dual-chamber pacing for sinus-node dysfunction. N Engl J Med 2002;346:1854–62.

61. Glotzer TV, Hellkamp MS, Zimmerman J, et al. Atrial high rate episodes detected bu pacemaker diagnostics predict death and stroke. Circulation 2003;107:1614–9.

62. Yusuf S, Camm AJ. Deciphering the sinus tachycardias. Clin Cardiol 2005;28:267–76.

63. Olshansky B, Sullivan RM. Inappropriate sinus tachycardia. Europace 2019;21:194–207.

64. Low PA, Sandroni P, Singer W, et al. Postural tachycardia syndrome – an update. Clin Auton Res 2002;12:107–9.

65. Olshansky B, Cannom D, Fedorowski A, et al. Postural orthostatic tachycardia syndrome (POTS):A critical assessment. Prog CV Dis 2020. https://doi.org/10.1016/j.pcad.2020.03.010.

66. Rodriguez-Manero M, Kreidieh B, Rifai MA, et al. Ablation of inappropriate sinus tachycardia.A systematic review of the literature. JACC Clin EP 2017;3:253–65.

67. Kusumoto FM, Schoenfeld MH, Barrett C, et al. 2018 AHA/ACC/HRS Guideline on the evaluation and management of patients with bradycardia and cardiac conduction delay. Circulation 2019;140:e382–482.

68. Mallidi HR, Bates M. Pacemaker use following heart transplantation. Ochsner J 2017;17:20–4.

69. Chin C-F, Messenger JC, Greenberg PS, et al. Chronotropic incompetence in exercise testing. Clin Cardiol 1979;2:12–8.

70. Wilkoff BL, Corey J, Blackburn D. A mathematical model of the cardiac chronotropic response. J Electrophysiol 1989;3:176–80.

71. Holden W, McAnulty JW, Rahimtoola SN. Characterization of heart rate response to exercise in the sick sinus syndrome. Br Heart J 1978;40:923–30.

72. Vallin HO, Edhag KO. Heart rate responses in patients with sinus node disease compared to controls: physiological implications and diagnostic possibilities. Clin Cardiol 1980;3:391–8.

73. Abbott JA, Hirschfeld DS, Kunkel FW, et al. Graded exercise testing in patients with sinus node dysfunction. Am J Med 1977;62:330–8.

74. Nerheim P, Birger-Botkin S, Piracha L, et al. Heart failure and sudden death in patients with tachycardia-induced cardiomyopathy and recurrent tachycardia. Circulation 2004;110(3):247–52.

75. Shinbane JS, Wood MA, Jensen DN, et al. Tachycardia-induced cardiomyopathy: a review of animal models and clinical studies. J Am Coll Cardiol 1997;29:709–15.

76. Umana E, Solares CA, Alpert MA. Tachycardia-induced cardiomyopathy. Am J Med 2003;114:51–5.

77. Nielsen JC, Thomsen PE, Højberg S, et al. On behalf of the DANPACE Investigators. A comparison of single-lead atrial pacing with dual-chamber pacing in sick sinus syndrome. Eur Heart J 2011;32:686–96.

78. Brandt NH, Kirkfeldt RE, Nielsen JC, et al. Single lead atrial vs dual chamber pacing in sick sinus syndrome: extended register-based follow-up in the DANPACE trial. Europace 2017;19:1981–7.

79. Jose AD, Collison D. The normal range and determinants odf the intrinsic heart rate in man. Cardiovasc Res 1970;4:160–7.

80. Benditt DG, Adkisson WO, Sutton R, et al. Ambulatory diagnostic ECG monitoring for syncope and collapse: an assessment of current clinical practice in the United States. PACE 2018;41(2):203–9.

81. Samson RA, Jolma CD, Zamora R. Normal values for corrected sinus node recovery time in adolescents. Pediatr Cardiol 1999;20:396–9.

82. January CT, Wann LS, Calkins H, et al. 2019 AHA/ACC/HRS focused update of the 2014 guideline for management of patients with atrial fibrillation. J Am Coll Cardiol 2019;140:e125–51.

83. Sutton R. Clinical trials in pacing for bradyarrhythmmias. J Interv Card Electrophysiol 2003;9:151–4.

84. Link MS, Hellkamp AS, Estes NA 3rd, et al. High incidence of pacemaker syndrome in patients with sinus node dysfunction treated with ventricular-based pacing in the Mode Selection Trial (MOST). J Am Coll Cardiol 2004;43:2066–71.

85. Lamas GA, Lee K, Sweeney M, et al. The Mode Selection Trial (MOST) in sinus node dysfunction: design, rationale, and baseline characteristics of the first 1000 patients. Am Heart J 2000;140:541-551.

86. Connolly SJ, Kerr CR, Gent M, et al. Effects of physiologic pacing versus ventricular pacing on the risk of stroke and death due to cardiovascular causes. Canadian Trial of Physiologic Pacing Investigators. N Engl J Med 2000;342:1385–91.

87. Tang ASL, Roberts RS, Kerr C, et al. Relationship between pacemaker dependency and the effect of pacing mode on cardiovascular outcomes. Circulation 2001;103:3081–5.

88. Skanes AC, Krahn AD, Yee R, et al. Progression to chronic atrial fibrillation after pacing: the Canadian trial of physiologic pacing. CTOPP investigators. J Am Coll Cardiol 2001;38:167–72.

89. Kerr CR, Connolly SJ, Abdollah H, et al. Canadian Trial of Physiological Pacing: effects of physiological pacing during long-term follow-up. Circulation 2004;109:357–62.

90. Wilkoff B, Cook JR, Epstein AE, et al. Dual-chamber and VVI implantable defibrillator trial investigators. Dual-chamber pacingor ventricular back-up pacing in patients with an implantable defibrillator: the the Dual Chamber and VVI Implantable Defibrillator (DAVID) Trial. J Am Med Assoc 2002;24:3115–23.

91. Barold SS, Herweg B, Sweeney MO. Minimizing right ventricular pacing. Am J Cardiol 2005;95:966–9.

92. Olshansky B, Day J, McGuire M, et al. Inhibition of unnecessary RV pacing with AV search hysteresis in ICDs (INTRINSIC RV): Design and protocol. PACE 2005;28:62–6.

93. Sweeney MO, Bank AJ, Nash E, et al. Minimizing ventricular pacing to reduce atrial fibrillation in sinus node disease. N Engl J Med 2007;357:1000–8.

94. Andersen HR, Thuesen L, Bagger JP, et al. Prospective randomized trial of atrial versus ventricular pacing in sick-sinus syndrome. Lancet 1994;344:1523–8.

95. Andersen HR, Nielsen JC, Thomsen PE, et al. Long-term follow-up of patients from a randomised trial of atrial versus ventricular pacing for sick-sinus syndrome. Lancet 1997;350:1210–6.

96. Andersen H, Nielsen J. Single-chamber ventricular pacing is no longer an option for sick sinus syndrome. J Am Coll Cardiol 2004;43:2072–4.

97. Saksena S, Prakash A, Ziegler P, et al, DAPPAF Investigators. Improved suppression of recurrent atrial fibrillation with dual-site right atrial pacing and antiarrhythmic drug therapy. J Am Coll Cardiol 2002;40:1140–50.

98. Lau C-P, Tse H-F, Yu C-M, et al. Hill MRS, for the new indication for preventive pacing (NIPP) investigators. Am J Cardiol 2001;88:371–5.

99. Bailin SJ, Adler S, Giudici M. Prevention of atrial fibrillation by pacing in the region of Bachmann's biundle. J Cariovasc Electrophysiol 2001;12:912–7.

100. Kay GN, Ellenbogen KA, Giudici M, et al. The Ablate and Pace Trial: a prospective study of catheter ablation of the AV conduction system and permanent pacemaker implantation for treatment of atrial fibrillation. APT Investigators J Interv Card Electrophysiol 1998;2:121–35.

101. Akerstrom F, Rodriguz-Manero M, Pachon M, et al. Atrioventricular junction ablation in atrial fibrillation: Choosing the right patient and pacing device. J Atrial Fib 2015;8:32–8.

102. Pachon JC, Pachon EI, Pachon JC, et al. "Cardioneuroablation" – new treatment for neurocardiogenic syncope, functional AV block and sinus dysfunction using catheter RF-ablation. Europace 2005;7:1–13.

103. Aksu T, Golcuk E, Yalin K, et al. Simplified cardioneuroablation in the treatment of reflex syncope, functional av block, and sinus node dysfunction. Pacing Clin Electrophysiol 2016;39:42–53.

104. Qin M, Zhang Y, Liu X, et al. Atrial ganglionated plexus modification: a novel approach to treat symptomatic sinus bradycardia. Pacing Clin Electrophysiol 2017;3:950–9.

105. Aksu T, Guler TE, Bozyel S, et al. Medium-term results of cardioneuroablation for clinical bradyarrhythmias and vasovagal syncope: effects on qt interval and heart rate. J Interv Card Electrophysiol 2021;60:57–68.

106. Aksu T, Guler TE, Bozyel S, et al. Vagal responses during cardioneuroablation on different ganglionated plexi: is there any role of ablation strategy? Int J Cardiol 2019;304:50–5.

107. Huang HD, Tamarisa R, Mathur N, et al. Stellate ganglion block: a therapeutic alternative for patients with medically refractory inappropriate sinus tachycardia? J Electrocardiol 2013;46:693–6.

108. Taketani T, Wolf RK, Garrett JV. Partial cardiac denervation and sinus node modification for inappropriate sinus tachycardia. Ann Thorac Surg 2007;84:652–4.

109. Ho RT, Ortman M, Mather PJ, et al. Inappropriate sinus tachycardia in a transplanted heart—further insights into pathogenesis. Heart Rhythm 2011;8:781–3.

Epidemiology and Outcomes Associated with PR Prolongation

Larry R. Jackson II, MD, MHS*, Francis Ugowe, MD

KEYWORDS

- PR prolongation • Epidemiology • Outcome • First-degree AV Block

KEY POINTS

- First-degree AV block (PR prolongation) defined as a PR interval > 200 ms (0.2 seconds) is common in the general population with a prevalence of 1% to 6% depending on age.
- PR prolongation is associated with increased risk of adverse outcomes including atrial arrhythmias, heart failure, and mortality, particularly in older populations.
- Future studies are needed, specifically to risk stratify patients with PR prolongation who may be at increased risk of adverse outcome as well as a basic mechanistic understanding of the role of PR prolongation in cardiovascular disease.

INTRODUCTION/HISTORY/DEFINITIONS/BACKGROUND

The PR interval reflects the time of electrical impulse propagation from the onset of atrial depolarization to the onset of ventricular depolarization and represents timing from the onset of the P wave to the start of the QRS complex on the surface electrocardiogram. The normal PR interval ranges from 0.12 to 0.20 seconds (120–200 ms) with the upper limit of normal defined as a time interval of 0.20 to 0.22 seconds.[1] Most PR prolongation is due to delayed impulse conduction through the atrioventricular node, although conduction delay in the atrium and His-Purkinje system can contribute to PR prolongation.

The etiologies of PR prolongation include organic heart disease from ischemia, inflammatory and infiltrative diseases, medications, autonomic influences, and collagen vascular disorders as well as idiopathic causes in patients without a history of cardiovascular disease. Although PR prolongation has classically been considered a benign finding, many of the original studies analyzing outcomes in patients with PR prolongation are confounded by selection bias including enrollment of primarily healthy, young male subjects with low burden of comorbid medical conditions.[2–6] More contemporary analyses have linked PR prolongation with adverse outcomes including progression of conduction system disease, increased risk of atrial remodeling and atrial arrhythmias,[7,8] and increased risk of all-cause mortality.[9]

This review aims to discuss the epidemiology and adverse outcomes associated with PR prolongation as well as the impact of PR prolongation in specific populations including patients with coronary artery disease, heart failure with reduced ejection fraction, and neuromuscular disease.

DISCUSSION
Epidemiology of PR Prolongation

Epidemiologic data on the incidence of PR prolongation have been reported in classical analyses, which primarily analyzed younger, male populations with a low burden of comorbid medical illness. Mymin and colleagues presented 30-year

This article originally appeared in *Cardiac Electrophysiology Clinics*, Volume 13 Issue 4, December 2021.
Duke University Medical Center, DUMC Box 3860, 2301 Erwin Road, Durham, NC 27710, USA
* Corresponding author.
E-mail address: larry.jackson@dm.duke.edu
Twitter: @LarryRJacksonII (L.R.J.); @Ugowe_MD (F.U.)

0733-8651/23/© 2023 Elsevier Inc. All rights reserved.

follow-up data on 3983 healthy men enrolled in the Manitoba cohort.[3] The incidence of PR prolongation increased with age, and after adjustment for heart rate, was 1.13 per 1000 person-years over the entire study period. Hiss and colleagues documented PR prolongation of 0.21 and 0.22 seconds in approximately 2 per 1000 records. Similar to Mymin and colleagues, the frequency of longer PR intervals was noted in older participants.[10] In a second study by Hiss and colleagues analyzing the electrocardiographic findings in 122,043 individuals, 802 electrocardiograms (6.5 per thousand) were noted to have a PR interval greater than 0.20 seconds.[2] There was no significant difference in the incidence rate in subjects aged less than 50 years; the proportion of subjects older than 50 years were small and precluded a calculation of incidence and prevalence. Packard and colleagues analyzed electrocardiograms from 1000 young health aviators (mean age 23.7 years) with follow-up after 10 to 12 years from baseline recordings. The number of electrocardiograms demonstrating PR prolongation was low (N = 11/1000) overall and as such an incidence rate could be not calculated.[4] In a similar cohort of healthy young men, Erikssen and colleagues analyzed changes in the PR interval from baseline to 7 years follow-up in men with no history of cardiovascular disease. No differences were seen in the prevalence of PR prolongation at baseline and follow-up (5.4%) (**Table 1**).[11]

Contemporary analyses from community-based cohorts have provided epidemiologic data of PR prolongation, taking into account real-world populations that vary by race/ethnicity, socioeconomic status, and burden of comorbid medical disease. Perlman and colleagues performed an epidemiologic study of PR prolongation in Tecumseh, Michigan; PR prolongation was defined as 0.22 seconds or longer.[5] PR prolongation was detected in 95 of 4678 participants (2.0%) with similar rates between men and women. The prevalence rates of PR prolongation increased significantly after the sixth decade of life. The prevalence of organic heart disease was 20% (N = 19/95) with most of these patients being older than 60 years. Kwok and colleagues performed a systematic review and meta-analysis of studies on PR prolongation and adverse cardiovascular outcomes. A total of 400,750 participants from 14 studies conducted in the United States, Europe, and Asia between the years of 1972 and 2011.[12] The prevalence of PR prolongation ranged between 2% and 14% across 7 studies with a mean prevalence of 7%. The definition of PR prolongation varied across studies from greater than 196 ms to greater than 220 ms.

Racial and ethnic differences in PR interval measurements have been documented in community cohorts. Santhanakrishnan and colleagues documented racial differences in electrocardiographic characteristics from Asians and Whites from 2 large community-based cohorts: Whites from the Framingham Heart Study and Asians from the Singapore Longitudinal Aging Study. Longer PR intervals were documented in Asian men and women compared to White men and women (β estimate 5.0 ± 1.4 ms and 6.6 ± 0.9 ms, both $P < .0006$) after adjustment for potential confounders including age, blood pressure, antihypertensive therapy, heart rate, body mass index, and diabetes mellitus.[13] In a study of racial and ethnic electrocardiogram predictors of atrial fibrillation and its impact on ischemic stroke in the Atherosclerosis Risk in Communities study, Blacks demonstrated statistically longer PR intervals than whites (defined as longer than the 95th percentile in the entire study population) in both the unadjusted and adjusted analysis.[14] In a comparison of the prevalence of first-degree atrioventricular block in African-American and Caucasian, Upshaw and colleagues analyzed 2123 electrocardiograms from patients aged 20 to 99 years. The overall prevalence of PR prolongation was 7.0% (N = 84/1201) and 6.9% (N = 64/922) among Caucasian and African Americans, respectively. PR prolongation was more prevalent in African-American patients compared with Caucasian patients in all age groups except for those patients in the eighth decade of life.[15] A limited number of studies have analyzed the incidence and prevalence of PR prolongation in Asian populations. Du and colleagues analyzed the prevalence of PR prolongation among a rural cohort of over 10,000 Chinese participants older than 40 years. In this cross-sectional study, the prevalence of PR prolongation, defined as a PR interval greater than 0.2 seconds, was 3.4% (95% confidence interval [CI], 3.9%–3.8%).[16] Men had a higher prevalence than women (5.1% vs 2.2%, $P < .001$). Independent risk factors associated with PR prolongation in this cohort included age, male sex, height, and systolic blood pressure. In a Japanese cohort from the National Integrated Project for Prospective Observation of Non-communicable Disease And its Trends in the Aged (NIPPON DATA), over 9000 community-dwelling participants, the prevalence of PR prolongation was 1.9% (N = 180/9051).[17]

Future epidemiologic studies are needed to understand the incidence and prevalence of PR prolongation in patients of Hispanic ethnicity and additional underrepresented racial and ethnic groups. In addition, caution should be taken

Table 1
Epidemiologic Studies of PR Prolongation

	Cohort Location	Study Design; Year	Participants	Findings
Du et al.[16]	Rural areas of Liaoning Province, China	Cross-sectional study from September 2017 to May 2018	10,926 participants aged ≥40 y (85.3% of those who were eligible)	• Prevalence of first-degree AV block (>0.20s) was 3.4% (95% CI, 3.0%–3.8%)
Erikssen et al.[11]	Male employees in 5 major companies and governmental agencies in Oslo, Norway	Cross-sectional cardiovascular survey. Follow-up 7 y	1832 healthy men aged 40–59 y	• Baseline and follow-up prevalence of prolonged PR (≥0.22 s)
Hiss et al.[2]	United States Air Force School of Aerospace Medicine, Headquarters Aerospace Medical Division	Prospective cohort study	122,043 healthy male subjects. Predominantly aviators and cadet applicants	• 6.5 electrocardiograms per thousand (N = 802/122,043) were noted to have a PR interval >0.20 s.
Johnson et al.[37]	United States Air Force School of Aerospace Medicine, Headquarters Aerospace Medical Division	Cross-sectional survey	67,375 electrocardiograms in asymptomatic subjects	• Incidence of first-degree AV block in the total surveyed population was 5.2 per thousand and did not change significantly in different age groups
Mymin et al.[3]	Manitoba Province, Canada	Population-based cohort with 30-y longitudinal starting on July 1st, 1948	3983 healthy men enrolled in the Manitoba cohort	• The incidence of PR prolongation increased with age, and after adjustment for heart rate, was 1.13 per 1000 person-years
Nikolaidou et al.[38]	Consecutive patients with suspected heart failure were referred to a community clinic in the United Kingdom between 2001 and 2014	Prospective cohort study; 2017	1420 patients with HeFREF; 1094 HeFNEF; 1150 no HeF	• The prevalence of first-degree heart block (heart rate corrected PR interval > 200 ms) was higher in patients with heart failure (21% HeFRF, 20% HeFNEF, 9% without heart failure).

(continued on next page)

Table 1
(continued)

	Cohort Location	Study Design; Year	Participants	Findings
Packard et al.[4]	United States Naval School of Aviation Medicine, Naval Air Station, Pensacola, Florida	Prospective cohort study; 10 y follow-up. Published in 1951	1000 young healthy aviators from July 1940 to March 1942	• No formal incidence or prevalence calculation was made but 11/1000 electrograms demonstrated PR prolongation (PR > 0.2 s)
Perlman et al.[5]	Prospective Epidemiology study of chronic disease including cardiovascular disease in Tecumseh, Michigan	Prospective cohort study; 1971	N = 4678	• PR prolongation was detected in 95 of 4678 electrocardiograms in participants older than 20 y • PR prolongation was not observed in participants younger than 20 y • Among the 95 persons with PR prolongation, there was no excess incidence of death or new events of coronary heart disease
Upshaw Jr. et al.[15]	Caucasian and African patients (inpatients, outpatients, and the emergency department) attending Piedmont Hospital in Atlanta, GA	Prospective cohort study; 2004	N = 2123	• First-degree atrioventricular block was more prevalent in African-American patients compared to Caucasian patients. • The prevalence of first-degree AV block began to increase at the age of 50 y in both groups

when interpreting the association of race, which is largely a social construct, and PR prolongation.

PR Prolongation and Adverse Outcomes

PR interval prolongation has historically been considered a low-risk rhythm disturbance of little consequence in healthy, asymptomatic individuals.[3–5,11,18] However, more recent analyses from large, longitudinal cohort studies have failed to show any meaningful connection between PR prolongation and adverse outcomes in healthy participants. For example, Aro and colleagues examined the electrocardiograms of 10,957 individuals (aged 30–59 years) recorded between 1966 and 1972, and followed prospectively for 30 ± 11 years in the Finnish Social Insurance Institution's Coronary Heart Disease Study (CHD Study).[1] They observed that PR prolongation was not associated with an increased risk of stroke, atrial fibrillation, heart failure, or mortality, even after multivariable adjustment and subgroup analyses.[1] On the contrary, in an analysis of 2722 participants from the Health, Aging, and Body Composition Study (aged 74 ± 3 years, 49.1% men), Mangani and colleagues observed that after multivariate adjustment that PR interval prolongation was associated with a 46% increased risk of incident heart failure (95% CI, 1.11–1.93), but was not associated with increased all-cause mortality.[8]

There are several possible explanations for the inconsistencies in observations between prolonged PR interval and outcomes. Researchers have suggested that earlier studies may have suffered from important limitations such as confounding, small sample sizes, inconsistent populations, inadequate follow-up periods to detect outcomes, and insufficient event ascertainment.[12] Yet, although the significance of PR prolongation in healthy populations remains unclear, there are a preponderance of studies that demonstrate PR prolongation in older individuals may portend an overall increased risk of morbidity and mortality, possibly as a signal of subclinical cardiovascular disease.[19] For instance, in a prospective cohort including 7575 individuals from the Framingham Heart Study (mean age, 47 years; 46% men), Cheng and colleagues observed that those with first-degree AV block are at a moderately elevated risk of all-cause mortality (hazard ratio [HR] 1.44; 95% CI, 1.09–1.91; P = .01), with an approximately 2-fold increased risk of future atrial fibrillation (HR 2.06; 95% CI, 1.36–3.12; P < .001), and about a three-fold increased risk of pacemaker implantation compared to patients without first-degree AV block (HR 2.89; 95% CI, 1.83–4.57; P < .001).[9] These findings were consistent even

after adjusting for traditional risk factors and excluding patients with intraventricular conduction abnormalities or who were on AV nodal-blocking medications.[9] Of note, roughly 27% of the patients with baseline first-degree AV block went on to develop second or third-degree AV block and/or complete heart block.[9]

Another illustration of this shift in understanding was demonstrated by Nielsen and colleagues[20] using a primary care cohort of more than 280,000 patients with a median follow-up of 5.7 years. Researchers observed that having a PR interval ≥200 ms was associated with an HR of 1.26 (95% CI, 1.17–1.35; P < .001) for atrial fibrillation compared with the reference group.[20] Interestingly, shorter PR intervals (<123 ms) were also associated with an elevated risk of developing AF with an HR of 1.21 (95% CI, 1.06–1.37; P = .004).[20] In a similar analysis, Park and colleagues showed that a prolonged PR interval signaled atrial fibrillation–related remodeling of the atria, greater left atrium size, a higher prevalence of hypertension, and persistent atrial fibrillation.[21] In addition, prolonged PR was also a predictor of recurrence of atrial fibrillation after radiofrequency ablation (HR = 1.969; 95% CI, 1.343–2.886; P = .001).[21]

Further support was shown in a systematic analysis of 14 studies evaluating outcomes associated with prolonged PR intervals.[12] Kwok and colleagues examined the data of over 400,000 individuals gathered between 1972 and 2011.[12] Pooled data showed that prolonged PR interval was associated with an increased risk of left ventricular dysfunction and heart failure (risk ratio [RR] 1.39; 95% CI, 1.18–1.65), atrial fibrillation (RR 1.45; 95% CI, 1.23–1.71), and overall mortality (RR 1.24; 95% CI, 1.02–1.51).[12] Curiously, investigators did not find a significant association between prolonged PR and coronary disease, vascular events such as myocardial infarction and stroke, or cardiovascular mortality.[12]

From a pathophysiological standpoint, there are several theories as to the underlying multifactorial mechanism that links PR prolongation to adverse cardiovascular outcomes. Firstly, PR prolongation could simply be viewed as an ECG representation of aging and degeneration of the native conduction system. As atherosclerotic disease is closely correlated with advancing age, it is postulated that PR prolongation could possibly serve as a marker for advanced atherosclerosis and cardiovascular events.[22]

In addition, coronary artery disease could affect perfusion of the AV nodal artery, a branch of the right coronary artery in most individuals, thus manifesting as AV prolongation. Research has also suggested that PR prolongation is independently associated with abnormal vascular function and increased arterial stiffness.[22,23] Furthermore, PR prolongation could be a proxy of other alterations in the cardiovascular or neurohormonal/autonomic system that herald a worse overall prognosis.[22] Although the mechanistic effect of PR prolongation on outcomes has not been definitively described, it is evident that further research is needed to reinforce our knowledge on this question.

PR Prolongation in Special Populations

Coronary artery disease

As mentioned previously, PR prolongation has been shown to be strongly associated with coronary artery disease and other adverse cardiovascular events. For example, Chan and colleagues found that in patients with coronary atherosclerosis or equivalent disease that prolonged PR interval independently predicted cardiovascular death (HR 14.1; 95% CI, 3.8–51.4; $P < .001$), new-onset ischemic stroke (HR 8.6; 95% CI, 1.9–37.8; $P = .005$), and combined cardiovascular endpoints (HR 2.4; 95% CI, 1.30–4.43; $P = .005$), which included occurrences of any primary endpoints or congestive heart failure.[22] At an exploratory cut-off of PR interval > 162 ms, the PR was also found to be predictive of new-onset MI (HR 8.0; 95% CI, 1.65–38.85; $P = .010$; C-statistic 0.70, $P = .001$).[22] In a separate study of 205 patients with non-ST segment elevation MI or unstable angina, Nabati and colleagues observed that PR prolongation was associated with clinically significant coronary disease ($P = .024$) with a positive trend toward a higher frequency of left main or three-vessel disease, and higher Gensini scores (an intensity index for coronary artery disease).[24] Furthermore, Nabati and colleagues did not observe a difference when risk factors such as the presence of hypertension, diabetes, hyperlipidemia, or family history were compared.[24] In addition, Xue and colleagues found that in a cohort of 915 patients who had suffered an ST-elevation myocardial infarction that approximately 9.5% went on to develop PR interval prolongation.[25] Furthermore, after adjusting for possible confounders, PR interval prolongation was independently associated with worse outcomes (HR 5.37; 95% CI, 1.85–15.62; $P = .002$) and increased long-term death.[25]

In contrast, Holmqvist and colleagues observed conflicting findings in an analysis of 9637 patients with at least single vessel disease who had undergone coronary angiography between 1989 and 2010.[26] Investigators found that after adjusting for pertinent variables, that prolonged PR interval (in this study >162 ms) did not predict a significant difference in the risk of all-cause mortality, death/stroke composite, or composite of cardiovascular death or rehospitalization.[26] Curiously, instead they found a *decreasing* PR interval (10 ms decrements) was associated with these adverse cardiovascular endpoints.[26] Holmqvist and colleagues did however observe an association between all-cause mortality and PR prolongation in subgroup analysis of patients not on antiarrhythmic drugs.[26] Although there is not a clear explanation for these inconsistent findings, a possible signal exist pointing to increased risk in patients with alterations in AV conduction.

Heart failure

Heart failure is associated with extensive electrophysiological reconstruction of the cardiac conduction system resulting in both QRS and PR interval prolongation and the development of atrial fibrillation.[19] In a subgroup analysis of the Heart and Soul study including 938 patients with stable coronary disease, Crisel and colleagues found that patients with PR prolongation (mean age 73 ± 10 years) were more than twice as likely to be hospitalized for heart failure exacerbations or to die from cardiovascular causes.[27] Most of the data regarding the epidemiology of PR prolongation in patients with heart failure originates from device trials and subsequent analyses.[19] In a retrospective study of the Danish Pacemaker and ICD Register, Kronborg and colleagues observed that 47% of patients who underwent cardiac resynchronization therapy (CRT) implantation had first-degree AV block and that a long native PR interval was an independent predictor of all-cause and cardiac death.[28] Separately, in a subgroup analysis of CARE-HF, Gervais and colleagues observed that, even after adjusting for CRT, baseline PR prolongation and a longer PR interval at 3 months status post-CRT implantation (paced PR for the intervention group and native PR for the control group) was associated with increased all-cause mortality and heart failure hospitalization.[29] Atwater and colleagues observed that heart failure patients who had baseline PR prolongation and subsequently received CRT had a shorter survival free of left ventricular assist device implantation or heart transplant.[30] Researchers theorized that patients with PR prolongation at baseline diminished effective resynchronization relative to patients with normal PR intervals.[30] Furthermore, data from Olshansky and colleagues suggest that PR prolongation may be a modifiable risk factor, as those patients seemed to derive the most benefit from CRT implantation.[31] Further studies are needed on the epidemiology and clinical significance of PR prolongation in patients with heart failure in real-world populations outside of device trials.

Neuromuscular disease

Neuromuscular disorders are associated with a wide range of phenotypic expressions. Cardiac involvement is more commonly seen in myopathies and less so in diseases that affect nerves and communication. Cardiac involvement in myopathies oftentimes can take the form of cardiomyopathy, as well as arrhythmias and conduction disturbances. As it pertains to PR interval prolongation, there are several neuromuscular diseases that have been studied in this area. Given that many of these disorders are rare, the associations made are limited to case series and are observational in nature. For example, Petri and colleagues observed that patients with myotonic dystrophy type I, a disease known to effect multiple systems and lead to progressive muscle wasting and weakness, had a prevalence of first degree of AV block of approximately 28.2%, along with numerous other conduction abnormalities.[32] Conduction defects ranging from sinus bradycardia, to PR interval prolongation, to complete heart block have also been observed in patients with Emery-Dreifuss muscular dystrophy.[33] Emery-Dreifuss is recognized by a classic triad of (1) early joint contractures, (2) progressive muscle weakness and atrophy in the upper arms/lower legs, and (3) cardiac involvement, typically AV conduction disturbances and atrial arrhythmias.[34] Per the 2018 ACC/AHA/HRS Guideline on the Evaluation and Management of Patients With Bradycardia and Cardiac Conduction Delay, patients with PR prolongation and comorbid neuromuscular disease with or without symptoms, such as myotonic dystrophy type I, may be considered for permanent pacemaker placement because of the unpredictable evolution of conduction disease (class IIb recommendation; level of evidence C).[35] Understandably, because of the limited data and expansive clinical heterogeneity that exists, the management of cardiac disease in neuromuscular disorders is extremely difficult. Yet, efforts are being made to try and bridge this gap in knowledge to better care for these complex patients.[36]

SUMMARY

Our understanding of the prognostic significance of the PR interval continues to evolve. Contemporary analyses have repeatedly demonstrated the association of PR prolongation with adverse outcomes including increased risk of atrial arrhythmias, heart failure, and mortality, particularly in older patients.

Whether PR prolongation is a marker for adverse outcomes or itself involved in the causal pathways that lead to cardiac pathology remains to be seen. Future studies are needed to understand the mechanism underlying the pathophysiology associated with PR prolongation, methods to stratify at-risk patients, and optimal monitoring strategies, specifically in older patients who have the highest prevalence of PR prolongation. Identification of PR prolongation on an electrocardiogram should prompt clinicians to ask patients about the presence of pre-existing heart disease and a family history of heart disease. Older patients with PR prolongation and a history of heart disease should undergo further evaluation for causes of PR prolongation including assessing for coronary artery disease and LV systolic dysfunction, although the utility and cost-effectiveness of the additional diagnostic evaluation in asymptomatic patients with PR prolongation is unknown.

CLINICS CARE POINTS

- The incidence and prevalence of PR prolongation increases with age, especially after the sixth decade of life.
- Data from contemporary cohorts suggest a clear association with PR prolongation and adverse outcomes including increased risk of atrial arrhythmias and all-cause mortality.
- Clinicians should be cognizant of PR prolongation that is detected in older patients. In addition, considerations should be given to increased monitoring for future events, although the exact time interval and optimal strategy for monitoring older patients with PR prolongation are unknown.

DISCLOSURE STATEMENT

Dr Jackson has support provided by the Duke Center for Research to Advance Healthcare Equity (REACH Equity), which is supported by the National Institute on Minority Health and Health Disparities under award number U54MD012530. In addition, Dr Jackson receives honoraria from Medtronic and Biotronik Inc. Dr Francis Ugowe has no disclosures.

REFERENCES

1. Aro AL, Anttonen O, Kerola T, et al. Prognostic significance of prolonged PR interval in the general population. Eur Heart J 2014;35:123–9.

2. Hiss RG, Lamb LE. Electrocardiographic findings in 122,043 individuals. Circulation 1962;25:947–61.

3. Mymin D, Mathewson FA, Tate RB, et al. The natural history of primary first-degree atrioventricular heart block. N Engl J Med 1986;315:1183–7.

4. Packard JM, Graettinger JS, Graybiel A. Analysis of the electrocardiograms obtained from 1000 young healthy aviators; ten year follow-up. Circulation 1954;10:384–400.

5. Perlman LV, Ostrander LD Jr, Keller JB, et al. An epidemiologic study of first degree atrioventricular block in Tecumseh, Michigan. Chest 1971;59:40–6.

6. Rose G, Baxter PJ, Reid DD, et al. Prevalence and prognosis of electrocardiographic findings in middle-aged men. Br Heart J 1978;40:636–43.

7. Cheng M, Lu X, Huang J, et al. Electrocardiographic PR prolongation and atrial fibrillation risk: a meta-analysis of prospective cohort studies. J Cardiovasc Electrophysiol 2015;26:36–41.

8. Magnani JW, Wang N, Nelson KP, et al. Electrocardiographic PR interval and adverse outcomes in older adults: the Health, Aging, and Body Composition study. Circ Arrhythm Electrophysiol 2013;6:84–90.

9. Cheng S, Keyes MJ, Larson MG, et al. Long-term outcomes in individuals with prolonged PR interval or first-degree atrioventricular block. J Am Med Assoc 2009;301:2571–7.

10. Hiss RG, Lamb LE, Allen MF. Electrocardiographic findings in 67,375 asymptomatic subjects. X. Normal values. Am J Cardiol 1960;6:200–31.

11. Erikssen J, Otterstad JE. Natural course of a prolonged PR interval and the relation between PR and incidence of coronary heart disease. A 7-year follow-up study of 1832 apparently healthy men aged 40-59 years. Clin Cardiol 1984;7:6–13.

12. Kwok CS, Rashid M, Beynon R, et al. Prolonged PR interval, first-degree heart block and adverse cardiovascular outcomes: a systematic review and meta-analysis. Heart 2016;102:672–80.

13. Santhanakrishnan R, Wang N, Larson MG, et al. Racial differences in electrocardiographic characteristics and prognostic significance in whites versus Asians. J Am Heart Assoc 2016;5:e002956.

14. Soliman EZ, Prineas RJ, Case LD, et al. Ethnic distribution of ECG predictors of atrial fibrillation and its impact on understanding the ethnic distribution of ischemic stroke in the Atherosclerosis Risk in Communities (ARIC) study. Stroke 2009;40:1204–11.

15. Upshaw CB Jr. Comparison of the prevalence of first-degree atrioventricular block in African-American and in Caucasian patients: an electrocardiographic study III. J Natl Med Assoc 2004;96:756–60.

16. Du Z, Xing L, Lin M, et al. Prevalence of first-degree atrioventricular block and the associated risk factors: a cross-sectional study in rural Northeast China. BMC Cardiovasc Disord 2019;19:214.

17. Hisamatsu T, Miura K, Fujiyoshi A, et al. Long-term outcomes associated with prolonged PR interval in the general Japanese population. Int J Cardiol 2015;184:291–3.

18. Rajala S, Haavisto M, Kaltiala K, et al. ECG findings and survival in very old people. Eur Heart J 1985;6:247–52.

19. Nikolaidou T, Ghosh JM, Clark AL. Outcomes related to first-degree atrioventricular block and therapeutic implications in patients with heart failure. JACC Clin Electrophysiol 2016;2:181–92.

20. Nielsen JB, Pietersen A, Graff C, et al. Risk of atrial fibrillation as a function of the electrocardiographic PR interval: results from the Copenhagen ECG Study. Heart Rhythm 2013;10:1249–56.

21. Park J, Kim TH, Lee JS, et al. Prolonged PR interval predicts clinical recurrence of atrial fibrillation after catheter ablation. J Am Heart Assoc 2014;3:e001277.

22. Chan YH, Hai JJ, Lau KK, et al. PR interval prolongation in coronary patients or risk equivalent: excess risk of ischemic stroke and vascular pathophysiological insights. BMC Cardiovasc Disord 2017;17:233.

23. Chan YH, Siu CW, Yiu KH, et al. Abnormal vascular function in PR-interval prolongation. Clin Cardiol 2011;34:628–32.

24. Nabati M, Kalantari B, Dehghan Z, et al. Association between prolonged PR intervals and significant coronary artery disease in patients with non-ST elevation myocardial infarction and unstable angina. Res Cardiovasc Med 2020;9.

25. Xue Y, Shen J, Liu G, et al. Predictors, incidence, and prognostic significance of PR interval prolongation in patients with ST-segment elevation myocardial infarction. Coron Artery Dis 2020;31:606–12.

26. Holmqvist F, Thomas KL, Broderick S, et al. Clinical outcome as a function of the PR-interval-there is virtue in moderation: data from the Duke Databank for cardiovascular disease. Europace 2015;17:978–85.

27. Crisel RK, Farzaneh-Far R, Na B, et al. First-degree atrioventricular block is associated with heart failure and death in persons with stable coronary artery disease: data from the Heart and Soul Study. Eur Heart J 2011;32:1875–80.

28. Kronborg MB, Nielsen JC, Mortensen PT. Electrocardiographic patterns and long-term clinical outcome in cardiac resynchronization therapy. Europace 2010;12:216–22.

29. Gervais R, Leclercq C, Shankar A, et al. Surface electrocardiogram to predict outcome in candidates for cardiac resynchronization therapy: a sub-analysis of the CARE-HF trial. Eur J Heart Fail 2009;11:699–705.

30. Atwater BD, Emerek K, Sorensen PL, et al. PR Prolongation predicts inadequate resynchronization with biventricular pacing in left bundle branch block. Pacing Clin Electrophysiol 2019;42:1477–85.

31. Olshansky B, Day JD, Sullivan RM, et al. Does cardiac resynchronization therapy provide unrecognized benefit in patients with prolonged PR intervals? The impact of restoring atrioventricular synchrony: an analysis from the COMPANION Trial. Heart Rhythm 2012;9:34–9.

32. Petri H, Vissing J, Witting N, et al. Cardiac manifestations of myotonic dystrophy type 1. Int J Cardiol 2012;160:82–8.

33. Emery AEH. Emery–Dreifuss muscular dystrophy – a 40 year retrospective. Neuromuscul Disord 2000;10:228–32.

34. Ismail H, Raynor E, Zimetbaum P. Neuromuscular disorders and the role of the clinical electrophysiologist. JACC Clin Electrophysiol 2017;3:1069–79.

35. Kusumoto FM, Schoenfeld MH, Barrett C, et al. 2018 ACC/AHA/HRS Guideline on the evaluation and management of patients with bradycardia and cardiac conduction delay: a Report of the American College of Cardiology/American Heart Association Task Force on Clinical Practice Guidelines and the Heart Rhythm Society. Circulation 2019;140:e382–482.

36. Feingold B, Mahle WT, Auerbach S, et al. Management of cardiac involvement associated with neuromuscular diseases: a Scientific Statement from the American Heart Association. Circulation 2017;136:e200–31.

37. Johnson RL, Averill KH, Lamb LE. Electrocardiographic findings in 67,375 asymptomatic subjects. VII. Atrioventricular block. Am J Cardiol 1960;6:153–77.

38. Nikolaidou T, Pellicori P, Zhang J, et al. Prevalence, predictors, and prognostic implications of PR interval prolongation in patients with heart failure. Clin Res Cardiol 2018;107:108–19.

Left Bundle Branch Block

Characterization, Definitions, and Recent Insights into Conduction System Physiology

Margarida Pujol-López, MD[a,b], José M. Tolosana, MD, PhD[a,b,c],
Gaurav A. Upadhyay, MD[d], Lluís Mont, MD, PhD[a,b,c], Roderick Tung, MD[d],*

KEYWORDS

- Left bundle branch block • Electromechanical dyssynchrony • Cardiomyopathy
- Left bundle branch pacing

KEY POINTS

- The anatomy of the left bundle branch (LBB) has marked variability between individuals. There are variations in size, branching pattern, number, and location of fascicular subdivisions.
- Left bundle branch block (LBBB) patterns on ECG rmay be the result of conduction system block either at the His or proximal LBB, more distal nonspecific intraventricular conduction delay, or combinations of the two.
- LBBB implies electrical and mechanical ventricular dyssynchrony leading to left ventricular remodeling that may be treated with biventricular resynchronization therapy or physiologic pacing.
- Detailed activation mapping of the basal left septum has revealed that the site of block is most commonly localized within the left His fibers, rather than in the LBB itself.
- Improved correlation between intracardiac activation patterns and 12-lead ECG is necessary for clinical trials and to tailor pacing modalities toward the intrinsic pathophysiology of conduction disorder.

INTRODUCTION/BACKGROUND

Left bundle branch block (LBBB) is not a simple and generalized electrocardiogram (ECG) alteration in QRS pattern. It is associated with advanced conduction system and structural heart disease, and has important prognostic implications with regard to heart failure and mortality.[1] The complex pathophysiology underlying LBBB has emerged to the forefront because of three clinical observations: (1) variable definitions of LBBB that affects patient management, treatment, and prognosis; (2) differential response and nonresponse to cardiac resynchronization therapy (CRT) based on presence or absence of LBBB; and (3) conduction system pacing (CSP) that can correct electrical dyssynchrony in patients with LBBB but not in those with nonspecific intraventricular conduction delay.

The purpose of this review is to synthesize data regarding understanding of LBBB in humans. To offer patients a physiologic pacing via the conduction system, a renewed focus on LBBB

This article originally appeared in *Cardiac Electrophysiology Clinics*, Volume 13 Issue 4, December 2021.
[a] Arrhythmia Section, Cardiology Department, Institut Clínic Cardiovascular, Hospital Clínic de Barcelona, Universitat de Barcelona, C/ Villarroel 170, Barcelona, Catalonia 08036, Spain; [b] Institut d'Investigacions Biomèdiques August Pi i Sunyer, Barcelona, Catalonia, Spain; [c] Centro de Investigación Biomédica en Red Enfermedades Cardiovasculares, Madrid, Spain; [d] Center for Arrhythmia Care, Pritzker School of Medicine, University of Chicago, The University of Chicago Medicine, Heart and Vascular Center, 5841 South Maryland Avenue, Chicago, IL 60637, USA
* Corresponding author.
E-mail addresses: rtung1@medicine.bsd.uchicago.edu; rodericktung@arizona.edu

Cardiol Clin 41 (2023) 379–391
https://doi.org/10.1016/j.ccl.2023.03.003
0733-8651/23/

pathophysiology has surfaced. Because of a revival of interest in CSP, there has also been renewed interest in investigating LBBB. Recent work has highlighted variability in the site of block, activation patterns studied with electrocardiographic imaging, anatomic variability of the proximal conduction system, and newer CSP site modalities to either preserve or restore synchronization.

EPIDEMIOLOGY

In asymptomatic adults, including athletes, the estimated prevalence of LBBB ranges from 0.1% to 0.8% (0.43% for men and 0.28% for women).[2] Its prevalence increases steadily from less than 1% at age 50 to 6% by 80 years,[3] and almost never occurs in those less than 35 years of age. The incidence of LBBB was 3.2 per 10,000 per year for men and 3.7 per 10,000 per year for women in the general population.[4] The average age at LBBB diagnosis was 69.6 ± 10.0 years in men and 68.3 ± 10.9 years in women, and the incidence of LBBB increased progressively with age.[5]

There are several factors found to be associated with LBBB development (**Fig. 1**)[5–7]; however, LBBB can develop in the absence of risk factors. Studies have implicated several genetic mutations in association with LBBB, such as variations in connexin 43 (gap junction protein that collaborates in fast conduction velocity),[8] and current evidence also suggests that LBBB development could be modulated by genotype.[2] LBBB may also develop as an acquired mechanical complication of procedural interventions, such as surgical aortic valve replacement or transcatheter aortic valve replacement (TAVR), because of the anatomic proximity of the aortic valve with the penetrating His bundle and the proximal cardiac conduction system. It is also commonly observed in severe hypertrophic cardiomyopathy treated with septal myectomy because of excision of the basal septum, which houses the proximal and distal left bundle branch (LBB).

ANATOMY OF THE LEFT BUNDLE

The His bundle is the anatomic continuation of the atrioventricular (AV) node, and it provides the connection to the right bundle branch and LBB.[9] Both branches course toward the papillary muscles of their corresponding ventricles. The bundle of His is composed of two segments: the penetrating and branching portions.[10] The penetrating segment is related to the atrial part of the membranous septum, the central fibrous body, and the septal leaflet of the tricuspid valve. The LBB originates in the branching portion located inferior and apical in relation to the membranous septum.[11] Given its location, the larger the membranous septum, the lower the possibility that the aortic valve pathology involves this crucial part of the conduction system.[11]

At the crest of the muscular interventricular septum, the His bundle starts to divide into right and left branches. The right bundle originates after the penetrating bundle on the left side of the septum and courses back toward the right ventricle in a course that is superior to the LBB. The main

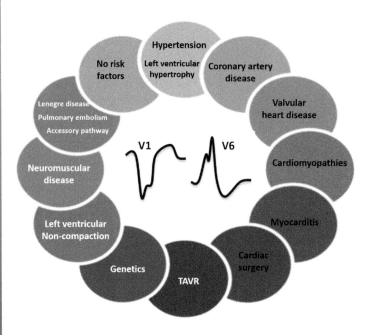

Fig. 1. Associated factors in the cause of left bundle branch block. TAVR, transcatheter aortic valve replacement.

LBB trunk extends inferiorly 10 to 15 mm toward the apex; it splits into three fascicles after which there are many subendocardial ramifications and interconnections. LBB trunk blood irrigation is supplied by the AV nodal artery (85%–90% is a branch of the right coronary artery)[12] and branches of left anterior descending coronary artery.[6]

The proximal left conduction system has marked variability between individuals. There are variations in size, number, location, and configuration of the subdivisions. Histopathologic investigations have suggested the presence of three primary fascicles[13]: (1) left anterior, (2) left septal or middle, and (3) left posterior (**Fig. 2**A). Durrer and colleagues[14] famously demonstrated three discrete endocardial regions that were synchronously excited 0 to 5 milliseconds after the start of the left ventricular activity potential. These areas increased rapidly in size and became confluent. The three areas of initial excitation could be assumed to correspond to the terminal areas of the three fascicles of the LBB.[15] The first areas in the left ventricle (LV) to be excited are[14]: high on the anterior paraseptal wall below the attachment of the mitral valve (left anterior fascicle), central on the left surface of the interventricular septum (left septal fascicle), and posterior paraseptal about one-third of the distance from apex to base (posterior fascicle ends). From each division of the LBB, their corresponding Purkinje networks emerge covering the subendocardium of the septum and the free wall of the ventricle.

The typical trifasicular diagrams (see **Fig. 2**A), however, are likely a simplified construct,[16] which may not necessarily encompass the intricacy and complex nature within the left-sided conduction system. Seminal illustrations from Tawara[9] highlight variability in size, width, bifurcation, and interconnectedness of the proximal system. Demoulin and Kulbertus[13,17] performed and illustrated dissections of the human conduction system and showed that only a minority exhibited discrete fascicles, and that plexiform patterns of Purkinje networks were more common. The conduction system is indeed vulnerable to focal fibrosis at the His or common left bundle, which is a possible mechanism for the development of LBBB, but distal to this location tremendous redundancy of the network is present.[16]

DEFINITIONS AND CRITERIA FOR TRUE LEFT BUNDLE BRANCH BLOCK

LBBB was first described on the ECG in 1909 by Eppinger[18] in studies in dogs; however, they interpreted the tracings as right bundle branch block (RBBB). In 1929, Barker and colleagues[19] concluded that ECGs that had been regarded as RBBB were the result of LBBB. In LBBB the impulse spreads first to the right ventricle (RV) via the right bundle branch and then to the LV via slow activation of the septum; this sequential activation lengthens the QRS to greater than or equal to 120 milliseconds. There are different electrocardiographic criteria to diagnose complete LBBB; some commonly used criteria include criteria by Bayés de Luna,[20] criteria by Strauss and coworkers,[21] and American College of Cardiology/American Heart Association/Heart Rhythm Society. **Table 1** shows the updated criteria proposed by American College of Cardiology/American Heart Association/Heart Rhythm Society in 2009 and restated in 2018.[22,23]

The criteria set that Strauss and colleagues[21] proposed in 2011 deserves specific mention. These more specific criteria for complete LBBB were defined to better predict response to CRT: QRS duration greater than or equal to 140 milliseconds (men) or 130 milliseconds (women); QS or rS in leads V1 and V2; and mid-QRS notching or slurring in greater than or equal to two of leads V1, V2, V5, V6, I, and aVL. They suggested the

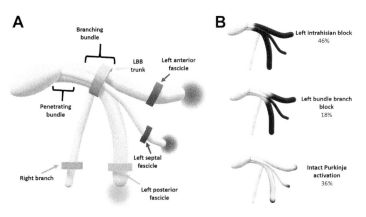

Fig. 2. Left bundle branch anatomy and sites of conduction block in patients with LBBB. (*A*) Histopathologic investigations confirmed the consistent presence of three fascicles constituting the left branch: anterior, septal, and posterior. (*B*) Patients with LBBB have three subtypes of conduction patterns: proximal left intrahisian block (46%), left bundle branch block (18%), and intact Purkinje activation without discrete conduction block (36%), most likely because of conduction slowing more distally or within the myocardium.[26]

Table 1
ECG criteria of complete left bundle branch block and hemiblocks

	Anterior Hemiblock	Posterior Hemiblock
Frontal axis	Left axis deviation: −45° to −90°	Right axis deviation: ≥100° (90° to 180°)
ECG	QRS <120 ms qR in lead aVL rS in leads in leads II, III, and aVF R-peak time in lead aVL ≥45 ms	QRS <120 ms rS in leads I and aVL qR in leads III and aVF

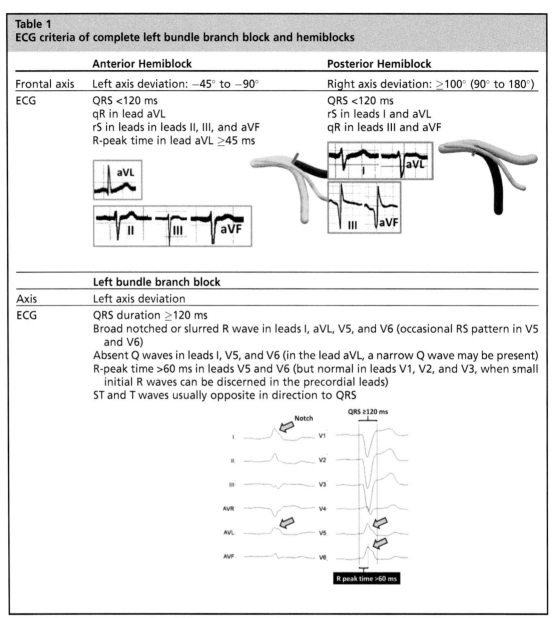

	Left bundle branch block
Axis	Left axis deviation
ECG	QRS duration ≥120 ms Broad notched or slurred R wave in leads I, aVL, V5, and V6 (occasional RS pattern in V5 and V6) Absent Q waves in leads I, V5, and V6 (in the lead aVL, a narrow Q wave may be present) R-peak time >60 ms in leads V5 and V6 (but normal in leads V1, V2, and V3, when small initial R waves can be discerned in the precordial leads) ST and T waves usually opposite in direction to QRS

Adapted from Kusumoto FM, Schoenfeld MH, Barrett C, et al. 2018 ACC/AHA/HRS Guideline on the Evaluation and Management of Patients With Bradycardia and Cardiac Conduction Delay: Executive Summary: A Report of the American College of Cardiology/American Heart Association Task Force on Clinical Practice Guidelines, and the Heart Rhythm Society. J Am Coll Cardiol. 2019;74(7):932-987 and Elizari MV, Acunzo RS, Ferreiro M. Hemiblocks revisited. Circulation. 2007;115(9):1154-63; with permission

higher QRS duration cutoff to avoid overdiagnosis of complete LBBB in patients with LV hypertrophy and left anterior fascicular block. The value of the Strauss criteria in improving the selection of potential CRT responders, however, has been mixed. These criteria were not independently associated with outcomes after adjustment for cause of the cardiomyopathy and QRS duration in some studies.[24]

Left Bundle Branch Block Patterns in Cardiac Resynchronization Therapy

Electrocardiographic LBBB patterns include patients with complete conduction block into or within the left bundle and patients with intact activation of the Purkinje system. That is, LBBB pattern can result from damage to the LBB itself, conduction delay within the fascicles or Purkinje fibers, or a combination of both.[25]

The site of LBBB has long been conceptualized as a result of diffuse and distal conduction system disease. By this paradigm, restoration of physiologic activation would inherently be difficult to achieve with single-site pacing stimulation. Electrophysiologic studies (EPS) performed by Upadhyay and colleagues[26] involving multielectrode recordings during interrogation of the basal left septum characterized that conduction block associated with the LBBB pattern is most commonly focal in nature and proximal, usually within the left-sided His fibers. The findings of complete disruption of the His-Purkinje activation were observed where atrial components were recorded synchronously with right-sided His activation measurements. Left-sided EPS has demonstrated two sites of conduction block in patients with LBBB pattern[27]: left intrahisian block (46%) and LBBB (18%), with the remainder demonstrating intact Purkinje activation (36%) (**Fig. 2**B; **Fig. 3**). These data were the first to demonstrate that focal left intrahisian block is the predominant lesion responsible for LBBB patterns and provides an explanation for corrective His pacing, in which a sufficient pacing stimulus can capture distal to the site of block and re-engage latent recruitable left Purkinje system fibers (**Fig. 4**). Importantly, corrective His pacing response was less frequently observed in those with more distal block in the left bundle, which paves the way for intraseptal fixation techniques to achieve left bundle area capture.

ELECTROMECHANICAL EFFECTS OF LEFT BUNDLE BRANCH BLOCK

His-Purkinje system tissue action potentials conduct rapidly at 1.5 m/s (1.3–1.7 m/s).[28] This network provides coupling between electrical excitation and mechanical contraction.[27] During LBBB, the electrical activation of the LV occurs as a result of transseptal activation, with myocardial cell-to-cell activation, which is comparatively slower. This leads to intraventricular and interventricular dyssynchrony along with a weaker and less effective resulting contraction.[29]

In terms of electrical dyssynchrony, RV activation occurs first, followed by activation of the LV usually at the level of the midseptum, where the rest of LV is activated in a homogeneous but delayed fashion, with the last site of activation in the lateral basal area.[25] **Fig. 5** shows the LBBB pattern of epicardial activation with electrocardiographic imaging. Auricchio and colleagues[30] showed that LV transeptal conduction time had a binary distribution with a border zone between 20 and 40 milliseconds in a study with three-dimensional contact and noncontact mapping; the patients with normal LV transeptal time (<20 milliseconds) represent 37%. These results were in line with the ones reported by Upadhyay and colleagues[26] showing that 36% of patients with LBBB pattern had intact Purkinje activation.

LBBB electrical dyssynchrony results in mechanical dyssynchrony. The ventricular septum is activated during isovolumetric contraction (before aortic valve opening), which stretches the posterior and lateral walls. These walls are then activated later in systole, with passive stretching of the septal wall. The dyssynchronous motion of the ventricular walls results in decreased contraction efficiency.[25,31] Characteristic noninvasive echocardiographic observations are as follows:

a. Septal flash (SF): An echocardiographic marker of LV dyssynchrony. It was described in 1974 as a "septal beak" with M-mode in patients with LBBB.[32] In 2009, Parsai and colleagues[33]

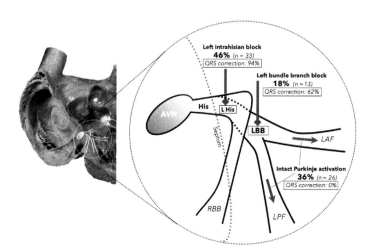

Fig. 3. Sites of conduction block and corresponding rate of LBBB correction with His bundle stimulation. RBB, right bundle branch. AVN, atrioventricular node; LAF, left anterior fascicle; LPF, left posterior fascicle. (*From* Upadhyay G, Cherian T, Shatz DY, et al. Intracardiac Delineation of Septal Conduction in Left Bundle-Branch Block Patterns. Circulation. 2019;139(16):1876-1888); with permission.)

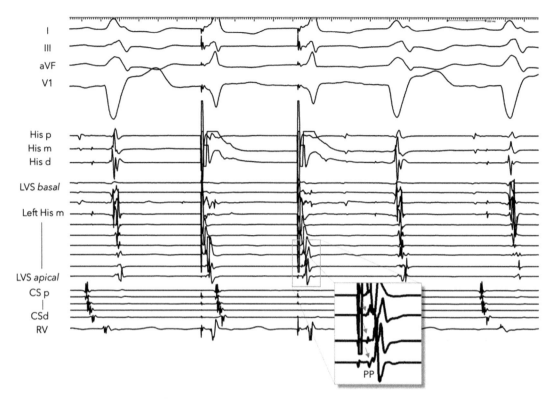

Fig. 4. Intracardiac recordings of left-intrahisian block during spontaneous complete LBBB pattern, which demonstrates recruitment of presystolic Purkinje activation during corrective pacing.

applied the concept of abnormal septal motion in CRT, as a marker of dyssynchrony in patients with LBBB. SF is a fast contraction and relaxation of the septum (septal thickening/thinning) occurring during the isovolumetric contraction period (within the QRS width). The prevalence of SF among LBBB patients is 45% to 63%.[34,35] The presence of SF has shown to be a robust predictor of CRT response (see **Fig. 5**).[36,37]

b. Apical rocking (AR): Short motion of the apex toward septum resulting from an early initial contraction of the interventricular septum and a subsequent lateral motion during the ejection because of the late contraction of the lateral wall; it generates a specific typical back-and-forth motion of the apex.[35]

c. Shorter filling and ejection time intervals, and longer isovolumetric time intervals because of

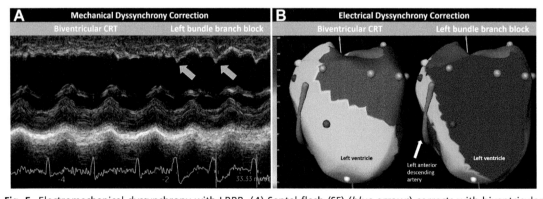

Fig. 5. Electromechanical dyssynchrony with LBBB. (*A*) Septal flash (SF) (*blue arrows*) corrects with biventricular CRT. (*Left*) Echocardiography in M-mode with CRT on shows no SF. (*Right*) In the same patient when CRT is off shows SF appearance. (*B*) Electrocardiographic imaging showing early activation in *red*, late activation in *blue*. *Right*, baseline activation with LBBB and late activation of the lateral left ventricle (in *blue*). *Left*, CRT normalizes the activation time and pattern (left ventricle in *red* and *green*).

delayed contraction of lateral wall causing late aortic valve opening.[2]

LV mechanical dyssynchrony pattern, characterized by AR and SF, is associated with a more favorable long-term survival after biventricular CRT. Both parameters are also indicators of an effective therapy. If corrected by CRT, visually assessed AR and SF were associated with reverse remodeling with a sensitivity of 84% and 79%, and specificity of 79% and 74%, respectively.[35]

CLINICAL SIGNIFICANCE OF LEFT BUNDLE BRANCH BLOCK
Prognosis

In the Framingham Study, newly acquired LBBB was most often a hallmark of advanced hypertensive or ischemic heart disease, or both.[1] Moreover, they found a significantly elevated risk of cardiovascular deaths (50% within 10 years of onset) among individuals with LBBB. Patients with LBBB have increased rates of cardiovascular mortality, sudden cardiac death, coronary artery disease, and heart failure.[2,38] It should be noted that patients without cardiovascular risk factors that develop LBBB at a younger age (<45 years) had better prognosis compared with those who developed LBBB during or after their fifth decade and had associated risk factors.[39]

Recent data published by Zegard and colleagues[40] showed that cardiac magnetic resonance could aid in risk-stratification of incidental LBBB; 57% of incidental LBBB had abnormal myocardial phenotype (LV ejection fraction [LVEF] <50%, dilation, hypertrophy, noncompactation, and/or fibrosis) with higher risk of total mortality and major cardiac events than patients with a normal myocardial phenotype and healthy control subjects (normal ECG and cardiac magnetic resonance). Moreover, in patients with incidental LBBB, myocardial fibrosis and LVEF less than 50% had additive effects on the risk of total mortality and total mortality/major adverse cardiac events.[40]

Left Ventricular Remodeling and Cardiomyopathy

LBBB induces loss of a large portion of septal contribution to LV function and results in substantial workload increase on the LV lateral wall.[36] This loss of septal work and increased workload on the lateral wall is a major stimulus to adverse LV remodeling. The dyssynchronous ventricular activation during LBBB leads to redistribution of circumferential shortening and myocardial blood flow and, in the long run, LV remodeling (decreasing LVEF and increasing LV volumes).[41]

LV remodeling by LBBB can be the primary cause of cardiomyopathy or contribute to worsen LV function in patients with subjacent cardiopathy. That is, conduction abnormalities may develop in patients with underlying cardiomyopathy caused by degeneration or fibrosis of the conduction system.[25] Patients with a mildly to moderately (36%–50%) reduced LVEF and LBBB have poor clinical outcomes that are significantly worse than those for patients without conduction system disease.[42]

Cardiac Resynchronization Therapy

CRT with biventricular pacing, or more recently with pacing via conduction system capture, has been shown to reverse the harmful effects of electromechanical dyssynchrony (see **Fig. 5**). It had been demonstrated that patients with LBBB benefit the most from biventricular CRT,[43] whereas no benefit or little benefit was observed in patients with a non-LBBB QRS pattern (RBBB or intraventricular conduction disturbances).[44] These consistent clinical findings highlight the need to subtype true LBBB pathophysiology from others. The mechanisms of the beneficial effect of CRT are complex and probably multifactorial. The correction of electrical dyssynchrony improves contractile function, which results in reversion of LV remodeling, alteration of sympathovagal balance, and induction of changes at the cellular level.

CRT results in a decrease in adverse remodeling and a decrease in mortality and hospitalization. However, it has been shown that the improvement is mainly observed in patients with LBBB pattern.[45] One of the continuing challenges in CRT is to decrease the proportion of nonresponders, usually reported to constitute approximately 30% of patients.[46] Inherent challenges with LV epicardial pacing via the venous system are anatomic limitations in the availability and course of coronary sinus branches, resulting in suboptimal lead location in about 2% to 5% of patients.[47] Notably, positions in the apex, middle cardiac vein, and anterior interventricular vein are associated with limited reverse remodeling. In this context His bundle pacing (HBP) and LBB area pacing (LBBAP) offer an alternative option as bailout strategies. Conduction via the His-Purkinje system pacing directly recruits the intrinsic specialized conduction system in contrast to biventricular CRT, which achieves nonphysiologic resynchronization with fusion of two (epicardial-LV and RV pacing) or three wavefronts with optimization with fusion optimized intervals.[48]

Episodic Left Bundle Branch Block

Episodic LBBB is transient or intermittent. Transient LBBB is an intraventricular conduction defect that subsequently returns to normal conduction. Intermittent LBBB refers to complexes showing LBBB and normally conducted beats in a single ECG tracing.[49] The most common cause of episodic LBBB is the change in heart rate (tachycardia or bradycardia).[50] Rate-dependent bundle branch block was described in 1963 as a form of phasic aberrant ventricular conduction in which there is inequality in the refractory periods of the bundle branches.[51] Bradycardia-related LBBB may be related to spontaneous diastolic depolarization of the LBB at slower heart rates, causing it to be refractory to the subsequently conducted impulse.[25]

Tachycardia-related LBBB occurs when the impulse arrives at the tissue that is still refractory. The prevalence of exercise-induced LBBB was 0.38%.[52] Individuals with exercise-induced LBBB have higher all-cause mortality when compared with those with normal exercise test results. However, exercise-associated LBBB patients are usually older and have more associated cardiovascular diseases.[52]

Apart from rate dependence, injury and ischemia are a cause of new-onset LBBB. Patients with a high clinical suspicion of ongoing myocardial ischemia and LBBB should be managed in a way similar to patients with ST-segment elevation myocardial infarction.[53] Electrocardiographic diagnosis of acute myocardial infarction is challenging in patients with LBBB. Specific ECG criteria (Sgarbossa criteria or Barcelona criteria[54]) may help in the detection of candidates for immediate coronary angiography. Other causes of episodic LBBB have been described, such as takotsubo cardiomyopathy, myocarditis, coronary fistulas, acute pulmonary embolism, drug-induced LBBB (propafenone, flecainide, trastuzumab, digitalis intoxication, phenothiazines or tricyclic antidepressants, chloroquine), Guillain-Barré syndrome, and pancreatitis.[50]

Left Bundle Branch Block Syndrome Associated with Pain or Dyspnea

Painful LBBB syndrome is a rare clinical entity characterized by chest pain attributed to LBBB in the absence of ischemia.[55] In these patients, a rate-related LBBB causes symptoms, such as chest pain or dyspnea,[56] which limits physical activity. The hypothesized mechanism is dyssynchrony and alteration of activation wavefront in the ventricles. Symptom spectrum ranges from self-limiting "walk-through" discomfort to severe debilitating pain.[55] CSP offers a new precise alternative to treat these patients who are conventionally treated with AV nodal blockers and right ventricular or biventricular pacemakers. Initial reports of LBBAP show promise to correct LBBB and relieve symptoms.[57]

The syndrome of painful LBBB should be considered after ruling out ischemia. Patients with clinical suspicion of ongoing myocardial ischemia and LBBB should be managed in a way similar to patients with ST-segment elevation myocardial infarction, regardless of whether the LBBB is previously known.[58] However, the presence of a (presumed) new LBBB does not always predict a myocardial infarction.[59] The Sgarbossa or Barcelona diagnostic algorithms can help in the diagnosis. The presence of concordant ST-segment elevation (ie, in leads with positive QRS deflections) seems to be one of the best indicators of ongoing infarction.[60]

Iatrogenic Left Bundle Branch Block after Aortic Valve or Septal Interventions

Aortic valve surgery or TAVR commonly traumatize the proximal conduction system because of their close anatomic relationship with the membranous septum at the junction of the non and right coronary cusps. The appearance of LBBB after TAVR reflects a proximal lesion of the LBB or within the left His fibers. New LBBB after TAVR incidence is approximately 25% (range, 5%–65%),[61] with most occurring intraprocedural or within 24 hours post-procedure. With newer generation valves, the incidence has decreased to 12% to 22%.[62] The incidence depends on clinical factors (preprocedural conduction abnormalities, prolonged QRS duration, female sex, previous coronary artery bypass graft, diabetes, and the amount of calcification of the aortic valve) and procedural characteristics (prosthesis implantation depth within the left ventricular outflow tract, self-expandable CoreValve).[62] Delayed high-degree AV block occurred in 8% patients with pre-existing LBBB, and 13% with new-onset LBBB.[63] Moreover, patients with new-onset persistent LBBB and a QRS duration greater than 160 milliseconds had a greater sudden cardiac death risk (hazard ratio, 4.78; $P = .006$).[64] In surgery, the incidence of LBBB following surgical aortic valve replacement is around 6.5%.[65] Surgical septal myectomy frequently leads to LBBB, up to 39%.[66]

CORRECTING LEFT BUNDLE BRANCH BLOCK WITH CONDUCTION SYSTEM PACING
Left Bundle Branch Pacing Versus His Bundle Pacing

The hypothesis for HBP to correct LBBB is that the pacing stimulus captures beyond an area of focal block and normalizes LBBB by direct recruitment

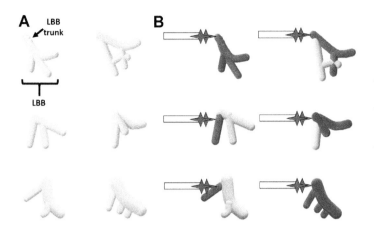

Fig. 6. Complex anatomy of the LBB. (*A*) Because of variability in the anatomy of the left bundle[13], pacing site depends on the interaction of factors, such as anatomy of the conduction system with its ramifications and divisions (showed in *B*), the depth of its location, and the thickness of the septum. Likelihood of pacing the branch, correcting LBBB, and the morphology of the paced QRS depends on all of this. (*B*) Lead simulating pacing the left branch; according to the arrangement and anatomy of the branch, the captured divisions and subdivisions are shown in *blue*.

of the LBB.[67] Previously this concept was attributed to the theory of longitudinal dissociation[68,69] and predestination of the Purkinje fibers within the His bundle, although prior work did study this with left-sided EPS. More recent investigation suggests that focal block may simply be present at the level of the anatomic left-sided His fibers.[26]

HBP has inherent limitations, which include challenging implant localization of the His bundle and deployment of the electrode in a small target zone. Higher thresholds above typical myocardial thresholds may result, which can lead to premature battery depletions. Furthermore, in about 10% to 30% of patients, LBBB may not be correctable by permanent HBP.[70] Left intrahisian block (46% of LBBB patterns) is the most likely to demonstrate QRS correction recruiting Purkinje fibers distal to the site of block. Importantly, it does not seem that patient with intact Purkinje activation (36%) are corrected with conduction system capture, because the delay is distal to the site of the pacing stimulus.[26]

LBBAP via deep intraseptal fixation was reported in 2017 as a novel pacing strategy to achieve CSP. The main advantages of LBBAP are: low and stable outputs,[71] a larger target zone for implant, and lower risk of block if progressive conduction system progresses. LBBAP can bypass conduction system pathology more distal to the left-sided His to produce physiologic activation.[15] Electrophysiologists should incorporate this intrinsic variability and fanlike arborization when performing pacing of the His-Purkinje conduction system (HBP or LBBAP). The ideal pacing site depends on the interaction between the anatomy of the conduction system (**Fig. 6**), the depth of the site of stimulation location, the thickness of the septum, and other factors. The His is a small target zone complicating the implant and having to be very precise. In addition, the location of the HBP lead may be closer to the aorta (**Fig. 7**). In contrast, the broad and arborized nature of the left bundle with fascicular ramifications provides a wider target area for permanent pacing.

LBBAP has been shown as an effective means to achieve physiologic pacing for patients for bradycardia and cardiac resynchronization for heart failure.[67,71,72] New implantation tools and

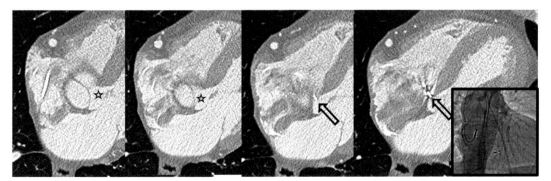

Fig. 7. His bundle pacing, close relationship of the tip of the lead with the aorta. The distance between the branching portion of the bundle of His from the aortic valve depends on the size of the membranous septum.[11] *Stars* point to the aorta; *white arrows* point to His bundle pacing lead.

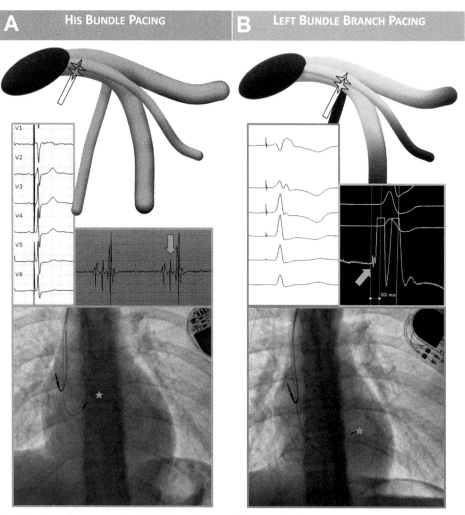

Fig. 8. Physiologic pacing strategies: HBP (*A*) and LBBAP (*B*). HBP obtains a very narrow QRS in the ECG with the lead in the upper septum (*orange star*) in the His area; electrogram shows (*orange arrow*) His signal. LBBAP obtains a right bundle branch block in the ECG; the lead is screwed more distal (*blue star*) than in the HBP position; electrogram shows (*blue arrow*) left bundle branch signal.

longer term data are necessary to define the role of HBP and LBBAP (**Fig. 8**).

SUMMARY

Although the anatomy of the LBB has marked variability between individuals, the penetrating His bundle and proximal left bundle and fascicular ramifications have emerged as targets for CSP to achieve physiologic conduction system capture. LBB block patterns on ECG may result from a spectrum of conduction disorders ranging from intraventricular conduction delay, complete or "true" conduction block, and combinations of the two. LBBB implies electrical and mechanical ventricular dyssynchrony leading to left ventricular remodeling that may be successfully treated with biventricular resynchronization therapy or CSP. Detailed activation mapping of the basal left septum has revealed that the site of block is most commonly localized within the left His fibers, rather than in the left bundle itself. HBP can circumvent proximal conduction disease and block when the stimulus strength is sufficient to capture tissue distal to the site block. LBBAP is a promising novel intraseptal fixation technique that can capture the arborized portion of the left conduction system and preserve or restore physiologic activation of the LV with lower and more durable thresholds. Improved correlation between intracardiac activation patterns and 12-lead ECG is necessary for clinical trials, which should tailor pacing modalities toward the pathophysiology that underlies individual conduction disorders.

CLINICS CARE POINTS

- LBBB has prognostic implications with regard to heart failure and mortality.
- LBBB implies electrical and mechanical ventricular dyssynchrony that may be treated with biventricular resynchronization therapy or conduction system pacing in patients with left ventricular dysfunction.
- Left ventricular remodeling caused by LBBB may be the primary cause of cardiomyopathy or contribute to worsen ventricular function in patients with underlying cardiomyopathy or coronary artery disease.
- Patients with high clinical suspicion of ongoing myocardial ischemia and LBBB should be managed in a way similar to ST-segment elevation myocardial infarction. Painful LBBB syndrome should be considered after ruling out ischemia.
- LBBAP is a promising novel intraseptal fixation technique that can capture the arborized portion of the left conduction system and preserve or restore physiologic activation of the left ventricle.

DISCLOSURE

M. Pujol-López is funded by the research grant Josep Font 2019, Hospital Clínic de Barcelona and Grant of the Catalan Society of Cardiology 2019 and 2020. J.M. Tolosana has received honoraria as a lecturer and consultant for Abbott, Boston Scientific, and Medtronic. G.A. Upadhyay has received honoraria as lecturer and consultant for Abbott, Biotronik, Medtronic, and Zoll Medical. L. Mont has received unrestricted research grants, fellowship program support, and honoraria as a lecturer and consultant from Abbott, Biotronik, Boston Scientific, LivaNova, and Medtronic. R. Tung has received speaking honorarium from Medtronic, Boston Scientific, Biotronik, and Abbott.

REFERENCES

1. Schneider JF, Thomas HE Jr, Kreger BE, et al. Newly acquired left bundle-branch block: the Framingham study. Ann Intern Med 1979;90(3):303–10.
2. Surkova E, Badano LP, Bellu R, et al. Left bundle branch block: from cardiac mechanics to clinical and diagnostic challenges. Europace 2017;19(8):1251–71.
3. Eriksson P, Hansson PO, Eriksson H, et al. Bundle-branch block in a general male population: the study of men born 1913. Circulation 1998;98(22):2494–500.
4. T Hardarson T, Arnason A, Elíasson GJ, et al. Left bundle branch block: prevalence, incidence, follow-up and outcome. Eur Heart J 1987;8(10):1075–9.
5. Imanishi R, Seto S, Ichimaru S, et al. Prognostic significance of incident complete left bundle branch block observed over a 40-year period. Am J Cardiol 2006;98(5):644–8.
6. Pérez-Riera AR, Barbosa-Barros R, de Rezende Barbosa MPC, et al. Left bundle branch block: epidemiology, etiology, anatomic features, electrovectorcardiography, and classification proposal. Ann Noninvasive Electrocardiol 2019;24(2):e12572.
7. Kumar V, Venkataraman R, Aljaroudi W, et al. Implications of left bundle branch block in patient treatment. Am J Cardiol 2013;111(2):291–300.
8. Ladenvall P, Andersson B, Dellborg M, et al. Genetic variation at the human connexin 43 locus but not at the connexin 40 locus is associated with left bundle branch block. Open Heart 2015;2(1):e000187.
9. Tawara S. Das Reizleitungssystem des Säugetierherzens (the conduction system of the mammalian heart). Jena: Gustav Fischer; 1906. 135–8 [149].
10. Lev M. Anatomic basis for atrioventricular block. Am J Med 1964;37:742–8.
11. Elizari MV. The normal variants in the left bundle branch system. J Electrocardiol 2017;50(4):389–99.
12. Frink RJ, James TN TN. Normal blood supply to the human His bundle and proximal bundle branches. Circulation 1973;47(1):8–18.
13. Demoulin JC, Kulbertus HE. Histopathological examination of concept of left hemiblock. Br Heart J 1972;34(8):807–14.
14. Durrer D, van Dam RT, Freud GE, et al. Total excitation of the isolated human heart. Circulation 1970; 41(6):899–912.
15. Cabrera JA, Porta-Sánchez A, Tung R, et al. Tracking down the anatomy of the left bundle branch to optimize left bundle branch pacing. J Am Coll Cardiol Case Rep 2020;2(5):750–5.
16. Fisher JD. Hemiblocks and the fascicular system: myths and implications. J Interv Card Electrophysiol 2018;52(3):281–5.
17. Kulbertus HE. The hemiblocks: a decade of study. Boehringer- Ingelheim Monogr 1979;1–69:11.
18. Eppinger H. Zur Analyse des Elektrokardiogramms. Wien Klin Wochenschr 1909;22:1091–8.
19. Barker PS, Macleod AG, Alexander J. The excitatory process observed in the exposed human heart. Am Heart J 1930;5:720–42.
20. Bayés de Luna A. Clinical electrocardiography: a textbook. 2nd edition. Armonk (NY): Futura Publishing Company Inc; 1998.
21. Strauss DG, Selvester RH, Wagner GS. Defining left bundle branch block in the era of cardiac resynchronization therapy. Am J Cardiol 2011;107(6):927–34.
22. Kusumoto FM, Schoenfeld MH, Barrett C, et al. 2018 ACC/AHA/HRS guideline on the evaluation and

management of patients with bradycardia and cardiac conduction delay: executive summary: a report of the American College of Cardiology/American Heart Association Task Force on Clinical Practice Guidelines, and the Heart Rhythm Society. J Am Coll Cardiol 2019;74(7):932–87.

23. Elizari MV, Acunzo RS, Ferreiro M. Hemiblocks revisited. Circulation 2007;115(9):1154–63.

24. Risum N, Tayal B, Hansen TF, et al. Identification of typical left bundle branch block contraction by strain echocardiography is additive to electrocardiography in prediction of long-term outcome after cardiac resynchronization therapy. J Am Coll Cardiol 2015;66(6):631–41.

25. Tan NY, Witt CM, Oh JK, et al. Left bundle branch block: current and future perspectives. Circ Arrhythm Electrophysiol 2020;13(4):e008239.

26. Upadhyay G, Cherian T, Shatz DY, et al. Intracardiac delineation of septal conduction in left bundle-branch block patterns. Circulation 2019;139(16):1876–88.

27. Tung R, Upadhyay G. Defining left bundle branch block patterns in cardiac resynchronization therapy: a return to His bundle recordings. Arrhythmia Electrophysiol Rev 2020;9(1):28–33.

28. Sugrue A, Bhatia S, Vaidya VR, et al. His bundle (conduction system) pacing: a contemporary appraisal. Card Electrophysiol Clin 2018;10(3):461–82.

29. Wiggers C. The muscular reactions of the mammalian ventricles to artificial surface stimuli. Am J Physiol 1925;73:346–78.

30. Auricchio A, Fantoni C, Regoli F, et al. Characterization of left ventricular activation in patients with heart failure and left bundle-branch block. Circulation 2004;109(9):1133–9.

31. Oh JK, Kane GC, Tajik AJ. The echo manual. Philadelphia: Wolters Kluwer; 2018.

32. Dillon JC, Chang S, Feigenbaum H. Echocardiographic manifestations of left bundle branch block. Circulation 1974;49(5):876–80.

33. Parsai C, Bijnens B, Sutherland GR, et al. Toward understanding response to cardiac resynchronization therapy. Eur Heart J 2009;30(8):940–9.

34. Ben Corteville B, De Pooter J, De Backer T, et al. The electrocardiographic characteristics of septal flash in patients with left bundle branch block. Europace 2017;19(1):103–9.

35. Stankovic I, Prinz C, Ciarka A, et al. Relationship of visually assessed apical rocking and septal flash to response and long-term survival following cardiac resynchronization therapy (PREDICT-CRT). Eur Heart J Cardiovasc Imaging 2016;17(3):262–9.

36. Calle S, Delens C, Kamoen V, et al. Septal flash: at the heart of cardiac dyssynchrony. Trends Cardiovasc Med 2020;30(2):115–22.

37. Doltra A, Bijnens B, Tolosana JM, et al. Mechanical abnormalities detected with conventional echocardiography are associated with response and midterm survival in CRT. JACC Cardiovasc Imaging 2014; 7(10):969–79.

38. Fahy GJ, Pinski SL, Miller DP, et al. Natural history of isolated bundle branch block. Am J Cardiol 1996; 77(14):1185–90.

39. Rabkin SW, Mathewson FA, Tate RB. Natural history of left bundle-branch block. Br Heart J 1980;43(2): 164–9.

40. Zegard A, Okafor O, de Bono J, et al. Prognosis of incidental left bundle branch block. Europace 2020;22(6):956–63.

41. Vernooy K, Verbeek X, Peschar M, et al. Left bundle branch block induces ventricular remodelling and functional septal hypoperfusion. Eur Heart J 2005; 26(1):91–8.

42. Witt CM, Wu G, Yang D, et al. Outcomes with left bundle branch block and mildly to moderately reduced left ventricular function. JACC Heart Fail 2016;4(11):897–903.

43. Zareba W, Klein H, Cygankiewicz I, et al. Effectiveness of cardiac resynchronization therapy by QRS morphology in the Multicenter automatic Defibrillator Implantation Trial-Cardiac Resynchronization Therapy (MADIT-CRT). Circulation 2011;123(10): 1061–72.

44. Cunnington C, Kwok CS, Satchithananda DK, et al. Cardiac resynchronisation therapy is not associated with a reduction in mortality or heart failure hospitalisation in patients with non-left bundle branch block QRS morphology: meta-analysis of randomised controlled trials. Heart 2015;101(18):1456–62.

45. Jastrzebski M, Baranchuk A, Fijorek K, et al. Cardiac resynchronization therapy-induced acute shortening of QRS duration predicts long-term mortality only in patients with left bundle branch block. Europace 2019;21(2):281–9.

46. Yu CM, Hayes DL. Cardiac resynchronization therapy: state of the art 2013. Eur Heart J 2013;34: 1396–403.

47. Gamble JHP, Herring N, Ginks M, et al. Procedural success of left ventricular lead placement for cardiac resynchronization therapy: a meta-analysis. JACC Clin Electrophysiol 2016;2(1):69–77.

48. Arbelo E, Tolosana JM, Trucco E, et al. Fusion-optimized intervals (FOI): a new method to achieve the narrowest QRS for optimization of the AV and VV intervals in patients undergoing cardiac resynchronization therapy. J Cardiovasc Electrophysiol 2014; 25:283–92.

49. Bauer GE. Transient bundle-branch block. Circulation 1964;29:730–8.

50. Bazoukis G, Tsimos K, Korantzopoulos P. Episodic left bundle branch block: a comprehensive review of the literature. Ann Noninvasive Electrocardiol 2016;21(2):117–25.

51. Schamroth L, Chesler E. Phasic aberrant ventricular conduction. Br Heart J 1963;25(2):219–26.

52. Stein R, Ho M, Machado Oliveira C, et al. Exercise-induced left bundle branch block: prevalence and prognosis. Arq Bras Cardiol 2011;97(1):26–32.

53. Collet JP, Thiele H, Barbato E, et al. 2020 ESC guidelines for the management of acute coronary syndromes in patients presenting without persistent ST-segment elevation. Eur Heart J 2021;42(14): 1289–367.

54. Di Marco A, Rodriguez M, Cinca J, et al. New electrocardiographic algorithm for the diagnosis of acute myocardial infarction in patients with left bundle branch block. J Am Heart Assoc 2020;9(14): e015573.

55. Shvilkin A, Ellis ER, Gervino EV, et al. Painful left bundle branch block syndrome: clinical and electrocardiographic features and further directions for evaluation and treatment. Heart Rhythm 2016; 13(1):226–32.

56. Prystowsky E, Padanilam BJ. Cardiac resynchronization therapy reverses severe dyspnea associated with acceleration-dependent left bundle branch block in a patient with structurally normal heart. J Cardiovasc Electrophysiol 2019;30(4):517–9.

57. Garg A, Master V, Ellenbogen KA, et al. Painful left bundle branch block syndrome successfully treated with left bundle branch area pacing. J Am Coll Cardiol Case Rep 2020;2(4):568–71.

58. Ibañez B, James S, Agewall S, et al. 2017 ESC guidelines for the management of acute myocardial infarction in patients presenting with ST-segment elevation. Eur Heart J 2018;39(2):119–77.

59. Chang AM, Shofer FS, Tabas JA, et al. Lack of association between left bundle-branch block and acute myocardial infarction in symptomatic ED patients. Am J Emerg Med 2009;27(8):916–21.

60. Lopes RD, Siha H, Fu Y, et al. Diagnosing acute myocardial infarction in patients with left bundle branch block. Am J Cardiol 2011;108(6):782–8.

61. Massoullié G, Bordachar P, Ellenbogen KA, et al. New-onset left bundle branch block induced by transcutaneous aortic valve implantation. Am J Cardiol 2016;117(5):867–73.

62. Auffret V, Puri R, Urena M, et al. Conduction disturbances after transcatheter aortic valve replacement: current status and future perspectives. Circulation 2017;136(11):1049–69.

63. Toggweiler S, Stortecky S, Holy E, et al. The electrocardiogram after transcatheter aortic valve replacement determines the risk for post-procedural high-degree AV block and the need for telemetry monitoring. JACC Cardiovasc Interv 2016;9(12): 1269–76.

64. Urena M, Webb JG, Eltchaninoff E, et al. Late cardiac death in patients undergoing transcatheter aortic valve replacement: incidence and predictors of advanced heart failure and sudden cardiac death. J Am Coll Cardiol 2015;65(5):437–48.

65. El-Khally Z, Thibault B, Staniloae C, et al. Prognostic significance of newly acquired bundle branch block after aortic valve replacement. Am J Cardiol 2004; 94(8):1008–11.

66. Cui H, Schaff HV, Nishimura RA, et al. Conduction abnormalities and long-term mortality following septal myectomy in patients with obstructive hypertrophic cardiomyopathy. J Am Coll Cardiol 2019; 74(5):645–55.

67. Zhang S, Zhou X, Gold MR. Left bundle branch pacing: JACC review topic of the week. J Am Coll Cardiol 2019;74(24):3039–49.

68. Narula OS. Longitudinal dissociation in the His bundle. Bundle branch block due to asynchronous conduction within the His bundle in man. Circulation 1977;56:996–1006.

69. Kaufmann R, Rothberger CJ. Beiträge zur entstehungsweise extrasystolischer allorhythmien. Z für die Gesamte Experimentelle Medizin 1919;9: 104–22.

70. Vijayaraman P, Chung MK, Dandamudi G, et al. His bundle pacing. J Am Coll Cardiol 2018;72(8): 927–47.

71. Huang W, Su L, Wu S, et al. A novel pacing strategy with low and stable output: pacing the left bundle branch immediately beyond the conduction block. Can J Cardiol 2017;33(12):1736.e1-3.

72. Huang W, Wu S, Vijayaraman, et al. Cardiac resynchronization therapy in patients with non-ischemic cardiomyopathy utilizing left bundle branch pacing. JACC Clin Electrophysiol 2020;6(7):849–58.

Bilateral Bundle Branch Block

Jasen L. Gilge, MD*, Benzy J. Padanilam, MD

KEYWORDS

- Bilateral bundle branch block • Left bundle branch block • Right bundle branch block
- Bundle branch block • Conduction system disorder

KEY POINTS

- Bilateral bundle branch block (BBBB) is an uncommon and underrecognized conduction abnormality.
- Electrocardiographic manifestation of BBB includes a right bundle branch block pattern in lead V1 (terminal R wave) and left bundle branch block pattern in leads I and aVL (absence of S wave).
- The presence of BBBB, although rare, may confer an increased risk of cardiovascular morbidity and mortality.
- Patients with BBBB may be a new subset of patients that could have a favorable response to cardiac resynchronization therapy.

INTRODUCTION

When electrocardiographic patterns of right bundle branch block (RBBB) and left bundle branch block (LBBB) occur alternatively, intermittently, or simultaneously in the same patient, a diagnosis of bilateral bundle branch block (BBBB) is considered.[1] Conduction system disease simultaneously affecting the left and right bundle branches may manifest a specific electrocardiogram (ECG) with an RBBB pattern of terminal R wave in lead V1 and an LBBB pattern in lead I and aVL showing no S wave (**Figs. 1 and 2**). This pattern was described as LBBB masquerading as RBBB in the 1950s.[2] Histologic studies of patients with BBBB have demonstrated extensive disease in both bundle branches, and electrophysiologic studies have suggested conduction block or delay in both bundle branches.[3–5] Although the pattern was originally described in the 1950s, renewed interest has been generated recently because of its adverse clinical prognosis and significance in cardiac resynchronization pacing.

DEFINITION AND PREVALENCE

Patients that exhibit the characteristic pattern of BBBB on ECG do not meet classical definitions for either LBBB or RBBB. According to current guidelines, they may be categorized as an intraventricular conduction delay (IVCD).[6] Although the professional society guidelines discourage use of terms like BBBB, it is only because of the paucity of clear anatomic and pathophysiologic basis for it.[6] An ECG pattern of complete RBBB (rSR or R) in lead V1 with an apparent LBBB pattern in lead I and aVL showing no S wave defines BBBB. However, in practice, physicians may label any wide QRS with a terminal R in V1 as RBBB, and 1 study estimated that 1.5% of ECGs described as having an RBBB actually had evidence of BBBB that was not recognized.[7] BBBB is thus underrecognized, and the true prevalence is uncertain. When evaluating the general population, IVCD, defined as QRS $\geq$ 110 milliseconds and not meeting LBBB or RBBB definitions, has been described to affect up to 0.6% of the population.[8] Although there is

This article originally appeared in *Cardiac Electrophysiology Clinics*, Volume 13 Issue 4, December 2021.

St Vincent Hospital, 8333 Naab Road, Suite 400, Indianapolis, IN 46260, USA

* Corresponding author.

E-mail address: Jasen.gilge@ascension.org

Cardiol Clin 41 (2023) 393–397

https://doi.org/10.1016/j.ccl.2023.03.011

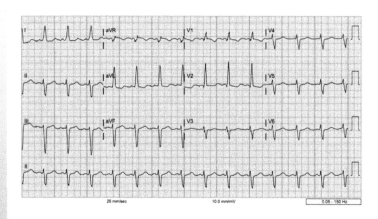

Fig. 1. BBBB ECG. Twelve-lead ECG showing BBBB. Features include QRS duration ≥ 120 milliseconds, a terminal R in lead V1 (RBBB pattern), and no S waves in lead I or aVL (LBBB pattern).

a paucity of data evaluating BBBB specifically, 1 study described the prevalence to be less than 0.01% of the general population.[9] Pastore and colleagues[10] evaluated 192 consecutive patients undergoing cardiac resynchronization therapy (CRT) and found that 7.8% of patients in this population had BBBB pattern on ECGs. Further population studies are needed to describe the true prevalence of BBBB.

PATHOPHYSIOLOGY

In 1954, Richman and Wolff[2] introduced the concept of masquerading bundle branch block where there is ECG evidence of RBBB in the precordial leads simultaneously with LBBB in the limb leads. Vectorcardiography in these patients revealed the initial vector was identical to that of an LBBB, but the remainder drastically differed. They further postulated that extensive septal and inferolateral left ventricular infarction drastically reduced posteriorly directed forces allowing the anteriorly directed forces of the right ventricle to produce an R′ in lead V1 while maintaining the typical LBBB appearance in lead I. Thus, they believed this ECG finding was truly an LBBB, which, as a result of myocardial infarction, was masquerading as an RBBB. However, subsequent histologic studies in patients with "masquerading bundle branch block" revealed extensive septal fibrosis with near complete destruction of the right bundle branch and to a lesser extent in the left bundle branch.[3,4] These histologic studies provided substantiation that the ECG manifestation is truly representative of disease of bilateral bundles and not myocardial infarction related. Furthermore, BBBB may occur in structurally normal hearts.[4] In 1955, Rosenbaum and Lepeschkin[1] reported a case series of alternating bundle branch block where patients exhibited ECGs with RBBB and, at other times, LBBB. They postulated that partial and intermittent interruption in both bundle branches produced alternating RBBB and LBBB in the same patient at varying times. This concept was later verified during electrophysiology studies of 7 patients by Wu and colleagues[11] in 1976 revealing an incomplete block in 1 bundle and intermittent block in the contralateral bundle.

RBBB

LBBB

BBBB

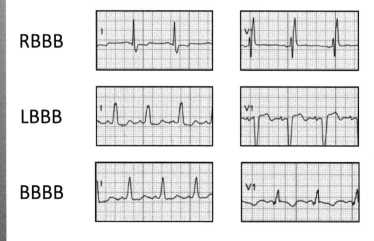

Fig. 2. Comparison of bundle branch blocks. Each of the 3 different forms of bundle branch block are depicted in leads I and V1. Note that BBBB meets ECG criteria for an RBBB in lead V1 while simultaneously satisfying criteria for an LBBB in lead I.

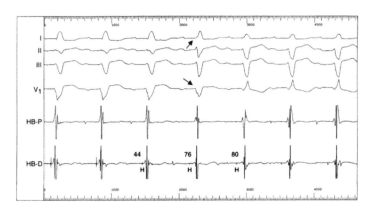

Fig. 3. Catheter-induced RBBB in a patient with underlying LBBB. Simultaneous His bundle tracing with limited surface ECG lead recordings was obtained at the time of accidental catheter-induced RBBB block. The first 4 beats exhibit an LBBB. Then, with catheter trauma to the right bundle branch, there is development of RBBB pattern in lead V1 and an LBBB pattern in lead I. Delay of conduction in both bundles results in prolongation of HV interval. (*arrows*) Timing of catheter-induced trauma. H, His bundle; HB-D, His bundle distal; HB-P, His bundle proximal. (*From* Padanilam BJ, Morris KE, Olson JA, et al. The surface electrocardiogram predicts risk of heart block during right heart catheterization in patients with preexisting left bundle branch block: implications for the definition of complete left bundle branch block. J Cardiovasc Electrophysiol. 2010;21(7):781 to 785. doi:10.1111/j.1540 to 8167.2009.01714.x; with permission)

Direct electrophysiologic evidence for the mechanism behind BBBB comes from studies with catheter-induced RBBB. Padanilam and colleagues[12] reported that patients with an ECG pattern of LBBB may develop transient complete heart block or RBBB in response to catheter trauma to the right bundle branch during right heart catheterization (**Fig. 3**). In that series of 27 patients, 9 developed RBBB on top of LBBB, suggesting BBBB. In a subsequent study of 50 patients by the same group, patterns of catheter-induced RBBB were evaluated in patients with normal, left fascicular blocks or LBBB at baseline.[7] Among the LBBB population, 7 out of 11 developed the BBBB pattern with catheter-induced RBBB. The remainder of the LBBB patients, and all patients with baseline normal or left fascicular block, developed a typical RBBB

(**Fig. 4**), providing evidence that BBBB pattern is specific to BBBB.[7] The terminal S wave in lateral leads represents the delayed RV depolarization in reference to LV depolarization in typical RBBB. When both right and left bundle branch conduction are delayed with left more than or equal to right, the terminal S wave in lateral leads may be absent.

Three-dimensional electroanatomic mapping of both ventricles during sinus rhythm has provided additional insight into the ventricular activation sequence in patients with conduction disease. In the setting of an LBBB, the apical anterolateral right ventricle is the earliest site to be activated with delayed transseptal conduction to the left ventricle with the lateral mitral annulus being the latest site of activation.[13,14] In RBBB, the left ventricular septum is the earliest site of ventricular

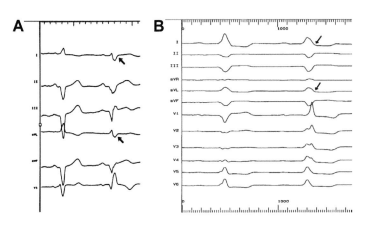

Fig. 4. Patterns of catheter-induced RBBB. (*A*) The baseline ECG exhibits features of a left anterior fascicular block. Following the first beat, catheter trauma to the right bundle branch results in an ECG typical for RBBB with a prominent S wave in lead I and aVL as depicted by the arrows. (*B*) The baseline ECG exhibits features of an LBBB. Following the first beat, catheter trauma to the right bundle results in ECG features typical of BBBB with terminal R wave in V1 and no S wave in lead I or aVL as depicted by the arrows. (*From* Tzogias L, Steinberg LA, Williams AJ, et al. Electrocardiographic features and prevalence of bilateral bundle-branch delay. Circ Arrhythm Electrophysiol. 2014;7(4):640 to 644. doi:10.1161/CIRCEP.113.000999;with permission)

activation with delayed transseptal conduction to the right ventricle with the outflow tract being the latest site of activation. In patients with BBBB, the first site of activation is the left ventricular septum with slow transeptal conduction to the right ventricle, similar to RBBB, but the conduction velocity to the lateral left ventricle is also dramatically delayed, as depicted in **Fig. 5**.[5,15]

CLINICAL IMPLICATIONS AND FUTURE PERSPECTIVES

Chronic bundle branch block of a single bundle typically does not progress to complete heart block.[16,17] However, the unique ECG manifestation of BBBB may have increased adverse outcomes. Tzogias and colleagues[7] reported that 8 out of 34 patients (24%) in their cohort required permanent pacemaker implantation (PPM) or implantable cardioverter-defibrillator (ICD) implantation. Thirty-eight percent of these patients also had an ejection fraction less than 40%. Another report cited 80% of patients with a BBBB had met a combined end point of death or PPM implantation during a 48-month follow-up period. Of the 80%, 41% died, whereas 39% required a PPM.[9] Although larger studies are needed to confirm the poor outcomes associated with BBBB, it is important to recognize the pattern and not group it under an IVCD diagnosis.

BBBB ECG is often read as RBBB in clinical practice, and such patients may not be considered for cardiac resynchronization.[7] The understanding of the underlying pathophysiology in BBBB with delayed LV activation similar to that in patients with LBBB pattern could help decisions regarding CRT. When measuring the extent of delayed left ventricular activation (Q-LV), BBBB patterns had similarly delayed Q-LV when compared with those with LBBB.[10] Based on studies showing prolonged Q-LV as an independent predictor of CRT response, BBBB patients may respond to CRT pacing better than patients with RBBB pattern.[18,19] Further studies of BBBB could help to further clarify the specificity of this ECG pattern, prognosis, and response to CRT.

CLINICS CARE POINTS

- The presence of alternating bundle branch blocks is a harbinger of severe conduction disease.
- When patients present with syncope and right bundle branch block, carefully inspect lead I for evidence of bilateral bundle branch block.
- When implanting a cardiac implantable electronic device in patients with bilateral bundle branch block and systolic congestive heart failure, consider cardiac resynchronization therapy.

DISCLOSURES

The authors of this article have no conflicts of interest or financial disclosures.

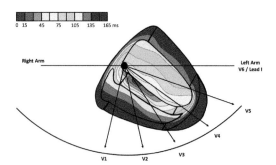

Fig. 5. Three-dimensional activation of the right and left ventricle in BBBB. Isochrones are represented here based on electroanatomic mapping data of both ventricles by Fantoni and colleagues.[5] The left ventricular septum is the first site of endocardial activation followed by delayed transseptal and left ventricular activation. The last sites of activation are the basal right ventricular and left ventricular free walls. The posterior-to-anterior activation produces the terminal R wave in lead V1 (RBBB pattern), whereas the right-to-left activation produces the dominant R wave and absence of S wave in leads I and aVL (LBBB pattern).

REFERENCES

1. Rosenbaum MD, Lepeschkin E. Bilateral bundle branch block. Am Heart J 1955;50:38–61.
2. Richman JL, Wolff L. Left bundle branch block masquerading as right bundle branch block. Am Heart J 1954;47:383–93.
3. Unger PN, Lesser ME, Kugel VH, et al. The concept of "masquerading" bundle-branch block and electrocardiographic-pathologic correlation. Circulation 1958;17:397–409.
4. Lenegre J. Etiology and pathology of bilateral bundle branch block in relation to complete heart block. Prog Cardiovasc Dis 1964;6:409–44.
5. Fantoni C, Kawabata M, Massaro R, et al. Right and left ventricular activation sequence in patients with heart failure and right bundle branch block: a detailed analysis using three-dimensional non-

fluoroscopic electroanatomic mapping system. J Cardiovasc Electrophysiol 2005;16:112–9.

6. Surawicz B, Childers R, Deal BJ, et al. AHA/ACCF/HRS recommendations for the standardization and interpretation of the electrogram. Part III: intraventricular conduction disturbances: a scientific statement from the American Heart Association Electrocardiography and Arrhythmias Committee, Council on Clinical Cardiology, the American College of Cardiology Foundation; and the Heart Rhythm Society: endorsed by the International Society for Computerized Electrocardiography2009. Circulation 2009;119:e235–40.

7. Tzogias L, Steinberg LA, Williams AJ, et al. Electrocardiographic features and prevalence of bilateral bundle-branch delay. Circ Arrhythm Electrophysiol 2014;7:640–4.

8. Aro AL, Anttonen O, Tikkanen JT, et al. Intraventricular conduction delay in a standard 12-lead electrocardiogram as a predictor of mortality in the general population. Circ Arrhythm Electrophysiol 2011;4:704–10.

9. Souza TG, Almeida RL, Targueta GP, et al. Abstract 14845: masquerading bundle branch block: an electrocardiographic marker of poor prognosis. Circulation 2015;132:A14845.

10. Pastore G, Maines M, Marcantoni L, et al. ECG parameters predict left ventricular conduction delay in patients with left ventricular dysfunction. Heart Rhythm 2016;13:2289–96.

11. Wu D, Denes P, Dhingra RC, et al. Electrophysiological and clinical observations in patients with alternating bundle branch block. Circulation 1976;53:456–64.

12. Padanilam BJ, Morris KE, Olson JA, et al. The surface electrocardiogram predicts risk of heart block during right heart catheterization in patients with preexisting left bundle branch block: implications for the definition of complete left bundle branch block. J Cardiovasc Electrophysiol 2010;21:781–5.

13. Rodriguez LM, Timmermans C, Nabar A, et al. Variable patterns of septal activation in patients with left bundle branch block and heart failure. J Cardiovasc Electrophysiol 2003;14:135–41.

14. Wyndam CR, Smith T, Meeran MK, et al. Epicardial activation in patients with left bundle branch block. Circulation 1980;61:696–703.

15. Xiao HB, Roy C, Gibson DG. Nature of ventricular activation in patients with dilated cardiomyopathy: evidence for bilateral bundle branch block. Br Heart J 1994;72:167–74.

16. McAnulty JH, Kauffman S, Murphy E, et al. Survival in patients with intraventricular conduction defects. Arch Intern Med 1978;138:30–5.

17. McAnulty JH, Rahimtoola SH. Chronic bundle-branch block clinical significance and management. J Am Med Assoc 1981;246:2202–4.

18. Singh JP, Fan D, Heist EK, et al. Left ventricular lead electrical delay predicts response to cardiac resynchronization therapy. Heart Rhythm 2006;3:128501292.

19. Zanon F, Baracca E, Pastore G, et al. Determination of the longest intrapatient left ventricular electrical delay may predict acute hemodynamic improvement in patients after cardia resynchronization therapy. Circ Arrhythm Electrophysiol 2014;7:377–83.

Congenital Heart Block

Leonard Steinberg, MD, BS[1]

KEYWORDS

- Heart block • Atrioventricular block • Congenital heart block • Structural heart disease
- Pacemaker • Cardiomyopathy • Prevention • Treatment

KEY POINTS

- The term congenital complete block (CCHB) defines conduction abnormalities diagnosed prenatally or in the 1st 27 days of life.
- The majority of CCHB occurs due to maternal autoimmune disorders or congenital structural heart disease.
- The diagnosis of CCHB imparts a high risk of fetal demise and perinatal mortality.
- Patients with CCHB are at risk for a progressively slowing junctional or ventricular escape rate, symptomatic bradycardia, left ventricular enlargement, cardiomyopathy, and sudden death.
- CCHB patients with symptomatic bradycardia or hemodynamic derangements should undergo placement of a permanent pacemaker.

One hundred twenty years have elapsed since Morquio[1] first reported heart block in several members of the same family. Since that time, congenital heart block has been reported and studied with increasing frequency. Still, owing to the rarity of this condition, there are few controlled trials and much not understood. Herein, relevant clinical information is provided on congenital complete heart block, including the different causes and mechanisms of disease; natural history and prognosis; and evaluation, treatment, and future directions.

The term congenital complete heart block (CCHB) has been used differently over time, introducing ambiguity into the literature. This term is often used synonymously with the terms isolated heart block (CCHB$_{ISO}$) or autoimmune heart block (CCHB$_{AI}$), but these 2 terms refer to smaller overlapping subsets. CCHB is now widely accepted to describe atrioventricular block (AVB) diagnosed in utero or in the first 27 days of life.[2] Patients presenting later in life tend to have a different array of clinical conditions underlying their AVB and a different prognosis.[3] CCHB$_{AI}$ refers specifically to the subset of CCHB with conduction abnormalities resulting from passive transfer of maternal antibodies. CCHB$_{ISO}$ refers to heart block in the absence of nontrivial structural abnormalities. Most of these patients have CCHB$_{AI}$.

Overwhelmingly, patients with CCHB present with complete AVB, which, with rare exceptions, is irreversible.[4,5] Patients presenting with PR prolongation and second-degree AVB also fit into the spectrum of congenital heart block.

MECHANISMS OF CONGENITAL HEART BLOCK

Patients with congenital heart block fall predominantly into 2 groups: those with CCHB$_{AI}$ and those with AVB secondary to congenital structural heart disease (CCHB$_{SHD}$). A small number of patients have purely genetic causes or no clear cause.

Autoimmune Congenital Heart Block

CCHB$_{AI}$ accounts for more than half of CCHB cases.[6] This condition—part of the spectrum of neonatal lupus—results from passive flow of maternal anti-Ro/SSA and anti-La/SSB autoantibodies across the placenta to the fetal circulation.

This article originally appeared in *Cardiac Electrophysiology Clinics*, Volume 13 Issue 4, December 2021.
Pediatric Cardiology, Children's Heart Center, Ascension St. Vincent, 8333 Naab Rd, Ste 320, Indianapolis, IN 46260, USA
[1] Present address: 10090 Hickory Ridge Drive, Zionsville, 46077.
E-mail address: lastein1@ascension.org

Cardiol Clin 41 (2023) 399–410
https://doi.org/10.1016/j.ccl.2023.03.002
0733-8651/23/© 2023 Elsevier Inc. All rights reserved.

cardiology.theclinics.com

These autoantibodies are the result of maternal autoimmune disease, although less than one-third of mothers with anti-Ro antibodies have a clinical diagnosis of an autoimmune disorder at the time of their pregnancy.[7] Conditions include Sjögren syndrome, lupus, and undifferentiated autoimmune syndrome. Population studies suggest the anti-Ro autoantibody occurs in 0.26% to 0.8% of women.[8,9] When no prior pregnancies have been affected, heart block occurs in only 2% to 5% of antibody-positive woman.[10] Only at the lower range of these estimates (0.26% incidence of anti-Ro and 2% risk of $CCHB_{AI}$) can one account for the reported incidence of $CCHB_{AI}$—approximately 1 in 25,000 infants.

There is mechanistic evidence for heart block with both the anti-Ro and anti-La autoantibodies,[11,12] but of the 2, the anti-Ro autoantibody is considered to be the more important.[13] There are 2 Ro antigens, a 52-kDa protein and a 60-kDa protein. The 60-kDa protein is easier to detect by immune assay, whereas the 52-kDa protein is more closely associated with the development of fetal heart block.[14]

Injury to the atrioventricular node likely occurs from 1 of 2 mechanisms. One postulate is that typically intracellular Ro antigens are found on the cell membrane and available to the circulating autoantibodies, thus triggering the inflammatory response.[15,16] Alternatively, autoantibodies may directly bind to L-type calcium channels.[17] These hypotheses are not mutually exclusive.[14] The resulting inflammatory cascade leads to apoptosis, fibrosis, and calcification.[16,18] Injury to the ventricular myocardium can occur as well, resulting in endocardial fibroelastosis (EFE) and/or fetal, infantile, or even late-onset dilated cardiomyopathy (DCM).[19,20] Autoimmune injury occurs in the 16th to 28th week of gestation.

The fact that almost all isolated CCHB is associated with maternal anti-Ro autoantibodies but heart block only occurs in only 2% to 5% of infants in affected mothers indicates that passive flow of autoantibodies is necessary but insufficient to effect injury to the conduction system. The last decade has witnessed the discovery of several fetal genetic markers for $CCHB_{AI}$ in anti-Ro antibody-positive mothers; the affected genes encode proteins regulating the inflammatory response.[21,22] These genetic predispositions partially explain the higher risk of autoimmune CCHB when a previous child has been affected. Mothers with a prior child with CCHB have 12.5% to 25% chance of having another child with CCHB. Those with a prior infant with neonatal lupus have 13% chance.[23,24] Higher levels of maternal autoantibody also confer additional risk.[24] Despite these advances in understanding,

there is no way yet to reliably predict which infants will develop heart block.

Infants may have other morbidities associated with transfer of autoantibodies. The most devastating of these is DCM, which occurs in 20% of infants with $CCHB_{AI}$ and carries a particularly poor prognosis.[20,25,26] EFE and other arrhythmias may be present as well. Congenital junctional tachycardia has been posited to be secondary to maternal autoantibodies in some cases.[14] Ascending aortic dilation has been increasingly recognized in these patients, but the aortic dimension seems to normalize over time.[27] Other affected systems variably include skin (photosensitive rash), liver (hepatic failure, elevated bilirubinemia, or asymptomatic hepatitis), and cell lines (anemia, neutropenia, or thrombocytopenia).[28] The constellation of these findings—with or without cardiac involvement—is referred to as neonatal lupus. The noncardiac manifestations are self-limited, typically resolving with clearance of the autoantibodies over the first 9 months of life.[7]

Other Forms of Congenital Complete Heart Block

$CCHB_{SHD}$ may account for as much as 42% of all CCHB cases.[2] AVB occurs most commonly in patients with left atrial isomerism (polysplenia syndrome) followed by ventricular inversion ("corrected" transposition).[29] AVB results from discontinuity of the electrical system.[14,30] Ventricular inversion is associated with mirror image positioning of the His and atrioventricular node and a prolonged course of the His bundle.[31] The site of AVB can be located above, below, or within the His.[32]

Some infants with CCHB have neither overt structural heart disease nor maternal autoantibodies. A portion of these infants may have $CCHB_{AI}$ with maternal autoantibodies levels too low to detect. Other cases may be due to genetic factors. Defects in SCN5A may cause CCHB from progressive cardiac conduction disorder, although these patients typically present as children or young adults.[33] TBX5 mutations cause Holt Oram syndrome characterized by heart block, atrial septal defects, and deformities of the thumb and forearm. In the absence of the full-blown syndrome, TBX5 as well as NKX2.5 can cause heart block, either in association with other structural heart disease or as an isolated finding.[34,35]

NATURAL HISTORY
Isolated Congenital Complete Heart Block

The natural history of fetal, neonatal, and childhood $CCHB_{ISO}$ is best revealed in an examination of previous registries. The results of these registries were recently well summarized.[36] Combined, the registries include more than 900 cases of CCHB. Cases are predominantly CCHB$_{AI}$. The overwhelming majority were diagnosed in utero. Among the six registries, in utero mortality ranged from 6% to 18% and perinatal mortality ranged from 2.3% to 14%, whereas total mortality ranged from 15% to 25%. Overall, 91 of 899 fetal cases died in utero. Of the remaining 820 cases (live births plus additional neonatal diagnosis) 70 died perinatally.[20,29,36–39] In the 3 registries with ~100% anti-Ro-positive mothers, the overall fetal/perinatal death rate in each study approached 20%.[20,36,38] Ten-year survival among liveborn infants approaches 90%.

Among 5 registries evaluating prognostic factors,[20,29,36–38] hydrops was universally associated with increased mortality. Other risk factors included slower ventricular rate,[20,29,37] earlier gestational age at detection,[20,37] pleural effusion,[36] prematurity,[38] and cardiomyopathy.[20,37] Cardiomyopathy has emerged as one of the most devastating comorbidities from CCHB$_{AI}$ and may present as DCM with decreased systolic function or as EFE. Both carry significant prognostic implications. The poor outcomes noted among patients with cardiomyopathy in the US registry of CCHB are corroborated by the results of prior studies.[20,25,26] Patients with CCHB$_{AI}$ with either DCM or EFE had a case fatality rate of 40%. The combination of DCM and EFE was universally fatal. The incidence of DCM may further increase in childhood and continues to carry a poor prognosis.[19,40]

An understanding of the natural history of CCHB in adolescents and adults is confounded by changing definitions of the term. Many patients included in published reports presented during childhood or adolescence and do not meet current criteria. Nevertheless, a few trends are worth mentioning. First, children with nonimmune isolated CCHB seem to fair better than those with autoimmune-mediated disease. Several studies in these patients demonstrate dramatically lower mortality, likely owing to the almost complete absence of DCM in this patient group.[3,19,25,41,42] This difference extends to the rate of pacemaker-mediated cardiomyopathy, which may be as high as 67% in CCHB$_{AI}$ but is almost never encountered in nonimmune CCHB$_{ISO}$.[43] Second, children diagnosed with CCHB fare better than infants and neonates, highlighting the likely difference in underlying disease processes and possibly pointing to a referral bias—with sicker patients presenting at an earlier age regardless of the underlying mechanism.

Adult patients trend toward gradual slowing of ventricular rate, development of mitral insufficiency, and left ventricular enlargement.[42,44] Michaëlsson and colleagues[44] prospectively studied 102 patients with isolated "congenital" complete heart block who were asymptomatic until at least 15 years of age. Sixteen developed mitral insufficiency, of whom 4 died. QT prolongation occurred as a new finding in adult patients and was associated with syncope and sudden death. Because of the unpredictable nature of these episodes, Michaelsson has proposed that all individuals with CCHB older than 15 years undergo placement of a permanent pacemaker.[45] Pacing has been shown to decrease mortality, normalize LV diastolic dimension, reverse LV dysfunction, and eliminate symptoms in multiple studies.[7,38,44,46–48]

Congenital Complete Heart Block in Structural Heart Disease

Fetuses and infants with CCHB$_{SHD}$ have a high mortality. In one study of 55 fetuses with CCHB, 29 had CCHB$_{SHD}$ and only 4 of those 29 survived.[49] Left atrial isomerism carries a particularly poor prognosis.[29,49–52] Among 59 patients with CCHB due to structural heart disease, left atrial isomerism accounted for 68% of cases and was associated with a neonatal mortality of 90%.[29] Mortality by age 3 months was 100% in this registry and has approached 100% in other studies as well.[50,51] Ventricular inversion accounts for an additional 14% of cases and was associated with a 25% neonatal mortality.[29]

EVALUATION AND TREATMENT

Evaluation and treatment of CCHB varies by age, with different recommendations for fetal, neonatal, childhood, and adult heart block largely based on case reports, small studies, registries, and expert opinion.

Evaluation

Evaluation of the fetus with or at risk of CCHB is primarily done by fetal ultrasonography and fetal echocardiography. Cardiac M-mode tracings are used to compare the rates and relationship of atrial and ventricular contraction, or Doppler can be used to evaluate the rates of mitral inflow and aortic outflow.

In addition to evaluation of cardiac rhythm, fetal echocardiography can provide a host of diagnostic and prognostic information to assist in pregnancy management and delivery planning. Identification of structural heart disease is key in planning for appropriate postnatal management. In addition, fetal ultrasonography allows for assessment of ventricular size and function, presence of hydrops, umbilical arterial Doppler, and Doppler of the umbilical vein and ductus arteriosus to provide a cardiovascular profile score.[53] A score less than 7 has been associated with poor prognosis.

Beyond echocardiography, fetal electrocardiography (ECG) and fetal magnetocardiography have been used to obtain fetal ECG.[54–56] These studies can diagnose atrioventricular conduction abnormalities and may provide incremental diagnostic and prognostic information; however, they are complicated and expensive to obtain and remain largely in the research realm.

Following delivery, most children with CCHB require a pacemaker early in life.[7] Those children without a pacemaker generally have adequate ventricular rates, normal left ventricular systolic function, and no symptoms of chronotropic incompetence. Continued follow-up for development of a pacing indication is required. Patients are typically seen every 6 months to every year with specific instructions provided to families to follow-up sooner if syncope or other symptoms develop. Beyond the history, primary modes of evaluation include the ECG, Holter monitor, and echocardiography. ECG is instrumental in assessing the ventricular escape rate and mechanism (junctional vs ventricular), as well as for evaluating the QT interval. Holter monitoring expands on this information by providing average daytime heart rates and by looking for pauses and significant QT prolongation at the slowest heart rates. Echocardiography is critical to assess for the development of ventricular dilation or dysfunction, mitral valve insufficiency, and for the presence of residual lesions in patients with congenital structural heart disease. Because of the nonspecificity of symptoms and the unpredictable nature of congenital heart block, consideration should be given to obtaining these objective measurements at each annual visit.

Treatment

Once third-degree heart block occurs, it is irreversible. Thus, a fetal treatment strategy starts with prevention, and prevention starts with screening. A scientific statement from the American Heart Association recommends weekly or every other week screening for fetuses of mothers known positive for SSA antibodies, and at least weekly screening for mothers who have had a prior infant with CCHB or neonatal lupus.[57] The goal is to catch conduction system injury at the level of first-degree or second-degree block and administer therapy to reverse or stabilize the severity. The value of this screening has been called into question for several reasons. First, the progression of heart block can be extremely rapid, progressing to CHB in less than 24 hours,[58] and necessitating extremely frequent screening. Second, recent data suggest that even without treatment, many infants with first- or second-degree AVB may not progress to complete AVB.[59] Finally and as discussed later, fluorinated corticosteroids, the agents typically proposed for reversal of CCHB, have not been shown to improve outcomes.

Multiple immunomodulators have been evaluated in the treatment of fetal CCHB$_{AI}$ (**Table 1**), but few of these agents have been subjected to rigorous testing. The most studied class of drugs is fluorinated corticosteroids. Early studies suggested great promise in improving outcomes by reversing the severity of heart block and by separately reversing or preventing cardiomyopathy.[60–62] The only prospective study on fetal steroid therapy in anti-Ro-exposed fetuses found no difference in outcome between 30 treated and 10 untreated fetuses but did suggest a role for dexamethasone in treating first- or second-degree AVB.[63] None of the 6 large registries of CCHB have provided support for the use of fluorinated corticosteroids.[20,29,36–39] A large meta-analysis of 747 patients from 9 studies, some of whom were included in the aforementioned registries, compared outcomes among at-risk fetuses exposed or not exposed to steroids.[64] Looking at the rate of live birth, overall survival, progression to complete AVB, need for cardiac pacing, and the frequency of other cardiac manifestations, no significant difference in any outcome was identified. Steroids have adverse fetal effects, including growth restriction and prematurity.[63] Nevertheless, steroid use remains prevalent in clinical practice. American Heart Association guidelines published in 2014 lists dexamethasone indicated as class IIb (worth considering) for the treatment of fetal first- or second-degree CCHB$_{AI}$.[57] In a 2018 survey of 49 physicians, 88% recommended steroids when second-degree AVB was detected in anti-Ro-positive mothers.[65] Continued use of dexamethasone may partially be due to a "Hail Mary" philosophy, recognizing the guarded prognosis associated with CCHB and the limited number of alternative, effective therapeutic options.

Intravenous immunoglobulin (IVIG) and plasmapheresis have both been evaluated in small studies; they may theoretically improve outcomes in at-risk infants by eliminating autoantibodies, decreasing placental transport of antibodies, or modulating the immune response.[66] Evaluated at

Table 1
Summary of published guidelines on the treatment of congenital complete heart block

Intervention	Indication	Age	Recommend	Evidence	Source
Heart rate screening	Prior pregnancy complicated by CCHB$_{AI}$ (at least weekly screening)	Fetal (weeks 16–28)	I	B	1
	Anti-Ro+ mother (weekly or every 2 wk)	Fetal (weeks 16–28)	IIa	B	1
Early delivery	CVP score <7, extreme bradycardia, endocardiofibroelastosis, LV dysfunction	Fetal	IIa	C	1
Sympathomimetics	HR <55 (or with associated hydrops, ventricular dysfunction, complex SHD)	Fetal	IIa	C	1
Dexamethasone	First- or second-degree AVB, anti-Ro+	Fetal	IIb	B	1
	Complete AVB, anti-Ro+	Fetal	IIb	B	1
Intravenous immunoglobulin	AVB any degree, anti-Ro+	Fetal	IIb	C	1
Chronotropic agents	Hydrops, very slow HR, shock	Neonate	IIa	C	1
Temporary pacing	Hydrops, very slow HR, shock	Neonate	IIa	C	1
Permanent pacing	Symptomatic bradycardia, complex ventricular ectopy, wide QRS ventricular dysfunction	Any age	I	B	2,3
	HR <55, (<70 if complex SHD)	Neonate, Infant	I	C	2
	HR <50, abrupt pauses >2 × cycle length	Child	IIa	B	2
		Adult	I	B	3
	Complex SHD and impaired hemodynamics due to loss of atrioventricular synchrony	Any age	IIa	C	2
	Asymptomatic CCHB	Child	IIb	C	2
		Adult	IIa	C	3

Table summarizes recommendations from various published guidelines on congenital complete heart block.
   Neonate less than 1 month old; infant, 1 to 12 mo; child 1 to 17 y; adults greater than 17 y.
   Strength: 1, therapy is recommended; IIa, reasonable; and IIb worth considering.
   Evidence: A, strong evidence/multiple randomized studies; 2, moderate evidence/single randomized study/registries; C, week evidence/expert opinion.
   Abbreviations: AVB, atrioventricular block; CCHB, congenital heart block; CVP, cardiovascular profile; HR, heart rate; LV, left ventricle; SHD, structural heart disease.
   Sources: 1, Diagnosis and treatment of fetal cardiac disease (2014)[66]; 2, ACC/AHA/HRS 2008 Guidelines for Device Based Therapy of Cardiac Rhythm Abnormalities[96]; 3, 2018 ACC/AHA/HRS Guideline on the Evaluation and Management of Patients With Bradycardia and Cardiac Conduction Delay.[6]

a dose of 400 mg/kg every 3 weeks, IVIG has not been shown to decrease the incidence of neonatal lupus.[67,68] Similarly, plasmapheresis has failed to demonstrate reversal of AVB or to clearly affect the natural history in autoimmune mothers.[69,70] Both IVIG and plasmapheresis are indicated as class IIb for the treatment of infants with CCHB$_{AI}$.[57]

Hydroxychloroquine, an inhibitor of Toll-like receptor ligation, has shown promise at reducing the risk of CCHB$_{AI}$ in autoimmune mothers. In the PROMISSE study, pregnant women with lupus or antiphospholipid antibody syndrome who took hydroxychloroquine had only a 1% risk of having a child with CCHB$_{AI}$.[71] The recently completed

PATCH trial prospectively evaluated 54 pregnancies in mothers with a prior pregnancy complicated by $CCHB_{AI}$. A dose of 400 mg daily was initiated before 10 weeks' gestation and continued throughout pregnancy. The 7.4% rate of CCHB was significantly less than that of historical controls.[72] There are no published guidelines on use of hydroxychloroquine in anti-Ro-positive woman. Nevertheless, the encouraging results from these studies provide reason to believe that hydroxychloroquine will be increasingly used in the prevention of $CCHB_{AI}$.

Beta agonists have been shown to increase heart rate and improve outcome in several small series and case reports.[73–76] However, there is some concern that the chronotropic benefits may be transient.[66,77] Terbutaline is the agent of choice. This agent is generally well tolerated but can cause maternal tachycardia, anxiety, and headaches.[66] Terbutaline is recommended as a class IIa agent (reasonable, see **Table 1**) for fetuses with a ventricular rate less than 55 bpm.[57]

Fetal (in utero) pacing has been attempted as a definitive mechanism to increase fetal heart rate. Trials of fetal pacing have met with poor outcomes. Fetal demise typically occurs shortly after the intervention.[41,78] Ongoing research in this area may eventually lead to the development of fetal pacemakers and improved outcomes.[79,80]

One problem for the fetus with CCHB is the propensity among obstetricians to deliver early and urgently to an unprepared cardiology, cardiothoracic, and neonatal team. Early delivery may be indicated for select infants with severe bradycardia, in whom postnatal interventions can improve prognosis. However, prematurity has been associated with decreased survival in infants with CCHB.[38] Early delivery only complicates the care of infants with congenital heart block, adding prematurity to the list of comorbidities, increasing metabolic demand in the face of impaired systemic output, and exacerbating the risk of early postnatal interventions. Delivery before 32 weeks has been associated with worse outcomes.[25] When possible, delay of delivery until 39 weeks is preferred.[57]

Postnatally, the only effective long-term therapy for CCHB is cardiac pacing. Guideline-directed indications for cardiac pacing in children were last addressed by a joint position paper from the American College of Cardiology, American Heart Association, and Heart Rhythm Society (ACC/AHA/HRS) in 2008[81] (see **Table 1**). The more recent ACC/AHA/HRS guidelines from 2018 did not address pacing in infants and children, although a separate position paper from the Pediatric and Congenital Electrophysiology Society (PACES) is expected soon.

Permanent pacing in any adult with CCHB is reasonable (class IIa) due to the unpredictable risk of syncope and sudden death. There is increasing consensus that asymptomatic adult patients with CCHB should undergo pacemaker placement.[45] In pediatric patients, strong evidence for these recommendations is lacking. The guidelines are largely based on small studies and registries, or on expert opinion. Indications for pacing are based on symptoms, heart rate or other ECG findings, and the presence of structural or functional heart disease.

Symptomatic irreversible bradycardia of any cause is a class I indication (recommended) for cardiac pacing. Syncope or apparent seizure suggests long pauses due to an unstable pacemaker mechanism or pause-dependent torsades de pointes and warrants prompt intervention. Other symptoms in childhood include fatigue, exercise intolerance, frequent nightmares or night terrors, and nocturnal enuresis in a previously continent child. These symptoms are nonspecific, sometimes resulting in premature pacemaker placement, but more commonly leading to a delay in pacing. Often symptoms are present from an early age and are either overlooked or accepted as the patient's baseline. Subconscious lifestyle modifications, such as avoiding athletics, are often dismissed as a personality quirk.

A wide complex escape rhythm implies an unstable pacing mechanism. Complex ventricular ectopy presents a high risk for sudden death. Both findings as well as ventricular dysfunction warrant pacemaker placement as a class I indication. The European Society of Cardiology guidelines also specify QT prolongation as a class I indication.[82]

In infants, a heart rate less than 55 (or 70 in the presence of hemodynamically significant structural heart disease) constitutes a class I indication for pacing. A heart rate less than 50 in children beyond the first year of life is a class IIa indication. Even in completely asymptomatic children with CCHB, normal systolic function, no symptoms, an adequate junctional rate, and normal QT interval, permanent pacing is considered a class IIb indication.

Pacing Therapy

The decision to implant a pacemaker in a newborn or child practically ensures a lifetime of cardiac pacing. The cumulative risks of pacing are higher both due to a higher procedural complication rate[83–85] and because of the sheer number of procedures required to maintain a lifetime of pacing. These factors alter the risk/benefit ratio and must be considered when contemplating pacing therapy.

The decision to pace is only the first of a long line of complex considerations to optimize patient care, particularly in small children. The site of pacing, route of pacing, and choice of which chambers to pace must all be considered. Pacing from the right ventricular (RV) apex or free wall is generally avoided because it may cause DCM or exacerbate a predisposition to developing it, particularly in patients with $CCHB_{AI}$.[86–90] Pacemaker-induced cardiomyopathy is reported in 7% of patients with obligate RV pacing.[91] Paradoxically, patients with $CCHB_{AI}$ have shown improvement in DCM following pacing therapy.[42] Although there is no one ideal site for RV pacing in all patients, there is general consensus that the apex should be avoided and that septal sites are preferable for transvenous leads in children.[92] Septal sites may also reduce the amount of lead slack necessary to account for somatic growth. His bundle pacing has not been evaluated in young patients. The high capture thresholds and increased rate of lead malfunction[93,94] suggest that His pacing is not yet suitable for pediatric patients, a group already prone to higher complication rates. For epicardial systems, pacing from the RV outflow and free wall were similarly associated with decreasing left ventricular function, whereas pacing from the LV apex or lateral wall was associated with restoration and maintenance of normal LV function.[92,95]

Single-chamber pacing is often preferred in infants and children because it decreases the lead burden and device complexity in a group prone to complications. In young patients with structurally normal hearts and normal function, single-chamber pacing has been shown to be equivalent to dual-chamber pacing, and pacemaker syndrome generally does not occur.[96–98] Patients with complex congenital heart disease and with significant ventricular dysfunction may benefit from dual-chamber pacing, and those with ventricular dysfunction should be considered for multisite or left ventricular-only pacing.[99] These considerations—particularly the need for LV pacing in small children—may drive the decision to implant an epicardial system. Most centers prefer epicardial pacing systems through at least in early childhood, if not longer. In patients with intracardiac shunts, epicardial pacing is always preferred due to the risk of systolic embolism.[100,101] Steroid-eluting epicardial leads have a performance profile similar to transvenous leads.[102] Although more invasive, epicardial systems can be used for similarly long periods, preserving venous access and with minimal additional risk of reinterventions.

Once a pacemaker has been placed, consideration of programming mode and lower rate is important. Programming slower, subphysiologic rates has been shown to reverse ventricular dysfunction while still preventing symptoms of bradycardia.[103,104] One proposed mechanism for improvement has been the periodic emergence of junctional escape rhythm, intermittently restoring intraventricular synchrony. However, patients receiving 100% ventricular pacing at the lower rate have also responded. In newborns with chronically low junctional rates, initiation of ventricular pacing at low rates with a gradual increase may minimize the risk of arrhythmia[99] or pacemaker-mediated cardiomyopathy.

SUMMARY

CCHB describes the presence of cardiac conduction abnormalities diagnosed in utero or within the first 27 days of life. Several causes may be responsible for this clinical presentation including maternal autoimmune disease, congenital structural heart defects, and genetic mutations. Of this heterogeneous group, the most prevalent and well-studied subgroup is those with $CCHB_{AI}$. This group is itself a subset of manifestations arising from neonatal lupus—a condition of immune-mediated injury to the cardiac conduction system, ventricular myocardium, and other fetal tissues by passive transfer of maternal autoantibodies to the Ro antigen.

Patients with CCHB are at risk for symptoms of chronotropic incompetence as well as for sudden death related to asystole or pause-dependent torsades de pointes. The natural history of the condition predicts gradually slowing ventricular rate, onset of symptoms, and sudden death. In utero risk factors include slower heart rates, hydrops, and cardiomyopathy. Postnatally, risk factors include slower heart rates, a wide complex escape rhythm, pauses, QT prolongation, mitral insufficiency, and cardiomyopathy. The presence of any of these findings warrants placement of a permanent pacemaker to relieve symptoms and prevent catastrophic events.

Looking forward, hydroxychloroquine shows promise in reducing the incidence of fetal AVB in those at risk. Genetic discoveries offer promise in identifying which pregnancies are at risk for developing $CCHB_{AI}$ and may help further elucidate the mechanism of injury. Refinement of device implantation tools and techniques may allow for reliable His bundle pacing in smaller patients. Emerging therapies for fetal heart block, including fetal cardiac pacing, may provide a novel therapeutic option and improve outcome. These and other unforeseen advances look to minimize the incidence and morbidity of CCHB.

CLINICS CARE POINTS

- Despite widespread use, fluorinated steroids have not been shown to clearly reduce risks of fetal progression to complete AV block and may add risk to the pregnancy.
- Early delivery of a fetus with CCHB is best avoided without specific indications such as extreme bradycardia LV dysfunction, or endocardial fibroelastosis.
- Frequent night terrors may be a symptom of nocturnal bradycardia in patients with congenital complete heart block.
- Epicardial pacing systems may have longevity similar to transvenous systems. Ideally, epicardial ventricular pacing should be performed from the LV apex or LV free wall.
- Single chamber pacing is non-inferior to dual chamber pacing in children with structurally normal hearts.

REFERENCES

1. Morquio L. Sur une maladie infantile et familiale characterisee par des modifications permanentes du pouls, des attaques syncopales et epileptiformes et la mort subite. Arch Med Enfants 1901; 4:467–75.
2. Brucato A, Jonzon A, Friedman D, et al. Proposal for a new definition of congenital complete atrioventricular block. Lupus 2003;12(6):427–35.
3. Villain E, Coastedoat-Chalumeau N, Marijon E, et al. Presentation and prognosis of complete atrioventricular block in childhood, according to maternal antibody status. J Am Coll Cardiol 2006; 48(8):1682–7.
4. Askanase A, Friedman D, Copel J, et al. Spectrum and progression of conduction abnormalities in infants born to mothers with anti-SSA/Ro-SSB/La antibodies. Lupus 2002;11(3):145–51.
5. De Raet J, Rega F, Meyns B. Late recovery of atrioventricular conduction after pacemaker implantation for complete heart block in congenital heart disease: fact or fluke? Acta Chir Belg 2010; 110(3):323–7.
6. Bordachar P, Zachary W, Ploux S, et al. Pathophysiology, clinical course, and management of congenital complete atrioventricular block. Heart Rhythm 2013;10(5):760–6.
7. Manolis AA, Manolis TA, Melita H, et al. Congenital heart block: Pace earlier (Childhood) than later

(Adulthood). Trends Cardiovasc Med 2020;30(5): 275–86.
8. Fritzler MJ, Pauls JD, Kinsella TD, et al. Antinuclear, anticytoplasmic, and anti-Sjogren's syndrome antigen A (SS-A/Ro) antibodies in female blood donors. Clin Immunol Immunopathol 1985;36(1): 120–8.
9. Satoh M, Chan EK, Ho LA, et al. Prevalence and sociodemographic correlates of antinuclear antibodies in the United States. Arthritis Rheum 2012; 64(7):2319–27.
10. Buyon JP, Hiebert R, Copel J, et al. Autoimmune-associated congenital heart block: demographics, mortality, morbidity and recurrence rates obtained from a national neonatal lupus registry. J Am Coll Cardiol 1998;31(7):1658–66.
11. Ambrosi A, Wahren-Herlenius M. Congenital heart block: evidence for a pathogenic role of maternal autoantibodies. Arthritis Res Ther 2012;14(2):208.
12. Gleicher N, Elkayam U. Preventing congenital neonatal heart block in offspring of mothers with anti-SSA/Ro and SSB/La antibodies: a review of published literature and registered clinical trials. Autoimmun Rev 2013;12(11):1039–45.
13. Ambrosi A, Sonesson SE, Wahren-Herlenius M. Molecular mechanisms of congenital heart block. Exp Cell Res 2014;325(1):2–9.
14. Brito-Zeron P, Izmirly PM, Ramos-Casals M, et al. The clinical spectrum of autoimmune congenital heart block. Nat Rev Rheumatol 2015;11(5): 301–12.
15. Wainwright B, Bhan R, Trad C, et al. Autoimmune-mediated congenital heart block. Best Pract Res Clin Obstet Gynaecol 2020;64:41–51.
16. Clancy RM, Buyon JP. More to death than dying: apoptosis in the pathogenesis of SSA/Ro- SSB/La-associated congenital heart block. Rheum Dis Clin 2004;30(3):589–602.
17. Xiao GQ, Hu K, Boutjdir M. Direct inhibition of expressed cardiac l- and t-type calcium channels by igg from mothers whose children have congenital heart block. Circulation 2001;103(11):1599–604.
18. Anderson RH, Wenick A, Losekoot T, et al. Congenitally complete heart block. Developmental aspects. Circulation 1977;56(1):90–101.
19. Udink ten Cate FE, Breur JM, Cohen MI, et al. Dilated cardiomyopathy in isolated congenital complete atrioventricular block: early and long-term risk in children. J Am Coll Cardiol 2001; 37(4):1129–34.
20. Izmirly PM, Saxena A, Kim MY, et al. Maternal and fetal factors associated with mortality and morbidity in a multi-racial/ethnic registry of anti-SSA/Ro-associated cardiac neonatal lupus. Circulation 2011;124(18):1927–35.
21. Ainsworth HC, Marion MC, Bertero T, et al. Association of natural Killer Cell Ligand Polymorphism

HLA-C Asn80Lys with the development of anti-SSA/Ro-associated congenital heart block. Arthritis Rheumatol 2017;69(11):2170–4.

22. Clancy RM, Marion MC, Kaufman KM, et al. Identification of candidate loci at 6p21 and 21q22 in a genome-wide association study of cardiac manifestations of neonatal lupus. Arthritis Rheum 2010;62(11):3415–24.

23. Izmirly PM, Llanos C, Lee LA, et al. Cutaneous manifestations of neonatal lupus and risk of subsequent congenital heart block. Arthritis Rheum 2010;62(4):1153–7.

24. Jaeggi E, Laskin C, Hamilton R, et al. The importance of the level of maternal anti-Ro/SSA antibodies as a prognostic marker of the development of cardiac neonatal lupuserythematosus a prospective study of 186 antibody-exposed fetuses and infants. J Am Coll Cardiol 2010;55(24):2778–84.

25. Jaeggi ET, Hamilton RM, Silverman ED, et al. Outcome of children with fetal, neonatal or childhood diagnosis of isolated congenital atrioventricular block: a single institution's experience of 30 years. J Am Coll Cardiol 2002;39(1):130–7.

26. Nield LE, Silverman ED, Taylor GP, et al. Maternal anti-Ro and anti-La antibody-associated endocardial fibroelastosis. Circulation 2002;105(7):843–8.

27. Radbill AE, Brown DW, Lacro RV, et al. Ascending aortic dilation in patients with congenital complete heart block. Heart Rhythm 2008;5(12):1704–8.

28. Lee LA. Neonatal lupus: clinical features and management. Paediatr Drugs 2004;6(2):71–8.

29. Lopes LM, Tavares GM, Damiano AP, et al. Perinatal outcome of fetal atrioventricular block: one-hundred- sixteen cases from a single institution. Circulation 2008;118(12):1268–75.

30. Dickinson DF, Wilkinson JL, Anderson KR, et al. The cardiac conduction system in situs ambiguus. Circulation 1979;59(5):879–85.

31. Lev M, Licata RH, May RC. The conduction system in Mixed Levocardia with ventricular inversion (corrected transposition). Circulation 1963;28:232–7.

32. Gillette PC, Busch U, Mullins CE, et al. Electrophysiologic studies in patients with ventricular inversion and "corrected transposition. Circulation 1979;60(4):939–45.

33. Baruteau AE, Kyndt F, Behr ER, et al. SCN5A mutations in 442 neonates and children: genotypephenotype correlation and identification of higher-risk subgroups. Eur Heart J 2018;39(31):2879–87.

34. Baruteau AE, Probst V, Abriel H. Inherited progressive cardiac conduction disorders. Curr Opin Cardiol 2015;30(1):33–9.

35. Xu YJ, Qiu XB, Yuan F, et al. Prevalence and spectrum of NKX2.5 mutations in patients with congenital atrial septal defect and atrioventricular block. Mol Med Rep 2017;15(4):2247–54.

36. Fredi M, Andreoli L, Bacco B, et al. First report of the Italian registry on Immune-mediated congenital heart block (Lu.Ne registry). Front Cardiovasc Med 2019;6:11.

37. Eliasson H, Sonesson SE, Sharland G, et al. Isolated atrioventricular block in the fetus: a retrospective, multinational, multicenter study of 175 patients. Circulation 2011;124(18):1919–26.

38. Levesque K, Morel N, Maltret A, et al. Description of 214 cases of autoimmune congenital heart block: Results of the French neonatal lupus syndrome. Autoimmun Rev 2015;14(12):1154–60.

39. Van den Berg NW, Slieker MG, van Beynum IM, et al. Fluorinated steroids do not improve outcome of isolated atrioventricular block. Int J Cardiol 2016;225:167–71.

40. Moak JP, Barron KS, Hougen TJ, et al. Congenital heart block: development of late-onset cardiomyopathy, a previously underappreciated sequela. J Am Coll Cardiol 2001;37(1):238–42.

41. Baruteau AE, Pass RH, Thambo JB, et al. Congenital and childhood atrioventricular blocks: pathophysiology and contemporary management. Eur J Pediatr 2016;175(9):1235–48.

42. Beaufort-Krol GC, Schasfoort-Van Leeuwen MJ, Stienstra Y, et al. Longitudinal echocardiographic Follow-Up in children with congenital complete atrioventricular block. Pacing Clin Electrophysiol 2007;30(11):1339–43.

43. Sagar S, Shen W-K, Asirvatham SJ, et al. Effect of long-term right ventricular pacing in young adults with structurally normal heart. Circulation 2010;121(15):1698–705.

44. Michaëlsson M, Jonzon A, Riesenfeld T. Isolated congenital complete atrioventricular block in adult life: a prospective study. Circulation 1995;92(3):442–9.

45. Michaelsson M, Riesenfeld T, Jonzon A. Natural history of congenital complete atrioventricular block. Pacing Clin Electrophysiol 1997;20(8 Pt 2):2098–101.

46. Breur JM, Udink Ten Cate FE, Kapusta L, et al. Pacemaker therapy in isolated congenital complete atrioventricular block. Pacing Clin Electrophysiol 2002;25(12):1685–91.

47. Glatz AC, Gaynor JW, Rhodes LA, et al. Outcome of high-risk neonates with congenital complete heart block paced in the first 24 hours after birth. J Thorac Cardiovasc Surg 2008;136(3):767–73.

48. Sholler GF, Walsh EP. Congenital complete heart block in patients without anatomic cardiac defects. Am Heart J 1989;118(6):1193–8.

49. Schmidt KG, Ulmer HE, Silverman NH, et al. Perinatal outcome of fetal complete atrioventricular block: a multicenter experience. J Am Coll Cardiol 1991;17(6):1360–6.

50. Garcia OL, Metha AV, Pickoff AS, et al. Left isomerism and complete atrioventricular block: a report of six cases. Am J Cardiol 1981;48(6):1103–7.

51. Phoon CK, Villegas MD, Ursell PC, et al. Left atrial isomerism detected in fetal life. Am J Cardiol 1996; 77(12):1083–8.

52. Taketazu M, Lougheed J, Yoo S-J, et al. Spectrum of cardiovascular disease, accuracy of diagnosis, and outcome in fetal heterotaxy syndrome. Am J Cardiol 2006;97(5):720–4.

53. Hofstaetter C, Hansmann M, Eik-Nes SH, et al. A cardiovascular profile score in the surveillance of fetal hydrops. J Matern Fetal Neonatal Med 2006;19(7):407–13.

54. Chia EL, Ho TF, Rauff M, et al. Cardiac time intervals of normal fetuses using noninvasive fetal electrocardiography. Prenatal Diagn 2005;25(7):546–52.

55. Gardiner HM, Belmar C, Pasquini L, et al. Fetal ECG: a novel predictor of atrioventricular block in anti-Ro positive pregnancies. Heart 2007;93(11): 1454–60.

56. Wakai RT, Leuthold AC, Cripe L, et al. Assessment of fetal rhythm in complete congenital heart block by magnetocardiography. Pacing Clin Electrophysiol 2000;23(6):1047–50.

57. Donofrio MT, Moon-Grady AJ, Hornberger LK, et al. Diagnosis and treatment of fetal cardiac disease: a scientific statement from the American Heart Association. Circulation 2014;129(21):2183–242.

58. Cuneo BF, Sonesson SE, Levasseur S, et al. Home Monitoring for fetal heart rhythm during anti- Ro pregnancies. J Am Coll Cardiol 2018;72(16): 1940–51.

59. Jaeggi ET, Silverman ED, Laskin C, et al. Prolongation of the atrioventricular conduction in fetuses exposed to maternal anti-Ro/SSA and anti-La/SSB antibodies did not predict progressive heart block. A prospective observational study on the effects of maternal antibodies on 165 fetuses. J Am Coll Cardiol 2011;57(13):1487–92.

60. Jaeggi ET, Fouron JC, Silverman ED, et al. Transplacental fetal treatment improves the outcome of prenatally diagnosed complete atrioventricular block without structural heart disease. Circulation 2004;110(12):1542–8.

61. Saleeb S, Copel J, Friedman D, et al. Comparison of treatment with fluorinated glucocorticoids to the natural history of autoantibody-associated congenital heart block: retrospective review of the research registry for neonatal lupus. Arthritis Rheumatol 1999;42(11):2335–45.

62. Tsuboi H, Sumida T, Noma H, et al. Maternal predictive factors for fetal congenital heart block in pregnant mothers positive for anti-SS-A antibodies. Mod Rheumatol 2016;26(4):569–75.

63. Friedman DM, Kim MY, Copel JA, et al. Prospective evaluation of fetuses with autoimmune-associated congenital heart block followed in the PR Interval and Dexamethasone Evaluation (PRIDE) Study. Am J Cardiol 2009;103(8):1102–6.

64. Hoxha A, Mattia E, Zanetti A, et al. Fluorinated steroids are not superior to any treatment to ameliorate the outcome of autoimmune mediated congenital heart block: a systematic review of the literature and meta-analysis. Clin Exp Rheumatol 2020;38(4):783–91.

65. Clowse MEB, Eudy AM, Kiernan E, et al. The prevention, screening and treatment of congenital heart block from neonatal lupus: a survey of provider practices. Rheumatology (Oxford) 2018; 57(suppl_5):v9–17.

66. Saxena A, Izmirly PM, Mendez B, et al. Prevention and treatment in utero of autoimmune-associated congenital heart block. Cardiol Rev 2014;22(6): 263–7.

67. Friedman DM, Llanos C, Izmirly PM, et al. Evaluation of fetuses in a study of intravenous immunoglobulin as preventive therapy for congenital heart block: Results of a multicenter, prospective, open-label clinical trial. Arthritis Rheum 2010; 62(4):1138–46.

68. Pisoni C, Brucato A, Ruffatti A, et al. Failure of intravenous immunoglobulin to prevent congenital heart block: findings of a multicenter, prospective, observational study. Arthritis Rheum 2010;62(4): 1147–52.

69. Buyon J, Roubey R, Swersky S, et al. Complete congenital heart block: risk of occurrence and therapeutic approach to prevention. J Rheumatol 1988; 15(7):1104–8.

70. Ruffatti A, Cerutti A, Favaro M, et al. Plasmapheresis, intravenous immunoglobulins and bethametasone - a combined protocol to treat autoimmune congenital heart block: a prospective cohort study. Clin Exp Rheumatol 2016;34(4): 706–13.

71. Buyon JP, Kim MY, Salmon JE. Predictors of Pregnancy Outcomes in patients with lupus. Ann Intern Med 2016;164(2):131.

72. Izmirly P, Kim M, Friedman DM, et al. Hydroxychloroquine to prevent Recurrent congenital heart block in fetuses of anti-SSA/Ro-positive mothers. J Am Coll Cardiol 2020;76(3):292–302.

73. Chan AY, Silverman RK, Smith FC, et al. In utero treatment of fetal complete heart block with terbutaline. A case report. J Reprod Med 1999;44(4): 385–7.

74. Groves AM, Allan LD, Rosenthal E. Therapeutic trial of sympathomimetics in three cases of complete heart block in the fetus. Circulation 1995;92(12): 3394–6.

75. Matsushita H, Higashino M, Sekizuka N, et al. Successful prenatal treatment of congenital heart block with ritodrine administered transplacentally. Arch Gynecol Obstet 2002;267(1):51–3.

76. Yoshida H, Iwamoto M, Sakakibara H, et al. Treatment of fetal congenital complete heart block with

maternal administration of beta-sympathomimetics (terbutaline): a case report. Gynecol Obstet Invest 2001;52(2):142–4.

77. Robinson BV, Ettedgui JA, Sherman FS. Use of terbutaline in the treatment of complete heart block in the fetus. Cardiol Young 2001;11(6):683–6.

78. Assad RS, Zielinsky P, Kalil R, et al. New lead for in utero pacing for fetal congenital heart block. J Thorac Cardiovasc Surg 2003;126(1):300–2.

79. Nicholson A, Chmait R, Bar-Cohen Y, et al. Percutaneously injectable fetal pacemaker: electronics, pacing thresholds, and power budget. Annu Int Conf IEEE Eng Med Biol Soc 2012;2012:5730–3.

80. Zhou L, Chmait R, Bar-Cohen Y, et al. Percutaneously injectable fetal pacemaker: electrodes, mechanical design and implantation. Annu Int Conf IEEE Eng Med Biol Soc 2012;2012:6600–3.

81. Epstein AE, DiMarco JP, Ellenbogen KA, et al. ACC/AHA/HRS 2008 Guidelines for Device-Based therapy of cardiac rhythm abnormalities: a report of the American College of Cardiology/American heart association Task Force on practice Guidelines (Writing Committee to Revise the ACC/AHA/NASPE 2002 Guideline Update for implantation of cardiac Pacemakers and Antiarrhythmia devices): developed in collaboration with the American association for Thoracic Surgery and Society of Thoracic Surgeons. Circulation 2008;117(21):e350–408.

82. Brignole M, Auricchio A, Baron-Esquivias G, et al. 2013 ESC Guidelines on cardiac pacing and cardiac resynchronization therapy: the Task Force on cardiac pacing and resynchronization therapy of the European Society of Cardiology (ESC). Developed in collaboration with the European Heart Rhythm Association (EHRA). Eur Heart J 2013;34(29):2281–329.

83. Czosek RJ, Meganathan K, Anderson JB, et al. Cardiac rhythm devices in the pediatric population: utilization and complications. Heart Rhythm 2012;9(2):199–208.

84. Fortescue EB, Berul CI, Cecchin F, et al. Patient, procedural, and hardware factors associated with pacemaker lead failures in pediatrics and congenital heart disease. Heart Rhythm 2004;1(2):150–9.

85. Vos LM, Kammeraad JAE, Freund MW, et al. Long-term outcome of transvenous pacemaker implantation in infants: a retrospective cohort study. Europace 2017;19(4):581–7.

86. Manolis AS. The deleterious consequences of right ventricular apical pacing: time to seek alternate site pacing. Pacing Clin Electrophysiol 2006;29(3):298–315.

87. Cho SW, Gwag HB, Hwang JK, et al. Clinical features, predictors, and long-term prognosis of pacing-induced cardiomyopathy. Eur J Heart Fail 2019;21(5):643–51.

88. Kiehl EL, Makki T, Kumar R, et al. Incidence and predictors of right ventricular pacing-induced cardiomyopathy in patients with complete atrioventricular block and preserved left ventricular systolic function. Heart Rhythm 2016;13(12):2272–8.

89. Tantengco MV, Thomas RL, Karpawich PP. Left ventricular dysfunction after long-term right ventricular apical pacing in the young. J Am Coll Cardiol 2001;37(8):2093–100.

90. Di Salvo G, Issa Z, Manea W, et al. Left ventricular function and right ventricular pacing for isolated congenital heart block. J Cardiovasc Med (Hagerstown) 2013. https://doi.org/10.2459/JCM.0b013e3283613836.

91. Moak JP, Hasbani K, Ramwell C, et al. Dilated cardiomyopathy following right ventricular pacing for AV block in young patients: resolution after upgrading to biventricular pacing systems. J Cardiovasc Electrophysiol 2006;17(10):1068–71.

92. Karpawich PP, Singh H, Zelin K. Optimizing paced ventricular function in patients with and without repaired congenital heart disease by contractility-guided lead implant. Pacing Clin Electrophysiol 2015;38(1):54–62.

93. Sharma PS, Dandamudi G, Naperkowski A, et al. Permanent His-bundle pacing is feasible, safe, and superior to right ventricular pacing in routine clinical practice. Heart Rhythm 2015;12(2):305–12.

94. Zanon F, Svetlich C, Occhetta E, et al. Safety and performance of a system specifically designed for selective site pacing. Pacing Clin Electrophysiol 2011;34(3):339–47.

95. Silvetti MS, Di Carlo D, Ammirati A, et al. Left ventricular pacing in neonates and infants with isolated congenital complete or advanced atrioventricular block: short- and medium-term outcome. Europace 2015;17(4):603–10.

96. Horenstein MS, Karpawich PP. Pacemaker syndrome in the young: do children need dual chamber as the initial pacing mode? Pacing Clin Electrophysiol 2004;27(5):600–5.

97. Horenstein MS, Karpawich PP, Tantengco MV. Single versus dual chamber pacing in the young: noninvasive comparative evaluation of cardiac function. Pacing Clin Electrophysiol 2003;26(5):1208–11.

98. Karpawich PP, Perry BL, Farooki ZQ, et al. Pacing in children and young adults with nonsurgical atrioventricular block: comparison of single-rate ventricular and dual-chamber modes. Am Heart J 1987;113(2 Pt 1):316–21.

99. Chandler SF, Fynn-Thompson F, Mah DY. Role of cardiac pacing in congenital complete heart block. Expert Rev Cardiovasc Ther 2017;15(11):853–61.

100. DeSimone CV, Friedman PA, Noheria A, et al. Stroke or transient ischemic attack in patients with transvenous pacemaker or defibrillator and

echocardiographically detected patent foramen ovale. Circulation 2013;128(13):1433–41.

101. Khairy P, Landzberg MJ, Gatzoulis MA, et al. Transvenous pacing leads and systemic thromboemboli in patients with intracardiac shunts: a multicenter study. Circulation 2006;113(20):2391–7.

102. Cohen MI, Bush DM, Vetter VL, et al. Permanent epicardial pacing in pediatric patients: seventeen years of experience and 1200 outpatient visits. Circulation 2001;103(21):2585–90.

103. Chen C-A, Chang C-I, Wang J-K, et al. Restoration of cardiac function by setting the ventricular pacing at a lower range in an infant with congenital complete atrioventricular block and dilated cardiomyopathy. Int J Cardiol 2008;131(1):e38–40.

104. Janoušek J, Tomek V, Chaloupecký V, et al. Dilated cardiomyopathy associated with dual-chamber pacing in infants: Improvement through either left ventricular cardiac resynchronization or programming the pacemaker off allowing intrinsic normal conduction. J Cardiovasc Electrophysiol 2004;15(4):470–4.

Reversible Causes of Atrioventricular Block

Chiara Pavone, MD[a], Gemma Pelargonio, MD, PhD[a,b,*]

KEYWORDS

- Atrioventricular block • Reversibility • Bradycardia • Pacemaker implantation

KEY POINTS

- Reversible causes of atrioventricular block should always be taken into account to avoid unnecessary pacemaker implantation.
- The most common causes of reversible atrioventricular blocks include ischemic heart disease, electrolyte imbalances, and medications.
- A watchful waiting approach is suggested owing to the self-limiting nature of most reversible causes of atrioventricular block.
- The recurrence of an atrioventricular block after the resolution of the underlying cause may unmask a preexistent conduction disease.

INTRODUCTION

Atrioventricular (AV) blocks are caused by a variety of conditions, some of which may be potentially reversible. These include medications, electrolyte imbalances and infective, infiltrative or ischemic diseases of the heart. Recognition of such causes is fundamental in the diagnostic workup of AV blocks, since reversibility of the block does not have indication for pacemaker (PM) implantation.

According to the 2018 American Heart Association guidelines,[1] patients with an acute AV block attributable to a known reversible and nonrecurrent cause, who had complete resolution of the AV block with treatment of the underlying cause, should not receive permanent pacing (class III indication). It is, therefore, of major importance to recognize such forms, because appropriate medical therapy of the underlying cause may avoid the need for permanent pacing and its associated risks.[2]

Block reversibility can, however, be transient and disease recurrence and progression may pose an indication for PM implantation. Patient follow-up is necessary to evaluate disease progression.

EPIDEMIOLOGY

The prevalence of AV block depends mainly on its degree of presentation. First-degree AV blocks can be seen in about 2.1% of the population and, of these, about 30% resolve spontaneously. Mobitz I second-degree AV block is seen in 1% to 2% of the population, whereas Mobitz II is rarer (0.003%). Third-degree block affects 0.03% of the population and its presence generally suggests an underlying structural heart disease.[3]

AV block-related bradycardia can be either symptomatic or asymptomatic. Symptomatic bradycardia is an indication for PM implantation, so the detection of potentially reversible causes of AV block is strongly suggested.

MANAGEMENT

The management of AV blocks focuses on patient stabilization and the resolution of reversible causes.

Symptomatic bradycardia associated with hemodynamic instability should be treated with atropine, which can improve AV conduction, increase

This article originally appeared in *Cardiac Electrophysiology Clinics*, Volume 13 Issue 4, December 2021.
[a] Cardiovascular Sciences Department, Fondazione Policlinico Universitario Agostino Gemelli IRCCS, Largo Agostino Gemelli 8, Rome, Italy; [b] Cardiology Institute, Catholic University of the Sacred Heart, Rome, Italy
* Corresponding author. Cardiovascular Sciences Department, Fondazione Policlinico Universitario Agostino Gemelli IRCCS, Largo Agostino Gemelli 8, Rome, Italy.
E-mail address: gemma.pelargonio@policlinicogemelli.it

the ventricular rate, and lead to symptom improvement. Second-line drugs for the management of symptomatic bradycardia include isoproterenol, dopamine, dobutamine, and epinephrine. It is important to note that blocks that take place below the AV node, that is, within the His–Purkinje system, are worsened by an increasing atrial rate and must be suspected when faced with a patient whose clinical condition deteriorates after the administration of atropine or dobutamine.

In cases refractory to medical therapy, temporary pacing can be used as bridge to resolution of the AV block or PM implantation. Temporary pacing can be either transcutaneous or transvenous, although the latter is burdened with high rates of complications and lead dislodgment.[4]

AV block reversibility depends on the resolution of the underlying cause. These causes are most commonly ischemic heart disease, drug-related AV block, and infection.

ISCHEMIC DISEASE

Approximately 40% of all AV blocks are caused by ischemic heart disease.[5] An AV block of varying degree may develop in the context of both acute and chronic ischemic heart disease, with high degree AV block rates varying between 2.7% and 14.0%.[6] The incidences are higher in inferoposterior lesions compared with anterior ischemia.[7] Although less common, conduction blocks in the setting of anterior myocardial infarction are associated with a worse prognosis. In general, ischemia-associated AV blocks, especially high degree blocks, increase morbidity and mortality rates.[8,9]

Two main mechanisms are implied in ischemic AV blocks. On one hand, an ischemic insult to the myocardium causes an increase in vagal tone, which can contribute to the bradyarrhythmia. On the other hand, decreased perfusion of the AV node may transiently decrease its conduction capacity, thus resulting in a conduction block.[10]

The blood supply to the AV node is highly variable,[11] with the right coronary artery being the main arterial source in the majority of the population (90%). Alternatively, the AV nodal branch may arise either from the left circumflex artery or from penetrating branches of the left anterior descending artery. If the ischemic insult is distal to the AV node, patients might develop a block within the His–Purkinje system. The latter presents on the electrocardiogram (ECG) as a Mobitz type II second-degree AV block, sometimes associated to right and/or left bundle branch blocks. Such infra-Hisian blocks must be closely monitored, because they carry a high risk of progression to complete heart block.

Revascularization can reverse AV block rapidly in the majority of patients. Accordingly, the current American Heart Association guidelines suggest to wait at least 72 hours after revascularization before implanting a permanent PM. Although almost all high-grade AV blocks in the setting of an acute myocardial infarction may be reversible, non–myocardial infarction presentations, such as stable or unstable angina, have lower reversibility rates,[12] probably owing to the long-term establishment of fibrosis in the nodal area.

DRUGS

Although the real incidence of drug-related AV blocks is unknown, they represent an important cause of potentially reversible conduction blocks and must be always excluded. Patients must be interrogated regarding prescription drugs or possible suicidal attempts by drug ingestion. The mainstay of therapy in all drug-induced blocks is the suspension of the culprit drug and, when possible, the administration of an antidote. Decreasing drug absorption through activated charcoal or gastric lavage may sometimes be necessary. The most commonly involved drugs are beta blockers, followed by digoxin. Others include calcium channel blockers, benzodiazepines, and antiarrhythmic medications.[13]

The reversibility of the block varies greatly between patients and up to 50% will need a permanent PM, because drug-related AV block may unmask a preexistent underlying conduction disorder.[14] The use of drugs that act on the AV node should be evaluated carefully in patients with conduction abnormalities, especially when used in combination. PR interval prolongation should be monitored during treatment or, if such drugs are strictly necessary for the survival of the patient, permanent PM implantation can be taken into account.

Discontinuation of the culprit drug may reverse the AV block in 41% to 72% of patients. However, 27% to 56% of patients suffer AV block recurrence and may need permanent PM implantation.[13,15]

Drugs slow down AV nodal conduction through various mechanisms, which may sometimes coexist within the same drug. These act by:

1. Decreasing adrenergic tone, such as beta blockers, calcium channel blockers, or anesthetics (propofol);
2. Increasing parasympathetic tone, such as digoxin or acetylcholinesterase inhibitors;
3. Inhibiting AV node conduction, such as antiarrhythmics;

4. Inhibiting either calcium or sodium currents, both implicated in the conduction velocity of the AV node, such as antidepressants; and
5. Increasing adenosine levels, which inhibits node function, such as dipyridamole.

The main drugs involved in the pathogenesis of AV blocks are listed in **Table 1**.

Beta Blockers and Calcium Channel Blockers

Beta blockers are the most commonly involved drugs in the pathogenesis of AV blocks. Both oral and topic formulations, such as timolol eye drops for the treatment of glaucoma, can be implied.[16] Beta blockers and calcium channel blockers act by decreasing adrenal tone, which causes a decrease in automaticity in the sinoatrial node and conduction velocity in the AV node. The use of selective beta blockers such as metoprolol has been associated with less reversibility and higher permanent pacing rates compared with nonselective beta blockers.[13]

Beta blocker and calcium channel blocker overdose must be promptly treated by interrupting the culprit drug and administering an intravenous bolus of 3 to 10 mg of glucagon, followed by continuous infusion (2–5 mg/h). High-dose insulin (1 U/kg bolus and infusion at 0.5 mg/kg/h) has shown a positive effect on heart rate and a reduction in mortality.[17]

The use of intravenous calcium is suggested in the setting of symptomatic bradycardia caused by calcium channel blocker overdose.

Digoxin

Digoxin is commonly used for the treatment of atrial fibrillation and heart failure. It acts by increasing calcium availability in the myocardiocyte, thereby improving heart contractility, and by increasing parasympathetic tone. Digoxin has a very narrow therapeutic window and its levels should be monitored, especially in patients with advanced age, renal failure, and metabolic disorders. Blood digoxin levels must be kept between 0.8 and 2.0 ng/mL. Digoxin levels higher than 4 ng/mL are associated with severe side effects and increased mortality.[18]

The signs and symptoms of digitalis toxicity include hyperkalemia, AV blocks, and life-threatening ventricular tachyarrhythmias. Digoxin intoxication may also lead to accelerated junctional rhythms, characterized by a ventricular rate of 60 to 100 bpm. The first step in the management of digitalis intoxication is the correction of hyperkalemia, which sometimes requires the use of dialysis.

The use of digoxin-specific antibody (Fab) has shown benefits in the treatment of severe digitalis intoxication. Its dosage depends on the amount of digoxin ingested by the patient and its action is fast, with 80% to 90% of patients showing symptom improvement in less than 1 hour.[19]

Other Substances

Benzodiazepines may induce AV blocks by altering the L-type calcium current. Flumazenil can be useful in the management of patients with benzodiazepine overdose.[20]

The cardiotoxic effects of cocaine are well-established. Its consumption is related to increased risk of myocardial ischemia, which can be caused by a variety of mechanisms, including depression of myocardial contractility, myocardial inflammation and increased platelet aggregation.[21] Cocaine inhibits cardiac sodium channels and may cause AV blocks of varying degree, which are normally self-limiting and can be managed conservatively by waiting.[22]

Acute consumption of excessive amounts of alcohol can cause blocks in calcium and sodium currents, thereby leading to transient and reversible AV blocks. Patients normally spontaneously revert to sinus rhythm upon becoming sober.[23]

Table 1
Drugs implied in the pathogenesis of atrioventricular blocks

Antihypertensives	Antiarrhythmics	SNC Drugs	Toxic Agents
Beta blockers (systemic and topical)	Adenosine	Benzodiazepines	Cocaine
Calcium channel blockers	Digoxin	Tricyclic antidepressants	Alcohol
Clonidine	Class Ic: Flecainide, propafenone	Antipsychotic medications	Organophosphates
	Class III: Amiodarone, dronaderone, sotalol	Acetylcholinesterase inhibitors Anesthetics	Traditional medicine

Organophosphates are commonly used as insecticides owing to their cholinergic activity. Acute organophosphate intoxication can manifest as a variety of cardiac conduction abnormalities, ranging from sinus bradycardia to ventricular arrhythmias. There have been reports of complete AV blocks arising several hours after organophosphate intoxication; therefore, extended ECG monitoring is suggested in the management of these patients.[24] Atropine can be used to reverse organophosphate poisoning.

Other less common substances that may cause AV blocks include Chinese herbal remedies, such as aconite,[25] and indigenous medicines, such as "mad honey," which is produced from flowers of the *Rhododendron* genus.[26]

ELECTROLYTE ALTERATIONS

Electrolytes play an important role in the heart's conduction system. Hyperkalemia, hypermagnesemia, and hyponatremia are the most commonly involved electrolyte imbalances in the formation of AV blocks. An arterial blood gas analysis should be performed in all patients with a new-onset AV block.

Hyperkalemia

High serum potassium levels (>6.5 mEq/L) cause a variety of conduction defects, which can eventually lead, in later stages, to an AV block.[27] ECG abnormalities suggestive of hyperkalemia include peaked T waves, QT shortening, and other nonspecific conduction defects. Hyperkalemia must be suspected as the underlying cause, especially in patients with renal failure or in patients taking potassium-sparing diuretics, potassium supplements, and drugs acting on the renin–angiotensin–aldosterone system, such as angiotensin-converting enzyme inhibitors and sartans. Hyperkalemia-related AV blocks generally resolve with the correction of potassium levels.

Severe hyperkalemia must be corrected by administering:

- 10% calcium gluconate (10 mL), and
- Insulin (10 U bolus) and 5% dextrose (50 mL bolus).

Lower potassium levels can be managed by giving oral or rectal polystyrene sulfonate (Kayexalate).

Hypermagnesemia

Hypermagnesemia (serum magnesium of >2 mEq/L) can be caused by renal insufficiency, hemolysis, adrenal insufficiency, and lithium intoxication. Magnesium acts as a calcium antagonist; therefore, its excess in the serum may result in reversible cardiac conduction delays and AV blocks. Severe hypermagnesemia is managed with hemodialysis and intravenous calcium gluconate.

INCREASED VAGAL TONE

As stated elsewhere in this article, an increased parasympathetic tone results in a lower velocity of the electrical impulse through the AV node, so people with increased vagal tone are at higher risk of AV block. It is a benign phenomenon, normally transient, but can often recur. It can be either symptomatic or asymptomatic. A simultaneous slowing of the sinoatrial node rate may help us in differentiating vagally mediated AV blocks and intrinsic conduction abnormalities. Some triggering events for vagally mediated AV blocks include carotid sinus massage, tilt-induced syncope, swallowing or cough syncope, or acute reversible events like painful stimuli.

Highly trained athletes are known to be prone to both sinus bradycardia and AV conduction abnormalities. It was historically thought that an increased vagal tone was the sole entity responsible for such bradyarrhythmias. However, recent studies showed that, in the absence of parasympathetic stimulation, the sinus rate and the AV node conduction velocity are intrinsically slower in athletes compared with untrained individuals.[28]

An asymptomatic first-degree AV block is a common finding in such individuals, whereas higher degree AV blocks are rarer, with the degree of presentation being closely related to exercise intensity.[29] Because such changes are worsened during vagal-predominant states (ie, rest), blocks of varying degree have been shown to completely resolve with exercise testing and reappear after exercise interruption. In fact, during exercise, sympathetic activation temporarily reverses the vagal tone-associated block, which then quickly reappears with exercise termination.[30,31] Athlete detraining could be helpful in decreasing the basal vagal tone.

Patients with obstructive sleep apnea syndrome are at higher risk of bradycardia compared with the general population. Both sinus arrest and AV blocks have been documented in up to 50% of patients with obstructive sleep apnea syndrome.[32] Heart block is correlated with increased mortality in this population. Recurrent acute AV blocks can be reversed by administering nasal continuous positive airway pressure therapy.[33]

INFECTIOUS CAUSES

An infectious cause must be investigated in all patients presenting with an AV block. Several infective agents may cause conduction abnormalities, either through direct infection of the myocardium or via a local or systemic inflammatory process. The most commonly implied organisms are *Borrelia burgdorferi*, group A streptococcus, in the setting of acute rheumatic fever, Chagas disease, and others. Fever, c-reactive protein (CRP), procalcitonin, and other acute phase reactants can guide the suspicion toward an infective cause.

Arrhythmias are a common complication of myocardial inflammation. AV blocks can be found in around 1.7% of patients with myocarditis. The presence of high-degree AV blocks in myocarditis has been linked with a worse prognosis and increased mortality.[34]

Although the pathophysiological mechanism linking myocarditis and conduction abnormalities has not yet been fully elucidated, it is thought that the extent of myocardial edema, which can be evaluated through cardiac MRI, can correlate with both the type of presenting arrhythmia and its severity.

Lyme Disease

Lyme disease is caused by the spirochete *Borrelia Burgdorferi* and can be transmitted by the bite of an *Ixodes* tick. Its prevalence is characterized by a particular geographic distribution and its incidence is highest during the summer months. Lyme borreliosis is most commonly seen in forested areas, especially in North America (United States and Canada), in Scandinavia, and in middle-European countries, such as Germany or Austria.

The disease is characterized by 3 distinct phases with worsening clinical features. Cardiac involvement may appear during the second stage of the disease, 1 month after the tick bite or 2 to 5 weeks after the typical target-shaped rash. Lyme carditis affects up to 10% of patients, and prevalence is higher in men (3:1).[35] The most common cardiac presentations include AV block of varying degree, myopericarditis, and other less specific conduction delays. The characteristic AV block is normally self-limited and rarely requires permanent pacing, with most cases of high degree AV block resolving completely within 1 to 6 weeks. Lyme-related AV block must be suspected in all patients who live in or have visited endemic areas. The diagnosis is made through serology.[36]

Myocardial invasion by spirochetes leads to the formation of an inflammatory cell infiltrate (first macrophages and then lymphocytes), with a peculiar band-like pattern. This event can be followed by myocardial necrosis and fibrosis, which can lead to conduction abnormalities.[37]

Although no prophylactic antibiotic regimens have been shown to decrease the incidence of Lyme carditis in infected patients, current suggested antibiotic regimens for the treatment of Lyme disease include oral amoxicillin or doxycycline for mild presentations (ie, first-degree AV blocks), whereas higher degree AV blocks and other risk factors require hospitalization and intravenous ceftriaxone.

Corticosteroids or nonsteroidal anti-inflammatory drugs can help in the treatment of conduction abnormalities that do not resolve within 24 to 48 hours of antibiotic therapy.[38]

Rheumatic Fever

Rheumatic fever is a complication of group A streptococcus pharyngotonsillitis, which mainly affects the pediatric population. It can lead to a variety of symptoms, including arthritis, cardiac involvement, subcutaneous nodules, erythema marginatum, and Sydenham's chorea. An anti-streptolysin O titer is used to determine whether a patient has had a recent group A streptococcus infection.

Cardiac involvement typically takes place after multiple attacks of acute rheumatic fever, but it can also occur after the first event. Rheumatic heart disease is caused by an autoimmune process mediated by T cells, probably secondary to molecular mimicry mechanisms, and fibrinous repair of the inflammatory foci.[39] All 3 layers of the heart can be affected and, although valve endocarditis is the most typical presentation, conduction abnormalities are not uncommon.

First-degree AV block is one of the minor diagnostic criteria for the diagnosis of rheumatic fever and can be found in about 72% of patients.[40] Higher degree blocks are less common, with incidence rates ranging from 1.6% for second-degree blocks to 0.6% for complete heart blocks.[41] The duration of the heart block ranges from a few minutes to a few weeks. Treatment is based on penicillin and high-dose aspirin and, although presentation is variable, conduction abnormalities of all degrees are typically self-limiting and resolve spontaneously within few weeks.[42]

ENDOCARDITIS

Infective endocarditis is an inflammatory process involving the cardiac valves. Most cases of infective endocarditis are of bacterial origin, with *Staphylococcus aureus* being the most common causative organism. With the involvement of the periannular space, either owing to the formation of a periannular abscess or of a particularly large vegetation, the heart's conduction system can be affected, thus leading to the formation of an AV block.[43,44]

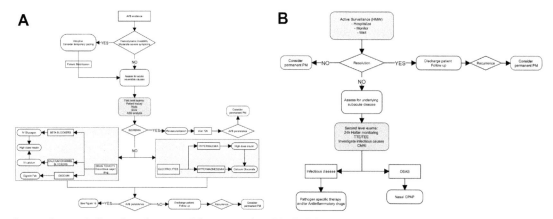

Fig. 1. Diagnostic flowchart for reversible causes of AV block. (*A*) Acute management of patients with AV blocks. (*B*) Management of AV blocks following patient stabilization. ABG, arterial blood gas; AVB, AV block; CMRI, cardiac magnetic resonance imaging; CPAP, continuous positive airway pressure; Fab, Digoxin specific antibody; HMW, Hospitalize, monitor, wait; OSAS, obstructive sleep apnea syndrome; TEE, transesophageal echocardiogram; TTE, transthoracic echocardiogram.

Duke's criteria are used in clinical practice for the diagnosis of infective endocarditis and transthoracic or transesophageal echocardiography can be useful in detecting large vegetations.

Antibiotic therapy is chosen based on the results of the culture and antibiogram and should not last less than 6 weeks. Particularly large valve vegetations may require surgery. There have been reports of AV block reversal following surgical removal of a vegetation.

HYPOTHERMIA

Extremely low body temperatures are associated to a variety of presentations. ECG findings include the presence of a prominent J (Osborn) wave and an array of arrhythmic presentations, including AV block of varying nature. The resolution of all rhythm abnormalities is typically seen after body temperature normalization, which can be done either through external or internal rewarming.

TRAUMA

According to a multicentric study by Yıldız and colleagues,[45] only 4 of 253 patients presenting with AV block were due to trauma. Blunt chest trauma can cause temporary conduction defects, which can present as AV blocks of varying nature and are normally self-limited.

FINAL CONCLUSIONS: WAITING IS KEY

AV blocks of varying degree are often caused by a range of acquired reversible conditions. These must be always kept in mind to identify who can benefit from permanent PM implantation and who can be managed conservatively. Careful patient selection for permanent pacing is mandatory to decrease both the risks associated to life-long device use and the relative costs. **Fig. 1** summarizes a stepwise approach toward possible reversible causes of AV block and their management.

AV block persistence despite reversal of the cause is an indicator of underlying conduction disorders and these patients may require permanent pacing owing to higher recurrence rates. However, because such conditions are often self-limiting, if the clinical conditions of the patient allow for it, a watchful waiting approach can be used for a good part of the population.

CLINICS CARE POINTS

- Temporary support measures (eg, atropine, dobutamine or transcutaneous pacing) can help manage symptomatic AV blocks while investigating for reversible causes.

- The worsening of clinical conditions after atropine administration should raise suspicion of lower blocks within the His–Purkinje system.

- Current guidelines suggest to wait for at least 72 hours after revascularization before permanent PM implantation in ischemic patients.

- Culprit drug suspension is the mainstay of drug-induced AV blocks, because some blocks may reverse spontaneously. When available, administer an antidote.

- Exclude electrolyte imbalances and, if present, correct them promptly.

DISCLOSURE

Conflict of interest: Dr C. Pavone has no conflict of interest for this article. Dr G. Pelargonio has no conflict of interest for this article.

REFERENCES

1. Kusumoto FM, Schoenfeld MH, Barrett C, et al. 2018 ACC/AHA/HRS guideline on the evaluation and management of patients with bradycardia and cardiac conduction delay: a report of the American College of Cardiology/American Heart Association Task Force on Clinical Practice Guidelines and the Heart Rhythm Society [published correction appears in J Am Coll Cardiol. 2019 Aug 20;74(7):1016-1018]. J Am Coll Cardiol 2019;74(7):e51–156.

2. Clémenty N, Fernandes J, Carion PL, et al. Pacemaker complications and costs: a nationwide economic study. J Med Econ 2019;22(11):1171–8.

3. Virani SS, Alonso A, Benjamin EJ, et al. Heart disease and stroke statistics-2020 update: a report from the American Heart Association. Circulation 2020;141(9):e139–596.

4. Brignole M, Auricchio A, Baron-Esquivias G, et al. 2013 ESC guidelines on cardiac pacing and cardiac resynchronization therapy: the Task Force on Cardiac Pacing and Resynchronization Therapy of the European Society of Cardiology (ESC). Developed in collaboration with the European Heart Rhythm Association (EHRA). Eur Heart J 2013;34(29): 2281–329.

5. Zoob M, Smith KS. The aetiology of complete heart-block. Br Med J 1963;2(5366):1149–53.

6. Auffret V, Loirat A, Leurent G, et al. High-degree atrioventricular block complicating ST segment elevation myocardial infarction in the contemporary era. Heart 2016;102(1):40–9.

7. Hreybe H, Saba S. Location of acute myocardial infarction and associated arrhythmias and outcome. Clin Cardiol 2009;32(5):274–7.

8. Kim HL, Kim SH, Seo JB, et al. Influence of second- and third-degree heart block on 30-day outcome following acute myocardial infarction in the drug-eluting stent era. Am J Cardiol 2014;114(11): 1658–62.

9. Kosmidou I, Redfors B, Dordi R, et al. Incidence, predictors, and outcomes of high-grade atrioventricular block in patients with ST-segment elevation myocardial infarction undergoing primary percutaneous coronary intervention (from the HORIZONS-AMI trial). Am J Cardiol 2017;119(9):1295–301.

10. Cardoso R, Alfonso CE, Coffey JO. Reversibility of high-grade atrioventricular block with revascularization in coronary artery disease without infarction: a literature review. Case Rep Cardiol 2016;2016: 1971803.

11. Arid JM, Armstrong O, Rogez JM, et al. Arterial vascularisation of the atrioventricular node. Surg Radiol Anat 2000;22(2):93–6.

12. Hwang IC, Seo WW, Oh IY, et al. Reversibility of atrioventricular block according to coronary artery disease: results of a retrospective study. Korean Circ J 2012;42(12):816–22.

13. Tisdale JE, Chung MK, Campbell KB, et al. Drug-induced arrhythmias: a scientific statement from the American Heart Association. Circulation 2020; 142(15):e214–33.

14. Osmonov D, Erdinler I, Ozcan KS, et al. Management of patients with drug-induced atrioventricular block. Pacing Clin Electrophysiol 2012;35(7):804–10.

15. Zeltser D, Justo D, Halkin A, et al. Drug-induced atrioventricular block: prognosis after discontinuation of the culprit drug. J Am Coll Cardiol 2004; 44(1):105–8.

16. Özcan KS, Güngör B, Osmonov D, et al. Management and outcome of topical beta-blocker-induced atrioventricular block. Cardiovasc J Afr 2015;26(6): 210–3.

17. Marino PL, Sutin KM. The ICU book. 3rd edition. Philadelphia: Lippincott Williams & Wilkins; 2007.

18. Supervía Caparrós A, Salgado García E, Calpe Perarnau X, et al. Immediate and 30 days mortality in digoxin poisoning cases attended in the Hospital Emergency Services of Catalonia, Spain. Mortalidad inmediata y a los 30 días en las intoxicaciones digitálicas atendidas en servicios de urgencias de Cataluña. Emergencias 2019;31(1):39–42.

19. Hauptman PJ, Blume SW, Lewis EF, et al. Digoxin toxicity and use of digoxin immune Fab: insights from a national hospital database. JACC Heart Fail 2016;4(5):357–64.

20. Anand K, Kumar M. Benzodiazepine overdose associated atrioventricular block. Anesth Essays Res 2013;7(3):419–20.

21. Kloner RA, Hale S, Alker K, et al. The effects of acute and chronic cocaine use on the heart. Circulation 1992;85(2):407–19.

22. Kariyanna PT, Jayarangaiah A, Al-Sadawi M, et al. A rare case of second degree Mobitz type II AV block associated with cocaine use. Am J Med Case Rep 2018;6(7):146–8.

23. van Stigt AH, Overduin RJ, Staats LC, et al. A heart too drunk to drive; AV block following acute alcohol intoxication. Chin J Physiol 2016;59(1):1–8.

24. Siegal D, Kotowycz MA, Methot M, et al. Complete heart block following intentional carbamate ingestion. Can J Cardiol 2009;25(8):e288–90.

25. Boehm KM, Yum E, Caraccio T. An overdose of aconite by a twenty-six-year-old woman. J Emerg Med 2011;41(3):298.

26. Silici S, Atayoglu AT. Mad honey intoxication: a systematic review on the 1199 cases. Food Chem Toxicol 2015;86:282–90.

27. Wogan JM, Lowenstein SR, Gordon GS. Second-degree atrioventricular block: Mobitz type II. J Emerg Med 1993;11(1):47–54.

28. Guasch E, Mont L. Diagnosis, pathophysiology, and management of exercise-induced arrhythmias. Nat Rev Cardiol 2017;14(2):88–101.

29. Bessem B, De Bruijn MC, Nieuwland W, et al. The electrocardiographic manifestations of athlete's heart and their association with exercise exposure. Eur J Sport Sci 2018;18(4):587–93.

30. Vidal A, Agorrody V, Abreu R, et al. Vagal third-degree atrioventricular block in a highly trained endurance athlete. Europace 2017;19(11):1863.

31. Hernández-Madrid A, Moro C, Marín Huerta E, et al. Third-degree atrioventricular block in an athlete. J Intern Med 1991;229(4):375–6.

32. Tilkian AG, Guilleminault C, Schroeder JS, et al. Sleep-induced apnea syndrome. Prevalence of cardiac arrhythmias and their reversal after tracheostomy. Am J Med 1977;63(3):348–58.

33. Becker H, Brandenburg U, Peter JH, et al. Reversal of sinus arrest and atrioventricular conduction block in patients with sleep apnea during nasal continuous positive airway pressure. Am J Respir Crit Care Med 1995;151(1):215–8.

34. Ogunbayo GO, Elayi SC, Ha LD, et al. Outcomes of heart block in myocarditis: a review of 31,760 patients. Heart Lung Circ 2019;28(2):272–6.

35. Fish AE, Pride YB, Pinto DS. Lyme carditis. Infect Dis Clin North Am 2008;22(2):275–vi.

36. Yeung C, Baranchuk A. Diagnosis and treatment of Lyme carditis: JACC review topic of the week [published correction appears in J Am Coll Cardiol. 2019 Nov 26;74(21):2709-2711]. J Am Coll Cardiol 2019; 73(6):717–26.

37. Montgomery RR, Booth CJ, Wang X, et al. Recruitment of macrophages and polymorphonuclear leukocytes in Lyme carditis. Infect Immun 2007; 75(2):613–20.

38. Wormser GP, Dattwyler RJ, Shapiro ED, et al. The clinical assessment, treatment, and prevention of Lyme disease, human granulocytic anaplasmosis, and babesiosis: clinical practice guidelines by the Infectious Diseases Society of America [published correction appears in Clin Infect Dis. 2007 Oct 1; 45(7):941]. Clin Infect Dis 2006;43(9):1089–134.

39. Kaplan MH, Bolande R, Rakita L, et al. Presence of bound immunoglobulins and complement in the myocardium in acute rheumatic fever. Association with cardiac failure. N Engl J Med 1964;271:637–45.

40. Hubail Z, Ebrahim IM. Advanced heart block in acute rheumatic fever. J Saudi Heart Assoc 2016; 28(2):113–5.

41. Filberbaum MB, Griffith GC, Solley RF, et al. Electrocardiographic abnormalities in 6,000 cases of rheumatic fever. Cal West Med 1946;64(6):340–6.

42. Malik JA, Hassan C, Khan GQ. Transient complete heart block complicating acute rheumatic fever. Indian Heart J 2002;54(1):91–2.

43. Graupner C, Vilacosta I, SanRomán J, et al. Periannular extension of infective endocarditis. J Am Coll Cardiol 2002;39(7):1204–11.

44. Sato M, Harada K, Watanabe T, et al. Right-sided infective endocarditis with coronary sinus vegetation causing complete atrioventricular block. Eur Heart J Cardiovasc Imaging 2020;21(3):345.

45. Şahin Yıldız B, Astarcıoğlu MA, Başkurt Aladağ N, et al. The frequency of type 2 second-degree and third-degree atrioventricular block induced by blunt chest trauma in the emergency department: a multicenter study. Ulus Travma Acil Cerrahi Derg 2015; 21(3):193–6.

Iatrogenic Atrioventricular Block

Christopher C. Cheung, MD, MPH[a], Shumpei Mori, MD, PhD[b],
Edward P. Gerstenfeld, MD, MS[a,*]

KEYWORDS

- Atrioventricular block • Complete heart block • Iatrogenic • Cardiac surgery • Transcatheter valve
- Catheter ablation

KEY POINTS

- Iatrogenic atrioventricular block can occur following cardiac surgery, transcatheter valve implantation, electrophysiologic procedures including catheter ablation of arrhythmias, and other percutaneous procedures.
- In patients undergoing transcatheter aortic valve replacement, predictors of heart block/pacemaker implantation include right bundle branch block, intraprocedural heart block, valve implantation depth, and valve type.
- In patients undergoing catheter ablation of arrhythmias, various strategies (pacing, cryotherapy, ablation from right coronary cusp) can minimize the incidence of inadvertent atrioventricular nodal injury.

INTRODUCTION

Iatrogenic atrioventricular (AV) block can occur in a variety of circumstances associated with cardiac surgical and catheter-based procedures. Specifically, surgical aortic valve and mitral valve repair or replacement carries an increased risk of conduction system injury and iatrogenic AV block due to tissue manipulation in close proximity to the intrinsic conduction system. More recently, transcatheter aortic valve replacement (TAVR) has become increasingly used in the management of aortic valve disease and can be associated with AV block requiring pacemaker implantation. Other cardiac procedures, including catheter ablation of arrhythmias, alcohol septal ablation, and percutaneous closure of ventricular septal defects, are also associated with iatrogenic AV block. In this article, we review the common causes of iatrogenic AV block, their etiology, and general management considerations.

ANATOMY

Iatrogenic AV block typically occurs with tissue manipulation or injury close to the compact AV node and AV conduction axis. When approached from the right atrium, the AV node is located at the apex of the triangle of Koch, defined inferiorly by the coronary sinus, posteriorly by the tendon of Todaro, and anteriorly by the septal tricuspid leaflet (**Fig. 1**). The tendon of Todaro, the thin fibrous structure running within the Eustachian ridge, eventually fuses into the central fibrous body. The AV node is located at the right atrial side of the central fibrous body and is comprised of the compact node and the inferior nodal extensions. The bundle of His, corresponding to the penetrating portion of the AV conduction axis, arises distal to the AV node and penetrates the central fibrous body at the infero-posterior margin of the AV portion of the membranous septum. Then, the AV conduction axis runs along the inferior

This article originally appeared in *Cardiac Electrophysiology Clinics*, Volume 13 Issue 4, December 2021.

[a] Section of Cardiac Electrophysiology, Division of Cardiology, University of California San Francisco, MU-East 4th Floor, 500 Parnassus Avenue, San Francisco, CA 94143, USA; [b] UCLA Cardiac Arrhythmia Center, University of California Los Angeles, Center of the Health Science, #46-131, 650 Charles E. Young Drive South, Los Angeles, CA 90095, USA

* Corresponding author. MUE-4th Floor, 500 Parnassus Avenue, San Francisco, CA 94147.

E-mail address: Edward.gerstenfeld@ucsf.edu

Cardiol Clin 41 (2023) 419–428
https://doi.org/10.1016/j.ccl.2023.03.009

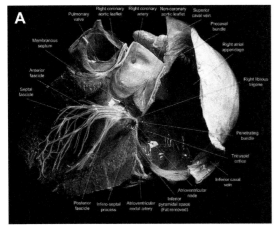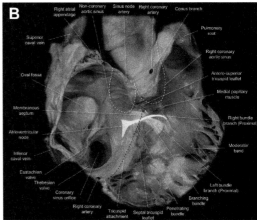

Fig. 1. Illustration of conduction system and surrounding structures from left posterior oblique (*A*) and right anterior oblique projection (*B*). Conduction system and surrounding structures from a left posterior oblique (*A*) and right anterior oblique (*B*) projection. The membranous septum is divided by the attachment of the septal tricuspid leaflet (*black dotted line*) into atrioventricular and interventricular portions (*B*). The oval fossa and the membranous septum are transilluminated separately. (*Courtesy of* UCLA Cardiac Arrhythmia Center, Wallace A. McAlpine MD collection, Los Angeles, CA; with permission)

margin of the membranous septum on the crest of the ventricular septum. The branching portion of the AV conduction axis gives rise to wide proximal left bundle branch before terminal bifurcation (pseudo-bifurcation) of the proximal right bundle branch. This wide branching portion is commonly found at the septal attachment of the septal tricuspid leaflet or proximal part of the interventricular portion of the membranous septum. The membranous septum is commonly located beneath the interleaflet triangle between the noncoronary and right coronary aortic sinuses. Therefore, the membranous septum is one of the fibrous components of the left ventricular outflow tract and deemed as a part of the central fibrous body with the right fibrous trigone, which anchors the medial part of the anterior mitral leaflet. The right fibrous trigone and its left-sided counterpart are key structures that allow fixation of a mitral annuloplasty ring or prosthesis into the medial part of mitral annulus during mitral valve surgery. Together, the proximity of the aortic root, left ventricular outflow tract, central fibrous body, and components of the triangle of Koch leads to a higher risk of injury or iatrogenic AV block with various cardiac surgical and catheter-based procedures.

CARDIAC SURGERY

AV block has been reported in various cardiac surgical procedures associated with tissue manipulation near sites of the intrinsic conduction system. Early reports over 4 decades prior reported the occurrence of heart block primarily after surgical aortic valve replacement.[1] Conduction distal to the penetrating bundle of His, corresponding to the nonbranching and branching bundles, is located at the inferior margin of the membranous septum and anatomically close to the septal base of the aortic root (see **Fig. 1**). Accordingly, aortic valve surgery may cause infra-Hisian AV block rather than intra-Hisian or nodal AV block.[2] In a previous report of 261 patients undergoing isolated aortic valve replacement, permanent pacemaker (PPM) implantation was required in 3% of patients, occurring both in patients with and without underlying conduction disease.[3] Recent reports have continued to identify a small but significant risk of iatrogenic AV block. In a European study of 159 patients undergoing isolated aortic valve replacement, PPM implantation was required in 6.9% of patients after prolonged periods of complete heart block lasting 7 days postoperatively.[4]

Patients undergoing mitral or tricuspid valve surgery, including valve replacement or repair, are also at risk for iatrogenic AV block. In a cohort of 391 patients undergoing mitral valve replacement or ring annuloplasty and without preoperative AV block, Berdajs and colleagues[5] reported any postoperative heart block (defined as first-, second-, and third-degree AV block) in up to 24% of patients. Complete heart block occurred in 4% of patients, with subsequent PPM implantation after a median of 4 days. In a recent cohort of 505 patients undergoing tricuspid valve surgery, 2.8% of patients developed postoperative complete heart block and underwent PPM implantation.[6]

Anatomically, the medial part of the anterior mitral leaflet/aortic-mitral continuity is fixed to the central fibrous body through the right fibrous trigone, with the infero-apical point of the right fibrous trigone corresponding to the infero-septal commissure of the mitral valve. The compact AV node is generally located at the right atrial aspect of the central fibrous body, posteroinferior to the membranous septum. Thus, surgical manipulation of the medial aspect of the anterior mitral leaflet, around the central fibrous body, carries a risk of damaging the compact AV node itself or penetrating bundle of His, to produce nodal or intra-Hisian block, respectively. Injury to the AV nodal artery may also occur within the inferior pyramidal space,[7] which contains the AV nodal artery.[8]

Notably, patients with endocarditis have a much higher rate of heart block requiring PPM implantation. This is typically due to the development of an aortic root abscess in close proximity to the conduction system. In previous reports of patients with aortic valve endocarditis undergoing valve replacement, complete heart block was present in up to 10% of patients.[9,10] In cases of tricuspid valve endocarditis, cohorts have reported up to one-third of patients requiring PPM implantation, as the tricuspid valve itself serves as a border of the triangle of Koch.[6]

Notably, patients with endocarditis have a much higher rate of heart block requiring PPM implantation. This is typically due to the development of an aortic root abscess in close proximity to the conduction system. In previous reports of patients with aortic valve endocarditis undergoing valve replacement, complete heart block was present in up to 10% of patients.[9,10] In cases of tricuspid valve endocarditis, cohorts have reported up to one-third of patients requiring PPM implantation, as the tricuspid valve itself serves as a border of the triangle of Koch.[6]

Predictors of Pacemaker Implantation

In a retrospective analysis of 1234 patients undergoing cardiac surgery without prior cardiac devices or indications for pacemaker or defibrillator, 1.6% of patients underwent PPM implantation in the postoperative period.[11] PPM implantation was most commonly performed for complete heart block (70%), with predictors of PPM requirement including left bundle branch block (LBBB), reoperation, and pulmonary hypertension.[11] In a retrospective analysis of 2446 cardiac surgeries in New Zealand, postoperative PPM implantation occurred in 4% of patients, with AV block on the preoperative electrocardiography (ECG; defined as first-degree or second-degree Mobitz type 1

AV block, and left or right bundle branch or bifascicular block, odds ratio [OR] 1.65, 95% confidence interval [CI] 1.08 to 2.53) and the type of surgery (valve surgery; OR 5.2, 95% CI 2.47–10.9) independently predictive of postoperative PPM implantation.[12]

In a large analysis of 77,882 patients undergoing aortic or mitral valve surgery in the United States between 1996 and 2014, the 1-year PPM implantation rate was 4.5% after mitral valve repair, 6.6% after aortic valve replacement, 9.3% after aortic valve replacement and mitral valve repair, 10.5% after mitral valve replacement, and 13.3% after aortic valve and mitral valve replacement. Most PPM implantations (80%) occurred during the index hospitalization. Older age, arrhythmia history, preoperative conduction disturbance, and concomitant surgical procedures were the strongest predictors for PPM implantation during the index hospitalization.[13]

Management Considerations

Complete heart block occurring early in the postoperative period may be due to multiple factors, including direct tissue injury, inflammation, or edema. Heart block or conduction delay due to tissue inflammation and edema may resolve with continued observation, and early PPM implantation may lead to excessive PPM implantation rates. In a retrospective study of 301 patients receiving PPM after cardiac surgery, late AV conduction recovery (defined as ventricular pacing <10% more than 1 month after implant placement) occurred in 12% of patients.[14] Female sex and transient presence of AV conduction postoperatively were independent predictors for conduction recovery.[14] In a systematic review of 10 studies evaluating PPM dependency or AV node recovery after cardiac surgery, pacemaker-dependency and AV node recovery occurred in 32% to 91% and 16% to 42% of patients, respectively.[15] Although there are no predictors of dependency/ recovery that were consistent across studies, it is reasonable to use a "watch-and-wait" strategy during the early postoperative period, particularly in cases where conduction system recovery might be anticipated. At some point, the cost of prolonged hospitalization must be weighed against the cost and long-term risk of PPM implantation.

In the 2018 American College of Cardiology (ACC)/American Heart Association (AHA)/Heart Rhythm Society (HRS) guideline on the evaluation and management of patients with bradycardia and cardiac conduction delay, PPM implantation is recommended before discharge in cases of postoperative AV block with persistent symptoms or hemodynamic instability (class 1 recommendation).[16] Although the timing of PPM implantation is likely to vary by the individual clinical situation, it is suggested that waiting 3 to 5 days after surgery for potential conduction system recovery is reasonable. Similarly, after mitral valve surgery, the ACC/AHA/HRS guidelines recommend PPM implantation before discharge in cases of new postoperative AV block with persistent symptoms or hemodynamic instability (class 1 recommendation), and after a 5- to 7-day waiting period after surgery.[16] A similar recommendation is also made for PPM implantation after tricuspid valve surgery (3–5 days). The risk of PPM implantation and suggested waiting period for resolution of AV block after various procedures is summarized in **Table 1**.

TRANSCATHETER AORTIC VALVE REPLACEMENT

TAVR is increasingly pursued in the management of aortic valve disease (severe aortic stenosis), particularly in patients at intermediate or high risk for cardiac surgical complications. Inadvertent conduction system injury can occur during TAVR. In the recent years, multiple studies have evaluated an array of transcatheter valve types, including both balloon-expandable (Edwards SAPIEN) and various self-expanding transcatheter valves. In the Placement of Aortic Transcatheter Valves (PARTNER) trial evaluating TAVR in patients with severe aortic stenosis who could not undergo surgery, 358 patients were randomized to TAVR versus standard care. Among 179 patients undergoing transcatheter implantation of an Edwards SAPIEN valve, PPM implantation rates were 3.4% at 30 days after TAVR, with no significant increase in PPM rates compared to standard care.[17] Similarly, in the PARTNER-2 trial, 2032 patients with severe aortic stenosis were randomized to transcatheter versus surgical aortic valve replacement. PPM implantation occurred at similar rates in both groups, with 8.5% of transcatheter and 6.9% of surgical patients undergoing device implantation within 30 days.[18]

Self-expanding valves appear to have a higher rate of PPM implantation after TAVR, potentially due to the deeper implantation depth and progressive radial force delivered by the self-expanding mechanism. In the U.S. CoreValve study, 795 patients with severe aortic stenosis were randomized to a self-expanding transcatheter valve (CoreValve) versus surgical aortic valve replacement. TAVR was associated with a PPM implantation rate of 19.8% versus 7.1% in the surgical group in the CoreValve study.[19] In a recent trial comparing the self-expanding valve to surgical valve replacement in patients at low surgical risk, patients undergoing TAVR received either the CoreValve (Medtronic; Minneapolis, MN), Evolut R

Table 1
Type of procedure and risk of permanent pacemaker implantation

Type of Procedure	Risk for PPM Implantation	Duration of Monitoring
Aortic valve surgery	3%–8.5%	3–5 d
Mitral valve surgery	1%–9%	5–7 d
Tricuspid valve surgery	2.3%–22%	3–5 d
Coronary artery bypass	2%–58%[a]	5–7 d
Transcatheter aortic valve replacement	2%–51% (by valve type)	1–2 d[b]
Catheter ablation of AV nodal re-entrant tachycardia	0.2%–2.3%	n/a
Catheter ablation of para-septal accessory pathway, atrial tachycardia, or premature ventricular complex	~2%	n/a
Alcohol septal ablation or surgical myomectomy	9%–14%	2–7 d[c]
Percutaneous ventricular septal defect closure	2%	n/a

Duration of monitoring prior to PPM implantation as per 2018 ACC/AHA/HRS guidelines and 2019 Journal of American College of Cardiology Scientific Expert Panel for conduction disturbances associated with TAVR.

[a] A wide range of conduction defects have been reported after coronary artery bypass surgery, likely due to a combination of degenerative disease of the heart, conduction system injury, or myocardial ischemia.

[b] Post-TAVR monitoring dependent on underlying risk factors (see Risk Groups in **Fig. 2**).

[c] Protocols for PPM implantation varied, but generally PPM was implanted when complete AV block was present for >24 h (although timing of actual implant was 2–7 d).

(Medtronic; Minneapolis, MN), or Evolut PRO (Medtronic; Minneapolis, MN) self-expanding, supraannular bioprosthesis. PPM implantation continued to occur frequently in 17% of patients undergoing TAVR.[20] In a study of 120 patients receiving the Lotus transcatheter valve system (Boston Scientific; Marlborough, MA), up to 29% underwent PPM implantation.[21] Similarly, in a study of 100 patients receiving the Direct Flow Medical transcatheter valve system (Direct Flow Medical Inc.; Santa Rosa, CA), PPM implantation occurred in 17% of patients.[22] In a European registry of 1000 patients receiving the self-expanding ACURATE neo transcatheter valve (Boston Scientific; Marlborough, MA), new PPM implantation occurred in 8.3% of patients.[23]

Predictors of Pacemaker Implantation

Similar to surgical aortic valve replacement, conduction system injury and subsequent PPM implantation is due to the close proximity of the bottom of the aortic root (virtual basal ring) to the conduction system (see **Fig. 1**A). Previous studies have reported the length of the membranous septum to be a surrogate for the distance between the aortic valve annulus and the bundle of His/conduction system. In a study of 73 patients undergoing TAVR and 29% receiving PPM, Hamdan and colleagues[24] identified the membranous septum length to be an independent predictor of high-degree AV block (OR 1.35, 95% CI 1.1–1.7) and subsequent PPM implantation (OR 1.43, 95% CI 1.1–1.8). When accounting for procedural characteristics, the difference between the membranous septum length and implantation depth was the strongest predictor for AV block (OR 1.4, 95% CI 1.2–1.7).[24] However, further studies have found that there can be substantial variation in aortic root anatomy, particularly in the location of the membranous septum relative to the virtual basal ring.[25,26] As such, PPM implantation may be dependent on the relationship between the implantation depth and the distance from the virtual basal ring to the inferior margin of the membranous septum, irrespective of membranous septum length itself.[25,26]

Preprocedural right bundle branch block (RBBB) is also a strong predictor of PPM implantation, as the TAVR prosthesis itself impinges on the proximal left bundle. In an analysis of 80 patients undergoing TAVR, preprocedural RBBB and prothesis type were both independently associated with the need for PPM implantation.[27] In a registry of 240 patients who received the Edwards SAPIEN transcatheter valve, 15% underwent PPM implantation, preprocedural RBBB, short membranous septum

length, and noncoronary cusp device-landing zone calcium volume together were strong predictors of PPM implantation (C-statistic 0.92, sensitivity 94%, specificity 84%).[28]

Patients undergoing TAVR may also develop progressive conduction block during the early postprocedural period. In a large observational study of 1064 patients undergoing TAVR in Switzerland, periprocedural high-degree AV block occurred in 9% of patients and delayed AV block in 7% of patients up to 8 days after the procedure. Delayed high-degree AV block occurred more commonly in men (OR 2.4, 95% CI 1.3–4.5) and in patients with conduction disorders after TAVR (OR 10.8, 95% CI 4.6–25.5).[29] Patients without conduction disturbances or with a stable ECG for 2 days or more did not develop delayed AV block.[29] In a meta-analysis of 17 studies and 11,788 patients, new-onset LBBB after TAVR was associated with a high risk of PPM implantation (risk ratio 2.18, 95% CI 1.28 to 3.70), and also cardiac death. However, periprocedural PPM implantation itself was not associated with all-cause mortality.[30]

In a single-center analysis of 467 patients undergoing self-expandable, mechanical, and balloon-expandable TAVR, high-grade conduction block developed in 14% of patients with a PR interval >240 msec and QRS duration $\geq$150 msec.[31] There were no episodes of high-grade conduction block in patients with a PR interval less than 200 msec and QRS duration less than 120 msec.[31] In an post-TAVR analysis of 611 patients excluding patients who had a PPM or received a PPM within 48 hours, 8.8% patients developed conduction block requiring PPM implantation 48 hours after TAVR.[32] Patients requiring PPM had PR and QRS prolongation by 40 msec and 22 msec, respectively. Independent predictors for conduction block included baseline RBBB (OR 3.56, 95% CI 1.07–11.77) and PR interval change (OR 1.31 per 10 msec increase, 95% CI 1.18–1.45).[32]

Management Considerations

Consideration for PPM implantation after TAVR must account for the preprocedural patient factors, implantation characteristics (valve positioning, membranous septum), and valve type (balloon-expandable vs self-expanding). Recently, the *Journal of the American College of Cardiology* Scientific Expert panel reviewed the general outline for the management of conduction disturbances after TAVR, dividing patients into 5 groups (**Fig. 2**).[33] Patients without pre-existing RBBB and with no new conduction disturbances (defined as first-degree AV block, RBBB, LBBB, or QRS$\geq$120 msec on ECG after TAVR) are at very

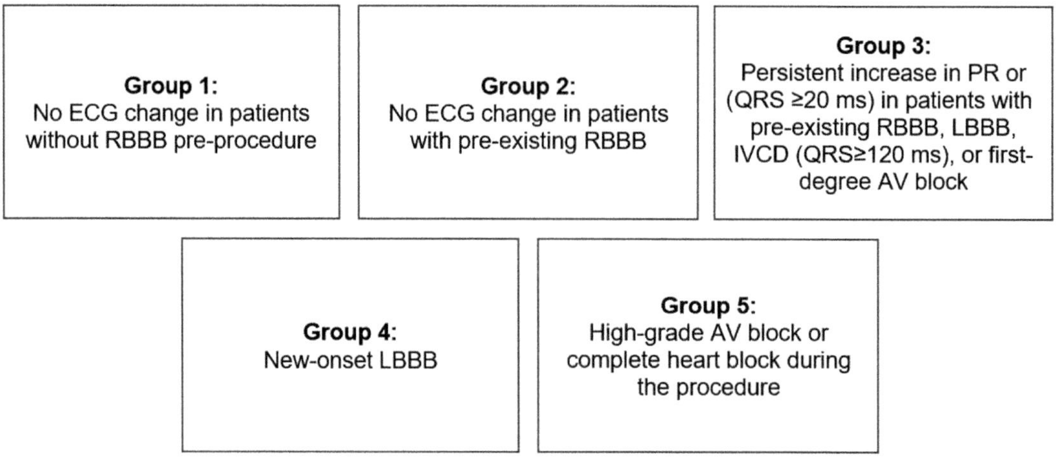

Fig. 2. Risk groups for conduction disturbances after transcatheter aortic valve replacement.

low risk for developing high-grade or complete heart block in the days after TAVR (group 1). Temporary pacing can be discontinued, and a 12-lead ECG can be repeated 24 hours after the procedure, with the patient discharged home if no ECG changes occur. In patients with pre-existing RBBB (group 2), temporary pacing is recommended for 24 hours, followed by repeat ECG for 2 days after TAVR. Patients with ECG changes, including a 20-msec increase in PR interval or QRS duration on ECG (postprocedural, or any day afterward), are considered to be at increased risk (group 3) and should have the temporary pacemaker left in situ for a longer period. Those with progressive ECG changes (continued increase in PR or QRS durations, PR>240 msec, or QRS>150 msec) are considered to be at higher risk for high-grade or complete AV block. Electrophysiologic study and/or pacemaker implantation before hospital discharge is reasonable in these patients. Among patients with new-onset LBBB (group 4) or high-grade or complete AV block during the TAVR procedure (group 5), temporary pacing should be continued during the first 24 hours, with close evaluation for recurrence of complete heart block or progressive conduction changes (PR or QRS duration) to prompt PPM implantation.

CATHETER ABLATION OF ARRHYTHMIAS

Catheter ablation of arrhythmias can result in inadvertent injury of the AV node or His bundle, due to the close proximity of the conduction system to sites of ablation in AV nodal re-entrant tachycardia (AVNRT), septal/paraseptal accessory pathways, paraHisian atrial tachycardia, and para-Hisian premature ventricular complexes.

In the ablation of AVNRT, the slow pathway region, usually corresponding to the rightward inferior nodal extension, is typically located inferiorly to the AV node, within the triangle of Koch (see Fig. 1B). Early studies reported rates of AV node injury requiring PPM implantation in 1.6% to 2.3% of patients.[34] However, contemporary studies have reported a significantly lower rate of AV block associated with slow pathway ablation, potentially related to the use of electroanatomic mapping and the option of cryotherapy ablation. In a retrospective study of 877 patients undergoing AVNRT ablation, AV block requiring pacemaker implantation occurred in 0.4% of patients.[35] Similarly, in a recent multicenter study of 1084 patients undergoing typical and atypical AVNRT radiofrequency ablation, transient and permanent AV block occurred in 0.2% of patients.[36]

Ablation of septal/paraseptal accessory pathways can also be associated with inadvertent AV nodal injury. In a study of 97 patients undergoing superoseptal, mid-paraseptal, and para-Hisian accessory pathway ablation, ablation was successful in 91%, but 2% of patients developed complete AV block requiring PPM implantation.[37] In 2 recent case series (53 and 14 patients, respectively) of mid-paraseptal and para-Hisian pathway ablation, given the availability of cryotherapy ablation or pacing techniques, there were no episodes of complete heart block or PPM implantation.[38,39] Atrial tachycardia may also arise from the para-Hisian region. In a retrospective review of 68 patients with focal atrial tachycardia, the arrhythmia was mapped and ablated in the right atrium, left atrium, and noncoronary cusp. Second- or third-degree AV block occurred in 14% of patients with radiofrequency ablation in the right atrium.[40] Similarly, ablation of premature ventricular complexes originating from the para-Hisian region carries the risk inadvertent conduction system injury.[41,42]

Management Considerations

Strategies to avoid inadvertent AV node injury during ablation include careful mapping from all adjacent structures, ablation from sites less likely to lead to AV block, and use of cryotherapy ablation catheters. Cryotherapy ablation catheters allow for testing of prospective sites using cryothermy (ice mapping), before delivery of the full cryotherapy lesion.[43] Once cryotherapy is initiated, the catheter typically sticks or freezes to the site of ablation, preventing motion and injury of nearby structures. Furthermore, the leading edge of cryotherapy is reversible, and thus, rapid identification of conduction system injury and immediate termination of cryotherapy can avoid sustained injury. Other reports have suggested the use of various pacing maneuvers to differentiate near- and far-field His signals to avoid inadvertent conduction system injury.[38] When mapping para-Hisian tachycardias from the right atrium, it is important to map adjacent structures, including the left atrium and noncoronary sinus of Valsalva, to determine the earliest site before performing ablation (see **Fig. 3**). If the earliest site remains at the right atrial septum, ablation superior (superoseptal) and distal (very small or absent A) to the bundle of His is safer than proximal or mid-paraseptal

ablation below the His bundle, as it is close to the penetrating bundle (bundle of His) and compact AV node, respectively. Furthermore, even if not the earliest signal, ablation from the noncoronary aortic sinus is much less likely to cause AV block as the fibrous trigone protects the penetrating bundle of His.[44,45] Similarly, for para-Hisian premature ventricular complexes, ablation from the right coronary sinus of Valsalva is less likely to cause AV block than ablation from the right side of the ventricular septum. In this setting, however, the ventricular arrhythmia cured from the right coronary aortic sinus itself may reflect that the focus is superior to the AV conduction axis, as shown in **Fig. 1B**.

OTHER PERCUTANEOUS PROCEDURES

Iatrogenic AV block can also be associated with various percutaneous cardiac procedures, including percutaneous alcohol septal ablation for the treatment of hypertrophic cardiomyopathy. In such cases, alcohol infusion into the septal branches of the left anterior descending artery to achieve septal infarction can also injury the right bundle branch and left anterior fascicle. Generally, alcohol septal ablation is associated with a substantially higher rate of complete heart block

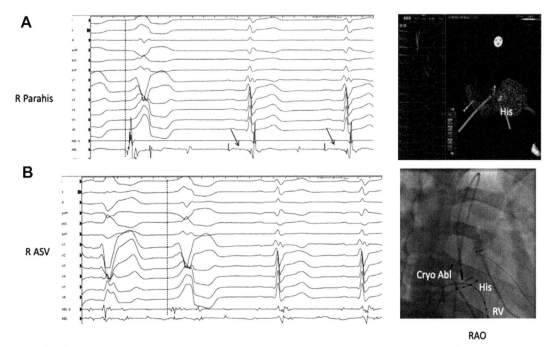

Fig. 3. Electroanatomic mapping of premature ventricular complexes in the para-Hisian region. (*A*) Electroanatomic mapping of a premature ventricular complex identified earliest activation at a para-Hisian site with far-field His signal (*arrow*) present during sinus rhythm. (*B*) Mapping of the aortic sinus by retrograde approach identified an equally early signal, with termination of the premature ventricular complex with cryoablation at this site. Abl, ablation; R ASV, right aortic sinus valve; R Parahis, right para-Hisian.

necessitating pacemaker implantation, approaching 22% in prior studies.[46] A baseline LBBB was the strongest predictor of complete heart block requiring PPM implantation. However, patients after alcohol septal ablation may have transient conduction disturbances due to edema and inflammation. In a study of 172 patients undergoing alcohol septal ablation, 20% of patients developed intraprocedural complete heart block, with 8.7% of patients developing delayed complete heart block within 1 to 6 days after alcohol septal ablation.[47] The ACC/AHA/HRS guidelines recommended PPM implantation before discharge in patients with second-degree Mobitz type II, high-grade, or complete AV block (class 1 recommendation), recognizing that PPM implantation occurred within 2 to 7 days after alcohol septal ablation.[16]

Transcatheter closure of ventricular septal defects has also been associated with reported conduction disease, with RBBB and left anterior hemiblock occurring in a proportion of cases. Complete heart block requiring PPM implantation occurred in the minority of patients (2%).[48]

SUMMARY

Iatrogenic AV block can occasionally occur in the context of cardiac surgical procedures, transcatheter valve procedures, catheter ablation of arrhythmias, and other percutaneous procedures. It is important to appreciate the anatomic proximity of the conduction system to understand the risks for periprocedural complete heart block and subsequent PPM implantation. Similarly, it is also important to recognize the patient, procedural, and anatomic risk factors for conduction system injury. Importantly, delayed conduction block can occur in patients undergoing TAVR, and select patients may benefit from prolonged observation or transvenous pacing. In contrast, patients undergoing valve surgery or transcatheter alcohol septal ablation procedures may have inflammation and edema, with resolution of conduction block during the recovery period.

CLINICS CARE POINTS

- After cardiac surgery, complete heart block can occur early in the post-operative period due to various factors, including direct tissue injury, inflammation, or edema. Although the timing of permanent pacemaker implantation varies according to the individual clinical situation, waiting 3 to 5 days after surgery (or 5 to 7 days after mitral valve surgery) is reasonable.

- In patients undergoing transcatheter aortic valve replacement, predictors of heart block and permanent pacemaker implantation include baseline right bundle branch block, intraprocedural heart block, implantation depth, and transcatheter valve type. A recent *Journal of the American College of Cardiology* Scientific Expert panel provides recommendations for observation and permanent pacemaker implantation in these various risk groups.

- In patients undergoing percutaneous catheter ablation, those undergoing AV nodal re-entrant tachycardia, septal/paraseptal accessory pathway, and para-Hisian arrhythmia ablation are at higher risk for inadvertent AV node injury. Various strategies (pacing maneuvers, cryotherapy ablation, ablation at coronary cusps) should be employed wherever possible.

DISCLOSURE

The authors have no relevant disclosures.

REFERENCES

1. Sanoudos G, Reed GE. Late heart block in aortic valve replacement. J Cardiovasc Surg 1974;15: 475–8.
2. Eksik A, Gul M, Uyarel H, et al. Electrophysiological evaluation of atrioventricular conduction disturbances in transcatheter aortic valve implantation with Edwards SAPIEN prosthesis. J Invasive Cardiol 2013;25:305–9.
3. Nardi P, Pellegrino A, Scafuri A, et al. Permanent pacemaker implantation after isolated aortic valve replacement: incidence, risk factors and surgical technical aspects. J Cardiovasc Med 2010;11:14–9.
4. Klapkowski A, Pawlaczyk R, Kempa M, et al. Complete atrioventricular block after isolated aortic valve replacement. Kardiol Pol 2016;74:985–93.
5. Berdajs D, Schurr UP, Wagner A, et al. Incidence and pathophysiology of atrioventricular block following mitral valve replacement and ring annuloplasty. Eur J Cardiothorac Surg 2008;34:55–61.
6. Herrmann FEM, Graf H, Wellmann P, et al. Atrioventricular block after tricuspid valve surgery. Int Heart J 2021;62:57–64.
7. Mori S, Nishii T, Takaya T, et al. Clinical structural anatomy of the inferior pyramidal space reconstructed from the living heart: three-dimensional visualization using multidetector-row computed tomography. Clin Anat 2015;28:878–87.
8. Kawashima T, Sato F. Clarifying the anatomy of the atrioventricular node artery. Int J Cardiol 2018;269: 158–64.

9. Adademir T, Tuncer EY, Tas S, et al. Surgical treatment of aortic valve endocarditis: a 26-year experience. Rev Bras Cir Cardiovasc 2014;29:16–24.

10. Yayla TE, Taylan A, Serpil T, et al. Surgical treatment of late aortic prosthetic valve endocarditis: 19 years' experience. Kardiochir Torakochirurgia Pol 2014;11:126–31.

11. Al-Ghamdi B, Mallawi Y, Shafquat A, et al. Predictors of permanent pacemaker implantation after coronary artery bypass grafting and valve surgery in adult patients in current surgical era. Cardiol Res 2016;7:123–9.

12. Wang TKM, Arroyo D, Martin A, et al. Permanent pacemaker implantation after cardiac surgery: rates, predictors and a novel risk score. N Z Med J 2018;131:88–91.

13. Moskowitz G, Hong KN, Giustino G, et al. Incidence and risk factors for permanent pacemaker implantation following mitral or aortic valve surgery. J Am Coll Cardiol 2019;74:2607–20.

14. Kiehl EL, Makki T, Matar RM, et al. Incidence and predictors of late atrioventricular conduction recovery among patients requiring permanent pacemaker for complete heart block after cardiac surgery. Heart Rhythm 2017;14:1786–92.

15. Steyers CM 3rd, Khera R, Bhave P. Pacemaker dependency after cardiac surgery: a systematic review of current evidence. PLoS One 2015;10:e0140340.

16. Kusumoto FM, Schoenfeld MH, Barrett C, et al. 2018 ACC/AHA/HRS guideline on the evaluation and management of patients with bradycardia and cardiac conduction delay: executive summary: a report of the American College of Cardiology/American Heart Association Task Force on Clinical Practice Guidelines, and the Heart Rhythm Society. Circulation 2019;140:e333–81.

17. Leon MB, Smith CR, Mack M, et al. Transcatheter aortic-valve implantation for aortic stenosis in patients who cannot undergo surgery. N Engl J Med 2010;363:1597–607.

18. Leon MB, Smith CR, Mack MJ, et al. Transcatheter or surgical aortic-valve replacement in intermediate-risk patients. N Engl J Med 2016;374:1609–20.

19. Adams DH, Popma JJ, Reardon MJ, et al. Transcatheter aortic-valve replacement with a self-expanding prosthesis. N Engl J Med 2014;370:1790–8.

20. Popma JJ, Deeb GM, Yakubov SJ, et al. Transcatheter aortic-valve replacement with a self-expanding valve in low-risk patients. N Engl J Med 2019;380:1706–15.

21. Meredith Am IT, Walters DL, Dumonteil N, et al. Transcatheter aortic valve replacement for severe symptomatic aortic stenosis using a repositionable valve system: 30-day primary endpoint results from the REPRISE II study. J Am Coll Cardiol 2014;64:1339–48.

22. Schofer J, Colombo A, Klugmann S, et al. Prospective multicenter evaluation of the direct flow medical transcatheter aortic valve. J Am Coll Cardiol 2014;63:763–8.

23. Mollmann H, Hengstenberg C, Hilker M, et al. Real-world experience using the ACURATE neo prosthesis: 30-day outcomes of 1,000 patients enrolled in the SAVI TF registry. Euro Interv 2018;13:e1764–70.

24. Hamdan A, Guetta V, Klempfner R, et al. Inverse relationship between membranous septal length and the risk of atrioventricular block in patients undergoing transcatheter aortic valve implantation. JACC Cardiovasc Interv 2015;8:1218–28.

25. Tretter JT, Mori S, Anderson RH, et al. Anatomical predictors of conduction damage after transcatheter implantation of the aortic valve. Open Heart 2019;6:e000972.

26. Mori S, Tretter JT, Toba T, et al. Relationship between the membranous septum and the virtual basal ring of the aortic root in candidates for transcatheter implantation of the aortic valve. Clin Anat 2018;31:525–34.

27. Koos R, Mahnken AH, Aktug O, et al. Electrocardiographic and imaging predictors for permanent pacemaker requirement after transcatheter aortic valve implantation. J Heart Valve Dis 2011;20:83–90.

28. Maeno Y, Abramowitz Y, Kawamori H, et al. A highly predictive risk model for pacemaker implantation after TAVR. JACC Cardiovasc Imaging 2017;10:1139–47.

29. Toggweiler S, Stortecky S, Holy E, et al. The electrocardiogram after transcatheter aortic valve replacement determines the risk for post-procedural high-degree AV block and the need for telemetry monitoring. JACC Cardiovasc Interv 2016;9:1269–76.

30. Regueiro A, Abdul-Jawad Altisent O, Del Trigo M, et al. Impact of new-onset left bundle branch block and periprocedural permanent pacemaker implantation on clinical outcomes in patients undergoing transcatheter aortic valve replacement: a systematic review and meta-analysis. Circ Cardiovasc Interv 2016;9:e003635.

31. Jorgensen TH, De Backer O, Gerds TA, et al. Immediate post-procedural 12-lead electrocardiography as predictor of late conduction defects after transcatheter aortic valve replacement. JACC Cardiovasc Interv 2018;11:1509–18.

32. Mangieri A, Lanzillo G, Bertoldi L, et al. Predictors of advanced conduction disturbances requiring a late (>/=48 H) permanent pacemaker following transcatheter aortic valve replacement. JACC Cardiovasc Interv 2018;11:1519–26.

33. Rodes-Cabau J, Ellenbogen KA, Krahn AD, et al. Management of conduction disturbances associated with transcatheter aortic valve replacement: JACC scientific expert panel. J Am Coll Cardiol 2019;74:1086–106.

34. Kalusche D, Ott P, Arentz T, et al. AV nodal re-entry tachycardia in elderly patients: clinical presentation and results of radiofrequency catheter ablation therapy. Coron Artery Dis 1998;9:359–63.

35. Chrispin J, Misra S, Marine JE, et al. Current management and clinical outcomes for catheter ablation of atrioventricular nodal re-entrant tachycardia. Europace 2018;20:e51–9.

36. Katritsis DG, Zografos T, Siontis KC, et al. Endpoints for successful slow pathway catheter ablation in typical and atypical atrioventricular nodal re-entrant tachycardia: a contemporary, multicenter study. JACC Clin Electrophysiol 2019;5:113–9.

37. Brugada J, Puigfel M, Mont L, et al. Radiofrequency ablation of anteroseptal, para-Hisian, and mid-septal accessory pathways using a simplified femoral approach. Pacing Clin Electrophysiol 1998; 21:735–41.

38. Luo S, Zhan X, Ouyang F, et al. Catheter ablation of right-sided para-Hisian ventricular arrhythmias using a simple pacing strategy. Heart rhythm 2019; 16:380–7.

39. Marazzato J, Fonte G, Marazzi R, et al. Efficacy and safety of cryoablation of para-Hisian and mid-septal accessory pathways using a specific protocol: single-center experience in consecutive patients. J Interv Card Electrophysiol 2019;55:47–54.

40. Lyan E, Toniolo M, Tsyganov A, et al. Comparison of strategies for catheter ablation of focal atrial tachycardia originating near the his bundle region. Heart Rhythm 2017;14:998–1005.

41. Kim J, Kim JS, Park YH, et al. Catheter ablation of parahisian premature ventricular complex. Korean Circ J 2011;41:766–9.

42. Yamashita S, Hooks DA, Hocini M, et al. Ablation of parahisian ventricular focus. HeartRhythm Case Rep 2015;1:64–7.

43. Skanes AC, Dubuc M, Klein GJ, et al. Cryothermal ablation of the slow pathway for the elimination of atrioventricular nodal reentrant tachycardia. Circulation 2000;102:2856–60.

44. Chokr MO, de Moura LG, Aiello VD, et al. Catheter ablation of the parahisian accessory pathways from the aortic cusps-experience of 20 cases-improving the mapping strategy for better results. J Cardiovasc Electrophysiol 2020;31:1413–9.

45. Pap R, Makai A, Szilagyi J, et al. Should the aortic root be the preferred route for ablation of focal atrial tachycardia around the AV node?: support from intracardiac echocardiography. JACC Clin Electrophysiol 2016;2:193–9.

46. Nagueh SF, Ommen SR, Lakkis NM, et al. Comparison of ethanol septal reduction therapy with surgical myectomy for the treatment of hypertrophic obstructive cardiomyopathy. J Am Coll Cardiol 2001;38: 1701–6.

47. Lawrenz T, Lieder F, Bartelsmeier M, et al. Predictors of complete heart block after transcoronary ablation of septal hypertrophy: results of a prospective electrophysiological investigation in 172 patients with hypertrophic obstructive cardiomyopathy. J Am Coll Cardiol 2007;49:2356–63.

48. Mongeon FP, Burkhart HM, Ammash NM, et al. Indications and outcomes of surgical closure of ventricular septal defect in adults. JACC Cardiovasc Interv 2010;3:290–7.

Systemic Diseases and Heart Block

Syed Rafay A. Sabzwari, MBBS, MD[a], Wendy S. Tzou, MD, FHRS, FACC[b],*

KEYWORDS

- Heart block • Atrioventricular node • Amyloidosis • Sarcoidosis • Systemic lupus erythematosus
- Rheumatologic disorders • Thyroid disorders • Muscular dystrophies

KEY POINTS

- Several systemic disorders can cause atrioventricular block largely because of infiltration, inflammation, or fibrosis of the conduction system owing to underlying disease process.
- Systemic disorders causing heart block can be broadly classified into infiltrative, rheumatologic, endocrine, and hereditary neuromuscular degenerative diseases.
- Infiltrative diseases like granulomas in sarcoidosis and amyloid fibrils in amyloidosis infiltrate the interstitial space including the atrioventricular nodal region causing heart block.
- Accelerated atherosclerosis leading to ischemia, vasculitis, myocarditis, and inflammatory infiltrates in rheumatologic disorders can lead to heart block.
- Myotonic, Becker, and Duchenne muscular dystrophies are inherited neuromuscular diseases that involve the myocardium in addition to the skeletal muscles and can cause progressive heart block.

INTRODUCTION

Several systemic disorders can cause atrioventricular (AV) block largely because of involvement of the myocardium and thereby the conduction system by infiltration, inflammation, or fibrosis owing to underlying disease processes (**Fig. 1**; **Table 1**). Conduction system disturbances may be permanent or transient, with conduction that is, intermittent or delayed. The underlying systemic disorder tends to govern overall presentation, as well as prognosis and management.

CLASSIFICATION

Infiltrative Disorders

Amyloidosis

Amyloidosis can result from a spectrum of diseases characterized by extracellular deposition of amyloid within various organs and tissues. Amyloid is formed from of a number of fibrillar proteinaceous components that misfold into abnormal cross β-sheet oligomers. This conformation results in characteristic gross pathologic and histologic features. The oligomers combine with proteoglycans to form amyloid infiltrates, which may be toxic. The heart is one of the organs that can be affected, and multiple clinical manifestations may result, including cardiomyopathy, arrhythmias, and conduction system disease. The majority of cardiac amyloidosis (CA) is caused by 1 of 2 proteins: transthyretin (ATTR) or light chain. Light chains are produced as a result of a proliferative hematologic disorder where plasma cells clone and produce excessive amounts of lambda and, less commonly, kappa light chains. Light chain amyloid deposition (AL or primary amyloidosis) underlies a significant proportion of amyloidosis presentations and is generally associated with worse prognosis compared with amyloidosis resulting from ATTR deposition, whether hereditary or nonhereditary (senile or wild type).

This article originally appeared in *Cardiac Electrophysiology Clinics*, Volume 13 Issue 4, December 2021.

[a] University of Colorado Anschutz Medical Campus, 12631 East 17th Avenue, Mail Stop B130, Aurora, CO 80045, USA; [b] Cardiac Electrophysiology, University of Colorado Anschutz Medical Campus, 12401 E 17th Avenue, MS B-136, Aurora, CO 80045, USA

* Corresponding author.

E-mail address: Wendy.Tzou@cuanschutz.edu

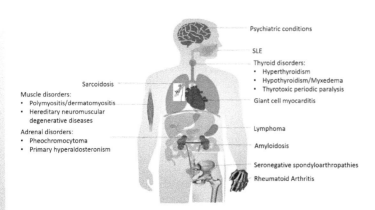

Fig. 1. Systemic diseases contributing to heart block.

Mechanism of heart block in cardiac amyloidosis
Unlike other inflammatory and infiltrative disorders, CA does not lead to myocardial scar formation. Amyloid fibrils deposit extracellularly throughout the heart, including in the valves and cardiac conduction system, thereby creating discontinuity and disarray between myocyte gap junctions that are critical for myocardial conduction. Additionally, amyloid deposition thickens the ventricle, producing restrictive physiology and marked diastolic dysfunction, and increased filling pressures that in turn lead to atrial dilation and atrial myopathy. Moreover, amyloid fibrils have direct toxic effect on myocardial cells, including increased calcium release owing to oxidative stress,[1] as demonstrated by impaired myocardial function and cell death in zebrafish resulting from exposure to AL light chains obtained from a patient with AL CA.[2] Also, perivascular amyloid infiltration leads to impaired vasodilation that causes continued ischemia to the myocardium, which can also affect the conduction system.[3]

Heart block in cardiac amyloidosis AV conduction block is more often seen than sinus node dysfunction, despite the extensive atrial involvement seen in CA. Traditionally, the electrocardiographic features associated with high-grade AV block include prolonged PR interval, and right and left bundle branch block. However, the pathology is mostly noted in the His–Purkinje system, even in the case of first-degree AV block with preserved conduction at the nodal level. Therefore, most studies have reported a prolonged HV interval in both ATTR and AL patients with CA.[4,5] The incidence of symptomatic AV block may be higher in ATTR CA owing to older age of presentation, particularly for those with senile ATTR, who also historically have had better overall survival compared with AL CA. No difference has been found in rates of high-grade AV block between patients with wild-type and hereditary ATTR CA overall.[6] However,

differences may exist based on the specific mutation among patients with hereditary TTR CA. For instance, Val122Ile compared with Thr60Ala mutation was associated with a lower prevalence of high-grade AV block at diagnosis ($P = 0.002$), although the incidence of high-grade AV block at follow-up was not different between the 2 mutations ($P = 0.15$).[6] Notably, the QRS duration tends to be normal, despite often diffuse amyloid infiltration of the bundle branches, and the mechanism is felt to be due to equal conduction delay in both bundle branches. This characteristic contrasts with other infiltrative diseases, where HV prolongation, usually more than 80 ms, is almost always associated with a widened QRS, and likely owing to a less homogenous involvement of the bundle branches.[4] For instance, in 1 series of 18 patients with advanced CA, the mean HV interval was 87 ± 27 ms.[7] In another study, the HV was prolonged (>55 ms) in all patients with CA, including 44% with a normal QRS duration (<100 ms). Reisinger and colleagues[4] also found, among 25% of patients with CA and first-degree heart block, that the His bundle deflection was greater than 30 ms, often with a notched or fragmented deflection. Importantly, the HV interval was prolonged (77 ± 18 ms) in 20 patients with a QRS of less than 120 ms, and even longer (88 ± 17 ms) in 5 patients with a QRS of greater than 120 ms. Hence it is important to note that a relatively narrow QRS does not exclude patients from having infranodal disease. Therefore, when evaluating patients with high-risk syncope even in the absence of conduction abnormalities on an electrocardiogram (EKG) (normal PR interval and QRS duration), further evaluation by an electrophysiologic study should be done to exclude the possibility of infra-Hisian disease.

Sarcoidosis
Sarcoidosis is a rare but increasingly recognized disease with a reported prevalence between

Table 1
Classification of systemic diseases causing heart block

A.	Infiltrative disorders		
	a.	Amyloidosis	
	b.	Sarcoidosis	
	c.	Tumors	
		i.	Primary tumors
		ii.	Metastatic tumors
B.	Rheumatologic disorders		
	a.	Dermatomyositis	
	b.	Polymyositis	
	c.	Systemic lupus erythematosus	
	d.	Systemic sclerosis	
	e.	Rheumatoid arthritis	
	f.	Giant cell myocarditis	
	g.	HLA B27 associated seronegative spondyloarthropathies	
C.	Endocrine disorders		
	a.	Thyroid gland	
		i.	Hyperthyroidism
		ii.	Hypothyroidism/ myxedema
		iii.	Thyrotoxic periodic paralysis
	b.	Adrenal gland	
		i.	Pheochromocytoma
		ii.	Hypoaldosteronism
D.	Hereditary neuromuscular degenerative diseases		
	a.	Myotonic dystrophy	
	b.	Becker muscular dystrophy	
	c.	Duchenne muscular dystrophy	
	d.	Kearns–Sayre syndrome	
	e.	Rare muscular dystrophies	
		i.	Scapuloperoneal dystrophy
		ii.	Erb's dystrophy
		iii.	Oculocraniosomatic syndrome
E.	Others		
	a.	Psychiatric conditions	

0.10% and 0.16% in the United States.[8,9] It is characterized by the deposition of noncaseating granulomas with associated inflammation and fibrosis that primarily affect not only the lungs, but can also involve all other organs. Cardiac sarcoidosis is under-recognized, because it can have a variety of manifestations, including absence of symptoms, cardiomyopathy, sudden cardiac death owing to ventricular arrhythmia, and high-grade AV block.[10] An evaluation of death certificates suggests that cardiac involvement is the leading cause of death in sarcoidosis.[11]

Mechanism of heart block in cardiac sarcoidosis The exact etiology of CS is unclear; however, it seems to result from an interplay between genetic, environmental, infectious, and immunologic factors. Polymorphism of HLA class II molecules, particularly HLA DQB*0601, and tumor necrosis factor (alpha), and particularly the TNFA2 allele, have been thought to form a potential genetic basis for CS.[12] The eventual immune response occurs owing to an interaction between immune-modulatory cells and various cytokines that lead to the characteristic noncaseating granuloma formation, which contains lymphocytes, macrophages, and epithelioid cells that fuse to form a multinucleated giant cell (**Fig. 2**). Cytokines involved include transforming growth factor beta, insulin-like growth factor 1, IL-4 and IL-5 that are subsequently responsible for fibrotic changes in the granuloma, leading to scarring.[13] CS can involve any cardiac structure, including the myocardium, valves, papillary muscles, coronary arteries, and pericardium. The inflammatory process often involves the interventricular septum and therefore can affect the AV node and His–Purkinje system, leading to heart block. Additionally, the inflammatory process and scar can involve the nodal artery causing ischemia to the AV node.[14]

Salient features and screening approach Complete AV block is one of the most common manifestations of CS, occurring at a younger age

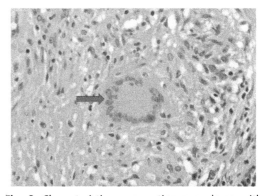

Fig. 2. Characteristic noncaseating granuloma with multinucleated giant cell (*arrow*) in cardiac sarcoidosis (hematoxylin-eosin stain, original magnification x 10). (*Adapted from* Patel B, Shah M, Gelaye A, Dusaj R. A complete heart block in a young male: a case report and review of literature of cardiac sarcoidosis. Heart Fail Rev. 2017;22(1):55-64; with permission)

compared with AV block from other causes. The prevalence of complete AV block in diagnosed CS is 23% to 30%.[14] Rosenthal and colleagues reported that 34% of patients aged less than 60 years presenting with AV block had underlying CS.[15] This incidence is higher than reported previously, likely owing to the use of advanced imaging modalities, including a PET scan with fluorodeoxyglucose and cardiac MRI (**Fig. 3**). Similar findings have been described in a retrospective study by Kandolin and colleagues who found that in patients less than 55 years of age, 19% (14/72) had CS as the cause of new, unexplained AV block. Notably, two-thirds of these patients had only cardiac involvement of sarcoidosis. No change in heart block was observed at 6 months of follow-up.[16]

CS should be considered in the differential diagnosis for younger patients (<60 years) with second-degree Mobitz II or third-degree AV block (class IIa).[17] Similarly, patients with biopsy-proven extracardiac sarcoidosis should be evaluated longitudinally for the development of cardiac involvement, including AV nodal conduction disease, by follow-up cardiac history (class I), EKG (class I), and echocardiogram (class IIa).[17] Subsequently, such patients who develop concerning symptoms (syncope/presyncope or palpitations) or abnormal EKG changes (pathologic Q waves, high-degree AV block, or bundle branch block) or an abnormal echocardiogram (regional wall motion abnormalities, wall aneurysm, basal septal thinning, left ventricular ejection fraction of <40%) should then undergo further evaluation with cardiac MRI or a PET scan with fluorodeoxyglucose (Class IIa).[17]

Diagnosis In 2014, the first international consensus recommendation for diagnosis of CS was released.[17] This consensus had 2 pathways to diagnosis. The first one is through histologic diagnosis from endomyocardial biopsy. The second pathway makes CS probable if there is histologically confirmed extracardiac sarcoidosis and 1 or more typical findings of CS are present, including high-grade AV block or nonischemic left ventricular systolic dysfunction unexplained by other causes (see **Fig. 3**).[17] With advancements in imaging techniques, the diagnosis of CS has improved. Echocardiography can show evidence of increased myocardial wall thickness, basal septal thinning, aneurysms, and wall motion abnormalities in a noncoronary distribution pattern. However, echocardiography can miss early stages or "silent CS". Cardiac MRI can identify areas of late gadolinium enhancement (LGE), which in the case of CS is patchy, midmyocardial or epicardial, and commonly involves the basal septum or lateral wall. Although cardiac magnetic resonance identifies mostly the presence of fibrosis, a PET scan with fluorodeoxyglucose can pick up regions with active inflammation owing to the presence of active proinflammatory macrophages that show a higher metabolic rate and glucose use (**Fig. 4**).[12,18]

Treatment of heart block In the inflammatory phase, Mobitz type II or third-degree heart block resulting from CS can potentially be reversed with immunosuppression, and treatment with corticosteroids is a Class IIa indication in the setting of newly diagnosed high-grade AV block and confirmed or probable CS.[17] Although there

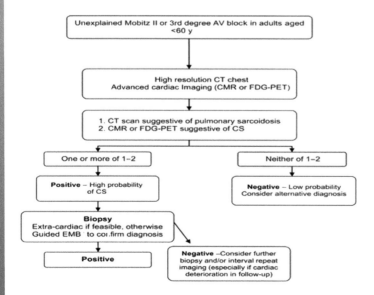

Fig. 3. Suggested algorithm for the investigation of patients with unexplained Mobitz II or third-degree AV block who are younger than 60 years. CMR, cardiovascular magnetic resonance; CS, cardiac sarcoidosis; CT, computed tomographic; ECG, electrocardiogram; EMB, endomyocardial biopsy; FDG-PET, ^{18}F-fluorodeoxyglucose–positron emission tomography. (*From* Birnie DH, Sauer WH, Bogun F, et al. HRS expert consensus statement on the diagnosis and management of arrhythmias associated with cardiac sarcoidosis. Heart Rhythm. 2014;11(7):1305-1323; with permission.)

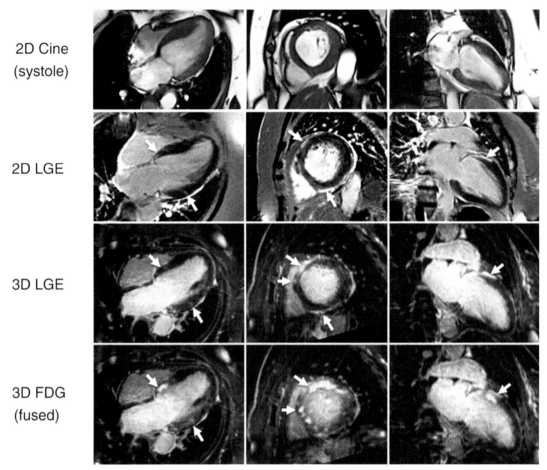

2D Cine (systole)

2D LGE

3D LGE

3D FDG (fused)

Fig. 4. Cardiac magnetic resonance images for respective 4-chamber, short-axis, and 2-chamber orientations showing systolic frame cine imaging and corresponding 2-dimensional (2D) late gadolinium enhancement (LGE) and 3-dimensional (3D) LGE scar imaging. White arrows indicate regions of abnormal LGE, consistent with mature scar. *Bottom* row shows 3D LGE images with fusion of 18F-labeled fluro-2-deoxyglucose (18F-FDG) positron emission tomography signal suggestive of active inflammation surrounding regions of established scar. (*From* White JA, Rajchl M, Butler J, et al. Active cardiac sarcoidosis: first clinical experience of simultaneous positron emission tomography–magnetic resonance imaging for the diagnosis of cardiac disease. Circulation.2013;127(22):e639-641; with permission.)

are no randomized trials to support this practice, a systematic review by Sadek and colleagues,[19] which included 10 articles in which 27 of 57 patients (47.4%) with AV block improved with corticosteroids to mostly normal AV conduction. Owing to lack of durable and reliable success in heart block recovery and unpredictable disease course, device implantation is still recommended as a Class IIa indication.[17] It is also worth mentioning that, owing to the risk of ventricular arrhythmias in CS, implantable cardioverter-defibrillator implantation is recommended in patients who require permanent pacing (class IIa recommendation), even in the absence of significant left ventricular systolic dysfunction.[17]

Tumors

Primary cardiac tumors are extremely rare, with a prevalence 0.02%, with the primary cardiac lymphomas comprising 1% to 2%. Secondary cardiac tumors owing to metastasis are more common, with a prevalence of 2.3% to 18.3% and represent 16% to 28% of extracardiac lymphomas.[20–24] AV block has accounted for up to 27% of clinical manifestations of primary cardiac lymphomas.[25–27] Metastatic tumors contributing to AV block include squamous cell cancers of the oral cavity, thyroid and uterus. Other reported metastatic tumors that may lead to AV block include bladder cancer, Merkel cell cancer, bronchogenic carcinoma (squamous cell and adenocarcinoma), and leiomyosarcoma.[28]

Mechanism of heart block Most tumors, and specifically metastatic tumors, involve the pericardium and myocardium; fewer than 5% involve the endocardium.[24,28] Because hematogenous spread is one of the modalities of metastases, the right atrium and right ventricle are commonly involved. Therefore, AV block has been attributed either to compression from mass effect or owing to direct infiltration of the AV node or the His–Purkinje system itself. Other mechanisms include those owing to metabolic derangements from renal involvement or directly through endocrine mechanisms leading to electrolyte abnormalities, particularly hypercalcemia. Moreover, many antineoplastic drugs can have adverse effects in the form of direct AV nodal blocking effect or from overall cardiotoxicity. These mechanisms have been discussed in Chiara Pavone and Gemma Pelargonio's article, "Reversible Causes of Atrioventricular Block," in this issue.

Rheumatologic Disorders

Mixed connective tissue disease
Mixed connective tissue disease is an autoimmune process with the combined features of multiple rheumatologic diseases, including systemic lupus erythematosus, systemic sclerosis, polymyositis, and rheumatoid arthritis (RA). It is associated with a high titer of anti-U1 ribonucleoprotein antibodies. Cardiac involvement in mixed connective tissue disease has been reported in 13% to 65% and can involve all components of the heart.[29] However, only one-fourth to one-third of the patients have symptomatic disease. Conduction disturbances have been noted in as many as 20% of patients in one of the largest series.[30]

Mechanism of heart block Although the pathophysiology of conduction disease in mixed connective tissue disease is not completely understood, 2 post mortem series suggest myocarditis as a mechanism, similar to what has been identified in other connective tissue diseases,[31,32] with pathologic changes noted in the myocardium mimicking those found in skeletal muscle in patients with polymyositis or dermatomyositis.

Dermatomyositis and polymyositis
Polymyositis and dermatomyositis are chronic muscle inflammatory disorders clinically characterized by muscle weakness and fatigue.[33,34] Cardiac involvement, including heart failure and conduction system abnormalities, has been seen in more than 70% of patients with polymyositis and confers an increased mortality risk.[35]

Mechanism of heart block Polymyositis and dermatomyositis are characterized by chronic

inflammatory infiltrates (primarily CD4+/CD8+ T cells), macrophages, and dendritic cells that infiltrate muscle fascicles and perivascular regions. This inflammatory pattern, although most studied in skeletal muscles, has also been identified in those with myocardial involvement. Inflammatory changes eventually produce cardiac myocyte degeneration and fibrosis.[36,37] Similar inflammatory changes and eventual contraction-band necrosis have been observed involving the cardiac conduction system on autopsy studies.[37,38] In other post mortem studies of patients with heart block, extensive fibrous replacement of the AV node, His bundle, and bundle branches have been reported.[38–40]

Salient features Cardiac involvement is often subclinical, and presentation delayed to a few years after the initial diagnosis of the rheumatologic condition. Most case reports describe a progressive course, evidenced by first-degree heart block, then subsequent development of hemi blocks and left bundle branch block.[41]

Giant cell myocarditis
Giant cell myocarditis (GCM) is a rare but aggressive and devastating disease characterized by rapidly progressing heart failure, ventricular arrhythmias, and conduction disease. In the 2 largest series of patients with GCM, complete heart block was noted in 5% to 31%.[42,43] The rate of death or transplant approximates 70% at 1 year after diagnosis.[44]

Mechanism of heart block GCM is an autoimmune, virus-negative myocarditis attributed to T-lymphocyte–mediated inflammation and is associated with systemic autoimmune disorder in approximately 20% of cases. Infiltration tends to diffusely involve the myocardium, including the AV node and His–Purkinje system, leading to heart block. Histologically, multinucleated giant cells with surrounding mononuclear inflammatory cells (predominantly T-cells) are observed. Acute inflammation eventually produces necrosis of cardiac myocytes. Although certain features are similar to cardiac sarcoidosis, including the identification of granulomas in a minority of patients with advanced disease, the overall disease course and presentation are usually more fulminant.[42]

Salient features and treatment Interestingly, more indolent presentations of AV block in GCM have been reported. Kandolin and colleagues[45] found that 6% of patients had biopsy-proven GCM when they studied 72 patients aged 18 to 55 years who had undergone pacemaker implantation for third-degree heart block. However, GCM individuals had worse 4-year outcomes, with 39% experiencing malignant ventricular arrhythmias, cardiac death, or transplantation. When compared with lymphocytic myocarditis, Davidoff and colleagues[46] reported AV block to be more common in GCM (60.0% vs 8.3%, respectively).

GCM is diagnosed by endomyocardial biopsy. Unlike sarcoidosis, the diagnostic yield of endomyocardial biopsy in GCM is relatively high owing to more widespread infiltration, ranging from 56% to 93%, depending on the biopsy protocol.[42,43]

The diagnosis of GCM along with CS should be strongly considered for adults less than 55 years of age presenting with high-degree AV block; unlike other myocarditis, expedient immunosuppressive treatment for GCM can alter the disease course by slowing or limiting its progression.[47,48] Continued immunosuppression is important as withdrawal of treatment can lead to fatal treatment relapse.[49]

Systemic lupus erythematosus, anti-RO/SSA, and anti-LA/SSB antibody

Adult complete heart block Although atrial fibrillation, sinus tachycardia, and atrial ectopic beats are the major arrhythmias noted in systemic lupus erythematosus, progressive AV conduction abnormalities can also be seen. High-grade AV block has been shown to be the presenting symptom in a few reported cases. Tselios and colleagues[50] reported a complete heart block incidence of 1% (out of 1366 patients) from a Toronto lupus clinic database.

Mechanism of heart block The exact etiology of complete heart block in systemic lupus erythematosus is not clear, but autoantibodies seem to be involved. Natsheh and colleagues[51] reported positive antinuclear antibody in all patients, anti-DNA in 84%, anti-La in 15%, and anti-Ro in 35% of patients. Evidence that these antibodies interact with the conduction system leading to complete heart block comes from studies showing that maternal anti-Ro and anti-La antibodies block L-type and T-type calcium channels in the fetal conduction system leading to congenital complete heart block. Recent data suggest that 2 types of mechanisms may exist for anti-Ro/SSA's role in adult complete heart block.[52,53]

1. Acquired: Formation of new anti-Ro antibodies is reported to account for this type, although data supporting this theory are mixed.[54–59] Regardless, 70% of adult patients with systemic lupus erythematosus and complete heart block reported to date have shown the presence of anti-Ro antibodies.[52]
2. Late progressive congenital form: More latent and subclinical immunomodulated effects

caused by maternal antibodies in utero have been observed, with first- or second-degree AV block observed in 2% to 5% of study populations, and progression to complete heart block only in adulthood.[60] Transient conduction defects have also been observed. Bergman and colleagues, demonstrated a 10% incidence of progression to first-degree AV block among children with a normal electrocardiogram within 1 month of birth, after prenatal exposure to anti-SSA/Ro52 antibodies.[61] Similarly, other studies have shown complete disappearance of first-degree AV block at birth over the ongoing years.[62] A Swedish nationwide retrospective study showed that 24.5% of 53 cases of isolated complete heart block of unknown origin had a seropositive mother for anti-Ro/SSA antibodies.[63] An infectious insult in adult life is postulated to act as the trigger for the manifestation of complete heart block in some cases.[52] This finding in turn implies that at least approximately 10% of adults with isolated complete heart block in the general population may have a seropositive mother, would not themselves be seropositive and therefore not respond to immunosuppressants.

Fig. 5 summarizes the assessment of complete heart block of unknown origin in adults with anti-Ro/SSA antibodies. However, the predominant antibody type in adult complete heart block is anti-DNA and not anti-Ro/SSA.[51] Besides, myocarditis in systemic lupus erythematosus consists of apoptosis of myocardiocytes leading to conduction system fibrosis in addition to ischemic heart disease associated nodal artery occlusive disease owing to vasculitis and accelerated atherosclerosis.[50,51,64,65] Moreover, in patients with systemic lupus erythematosus without cardiac involvement, antimalarial treatment of systemic lupus erythematosus can also contribute to cardiomyopathy as well as heart block as reviewed in Chiara Pavone and Gemma Pelargonio's article, "Reversible Causes of Atrioventricular Block," in this issue. In 1 series, 17 of 47 patients with biopsy-confirmed antimalarial cardiomyopathy had complete heart block, with majority of them requiring permanent pacemaker implantation.[66]

Salient features in adults As with systemic lupus erythematosus in general, complete heart block in systemic lupus erythematosus almost exclusively has been seen in females (94% cases) with a median age of 37 years (range, 12–63 years) at a median time of 10 years (range, 1–25 years) after systemic lupus erythematosus diagnosis.[51] However, in only 5 reported cases, syncope

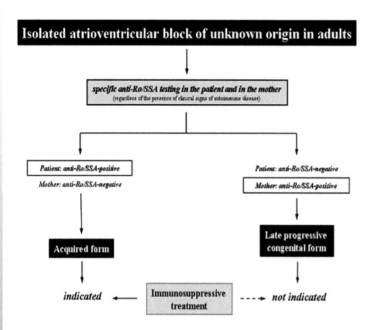

Fig. 5. Algorithm in assessment of complete heart block of unknown origin adults associated with anti-Ro/SSA antibodies. (*From* Lazzerini PE, Capecchi PL, Laghi-Pasini F. Isolated atrioventricular block of unknown origin in adults and anti-Ro/SSA antibodies: clinical evidence, putative mechanisms, and therapeutic implications. Heart Rhythm. 2015;12(2):449-454; with permission.)

owing to complete heart block was the initial manifestation leading to the diagnosis of systemic lupus erythematosus. In most of these cases, systemic manifestations of systemic lupus erythematosus usually took days to weeks to develop and in one case up to several years. An EKG before the development of complete heart block can be normal, but can also show evidence of first-degree and second-degree AV block as well as intraventricular conduction delays.[51] Owing to predominant involvement of the AV node and

His–Purkinje system the QRS in these patients is usually narrow (**Fig. 6**A).

Anti-Ro/SSA–associated AV block in adults in the absence of clinical autoimmune disease can represent 20% of all cases of isolated complete heart block of unknown origin.[52] **Fig. 6**A shows the EKG of a 29-year-old woman with positive anti-Ro/SSA antibodies who was noted to have sudden onset complete heart block in the absence of any signs or symptoms of systemic lupus erythematosus.[53] Hence, the possibility of this

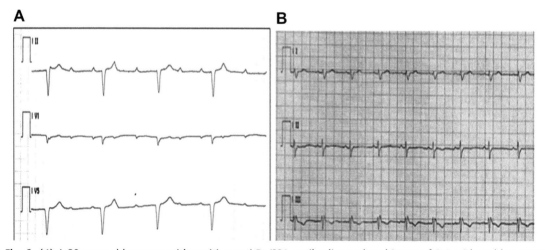

Fig. 6. (*A*) A 29-years-old woman with positive anti-Ro/SSA antibodies and no history of SLE with sudden onset complete heart block. (*B*) Normal AV conduction after 2 weeks of immunosuppressive therapy with prednisone. SLE, systemic lupus erythematosus. (*From* Lazzerini PE, Brucato A, Capecchi PL, et al. Isolated atrioventricular block of unknown origin in the adult and autoimmunity: diagnostic and therapeutic considerations exemplified by 3 anti-Ro/SSA-associated cases. HeartRhythm Case Rep. 2015;1(5):293-299; with permission.)

mechanism in patients with "idiopathic" complete heart block should be considered and accordingly should prompt investigation of anti-Ro antibodies in both the patient and mother. The results of this testing can help to categorize the patient's AV block as either acquired or late progressive. The timely institution of immunosuppressants will only help to treat the acquired form (see **Fig. 6**B), whereas the remainder might require implantation of a permanent pacemaker.

Neonatal complete heart block Since the 1980s, congenital complete heart block has been thought to be associated with maternal anti-Ro/SSA and anti-La/SSB antibodies not necessarily dependent on clinical evidence of maternal Sjogren syndrome and systemic lupus erythematosus.[67–69] Congenital complete heart block represents the most severe and representative effect of anti-Ro/SSA antibodies in the fetal heart and these antibodies account for 80% to 95% of congenital complete heart block in the absence of structural heart disease.[67,70] The risk of congenital complete heart block in first anti-Ro positive pregnancy is 1% to 2%, but it increases significantly to 12% to 20% with future pregnancies. It is thought that congenital complete heart block is a manifestation of a spectrum of progressively worsening heart block starting from first then second and eventually irreversible congenital complete heart block.[62,71]

Mechanism of heart block In comparison with the association of complete heart block to anti-Ro antibodies, data supporting an association of complete heart block with anti-La antibodies are less robust. Two studies suggested anti-La to be more associated with neonatal cutaneous lupus erythematosus than complete heart block; however, another study suggested anti-La antibodies increasing the risk of congenital complete heart block.[72–74] Hence, the consensus remains that congenital complete heart block can develop with either of the 2 antibodies or even in their absence. Although the exact mechanism is not known, there are a few theories proposed for development of complete heart block in neonates. (1) The inflammatory theory proposes inflammation-driven injury to the AV node owing to interaction between anti-Ro/SSA and specific antigens expressed in the fetal conduction system; (2) an electrophysiology theory based on experimental models, suggesting a rapidly occurring and fully reversing electrophysiologic interference demonstrated by anti-Ro/SSA on AV conduction; and (3) calcium-channel theory incorporates a unique pathophysiologic interaction between anti-Ro/SSA and fetal calcium channels, predominantly L-type Ca channels that are more predominant in neonates than adults for AV conduction owing to underdeveloped sarcoplasmic reticula, with decreased calcium storage and therefore greater dependence on transsarcolemmal calcium entry through L-type calcium channels.[62,71,75,76] Moreover, experimental studies have also suggested that IgG bind to L- and T-type calcium channels, thereby significantly inhibiting their currents.

Salient features in neonates Fetal monitoring in the peripartum period is usually recommended when the antibody titer is more than 8 enzyme-linked immunosorbent assay units in commercial laboratories. Neonates are most at risk for heart block during the first 18 to 24 weeks of gestation. However, the risk is less during the 26th to 30th weeks and very rare after 30 weeks of pregnancy. Second-degree AV block, mostly Mobitz type 1 owing to impaired AV node conduction, has a better prognosis with chance of reversibility based on a meta-analysis of 4 studies in which 24% of the patients recovered normal conduction regardless of therapy.[77]

Hickstein and colleagues[78] suggested immunoadsorption as a possible treatment for pregnant women with high titers of SSA antibodies. However, infants with complete heart block and particularly those with a heart rate of less than 50 beats/min before delivery may require a permanent pacemaker.[79] This is likely due to the involvement of His–Purkinje system in infants with complete heart block. As in adults, owing to the predominant involvement of the AV node and His–Purkinje system, the QRS duration usually remains normal.

Rheumatoid arthritis
AV nodal block in RA is very rare, but is usually complete.[80] The incidence is estimated to be 1 in 1000 to 1600 patients.[81,82]

Mechanism of heart block Patients with RA can have primary infiltration of the AV node by mononuclear cells consisting of lymphocytes, plasma cells, and histiocytes or rheumatoid granulomas. Continued inflammation in the AV node results in fibroelastosis.[83] Other mechanisms include AV nodal artery vasculitis, hemorrhage into a rheumatoid nodule, or extension of the inflammatory front from adjacent mitral or aortic valve. Villecco and colleagues noted antibodies directed against the conduction system more often than in RA patients with RBBB compared with those without (76% vs 21%).[83] It is also thought that the incidence might be higher in patients treated primarily with corticosteroids because there is a higher incidence of necrotizing arteritis in such patients.[84]

Salient features The majority of patients with complete heart block have established erosive, nodular RA with clinical features of extra-articular RA and high titers of rheumatoid factor. The progression from normal conduction to complete heart block can be sudden and permanent, although rare reports of spontaneous recovery exist.[80]

Systemic sclerosis

Complete heart block is very rare in systemic sclerosis, although lesser degrees of AV block can be more common, with first-degree AVB in 6% to 10%, and second- and third-degree AV block in up to 2% of patients.[85–88]

Mechanism of heart block AV block in systemic sclerosis is primarily owing to advanced fibrosis of the myocardium extending to the AV node, although selective fibrosis of the conduction system has not been established definitively.[89] Additionally, inflammatory involvement of the arterial blood supply and the conduction tissue can also play a role.[80] Volta and colleagues[90] showed that 25% of the patients with progressive systemic sclerosis had antibodies against the conduction system.

HLA B27 and seronegative ankylospondyloarthropathies

Seronegative spondyloarthropathies, which are primarily composed of ankylosing spondylitis and Reiter's syndrome, are characterized by a variable but strong association with immunogenetically important cell surface protein HLA B27, sacroiliitis, and an absence of rheumatoid factor.

Mechanism of heart block The primary mechanism underlying complete heart block is the same for aortic regurgitation in these patients and is due to an inflammatory process in the aortic root and the adjacent myocardium, which in turn leads to varying degrees of fibrosis.[91,92]

Salient features There has been an association of HLA B-27 and complete heart block noted even in the absence of clinical or radiographic evidence of rheumatic disease in 15% to 20% of men with complete heart block.[93] It is noteworthy that complete heart block in HLA B-27 predominantly involves the His bundle and is therefore associated with complete heart block owing to intra-His rather than infra-Hisian block, correlating with a normal PR interval. This finding is supported by a series of 12 patients with complete heart block and HLA B27 disease (8 having ankylosing spondylitis) who underwent an electrophysiologic study; only 1 patient had infra-Hisian block, whereas 10 patients

had supra-Hisian second- or third-degree AV block.[94]

Another important feature is the tendency of complete heart block to occur paroxysmally. Although consequences from the disease process overall might resolve without significant clinical sequelae, complete and long-lasting remission rarely occurs.[93,95,96]

Management Treatment is directed toward the underlying disease process and includes corticosteroids in the acute setting and eventual transition to disease-modifying antirheumatic drugs. In most rheumatologic disorders, by the time high-grade AV block is diagnosed, the disease process has advanced enough that complete or durable reversibility of AV block is unlikely. Therefore, patients often require permanent pacemaker implantation. However, those patients who are asymptomatic or without evidence of high-grade AV block can be monitored periodically in the form of either outpatient follow-up EKGs or Holter monitor. There are no specific guideline recommendations for the implantation of permanent pacemaker in rheumatologic disorders.

Endocrine disorders

Hyperthyroidism

Thyroid hormones have mechanism of action on the heart with mostly positive inotropic, chronotropic, and dromotropic responses leading to faster heart rates and improved cardiac output.[97–99] Although hyperthyroidism has been mostly known in relation to tachyarrhythmias, it has been rarely associated with heart block. Most reported cases have described other disease processes such as infectious disease, hypercalcemia, rheumatic fever or digitalis treatment concomitantly present with thyrotoxicosis; however, primary involvement with only thyrotoxicosis has also been reported.[100–102]

Mechanism of heart block Thyroid hormones effect sodium pump density and enhance the permeability of Na^+ and K^+ permeability within myocytes.[103,104] The exact mechanism of heart block in hyperthyroidism is not well-known. Data from case reports and autopsy studies describe potential pathophysiology, although the correlation of biochemical evidence of elevated T4 and T3 levels to postmortem histopathologic evidence is challenging owing to immediate postmortem decreases in T4 and fluctuating T3 levels.[102] Interstitial inflammation and focal myocarditis around the AV node have been noted, along with myocyte necrosis and hypertrophy, myocardial edema, and interstitial and perivascular fibrosis that can lead to AV nodal conduction abnormalities through direct injury or ischemic effects.[102,105] Ortmann and colleagues[102] described microscopic evidence of degenerative changes with vacuolization with negative immunohistochemical finding excluding necrosis (**Fig. 7**). Ischemic effects are likely augmented in the setting of baseline atherosclerotic coronary artery disease, which is found in the majority of patients with thyrotoxicosis, and in whom increased work of the heart can worsen ischemia to the conduction system and AV node in general. Finally, under the influence of excessive thyroid hormone levels, the autonomic nervous system has a reciprocal action of exacerbating hypervagatonia, which might have been present before hyperthyroidism, and may precipitate AV nodal conduction abnormalities.[106,107]

Treatment Treatment of thyroid storm involves administration of intravenous glucocorticoids, which can also help to decrease peri-AV nodal inflammation and thereby improve AV conduction. Additionally, antithyroid medication can eventually decrease circulating T4 and T3 levels, improving the constant myocardial proinflammatory state. Administration of beta-blockers such as propranolol in thyrotoxicosis, given especially when tachyarrhythmias are present, can in turn promote AV block. However, in patients with gradual and progressive perinodal fibrosis, glucocorticoids may not be effective in reversing AV block, and pacemaker implantation might be required.

Hypothyroidism and myxedema
Myxedema has been associated with AV block, as demonstrated through multiple case reports and histopathologic studies.[108–113] Given that AV block in this context can be reversible with thyroid replacement therapy, the yield of screening patients for hypothyroidism is particularly high.

Mechanism of heart block Various histopathologic changes in the myxedema heart have been identified that may increase risk of AV block, including interstitial edema, myocardial fibrosis, and mucinous vacuolization with positive periodic acid-Schiff staining. However, because some of these changes persist after resolution of AV block after treatment with thyroid replacement therapy, their exact contribution is not completely certain.[114,115] As is true in the context of other systemic processes that lead to increased myocardial oxygen demand, ischemia to the AV node may be enhanced in the presence of underlying coronary artery disease. Significant interstitial edema may also lead to mechanical compression of the AV node. Possibly most relevant, thyroid hormones have direct and indirect stimulatory effects, the latter mediated through increased catecholamines, on AV nodal conduction; in the setting of insufficient thyroid hormone levels, bradycardia and AV block can therefore result, as well as be effectively treated with thyroid replacement therapy.[116,117]

Salient features The clinical presentation of myxedema can be very insidious, especially in the elderly. Given the therapeutic reversibility of heart block in myxedema, the presentation of heart block of an unclear etiology should warrant screening for thyroid status particularly if clinical signs are also suggestive of thyroid dysfunction. Complete heart block in a small subset of patients might not reverse despite thyroid replacement, which may result from extensive myocardial fibrosis to prolonged thyroid deficiency.[117]

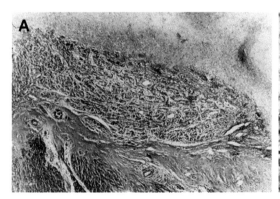 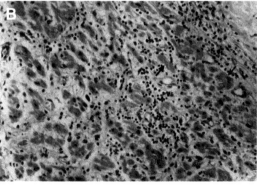

Fig. 7. (*A*) Penetrating His bundle shows interstitial edema and mixed infiltrate. Inflammation cells are also seen in the fibrous body close to the bundle (stain: hematoxylin and eosin; original magnification ×25). (*B*) Absence of necrosis of the His bundle myocytes. Degenerative changes with vacuolization (↑) and mixed interstitial inflammation. (*Adapted from* Ortmann C, Pfeiffer H, Du Chesne A, Brinkmann B. Inflammation of the cardiac conduction system in a case of hyperthyroidism. Int J Legal Med. 1999;112(4):271-274; with permission.)

Pheochromocytoma

Pheochromocytoma is a rare but potentially life-threatening tumor of the adrenal medulla with an incidence of 1 in 100,000.[118] It is characterized by excessive secretion of norepinephrine, epinephrine, and dopamine leading to imbalances in the autonomic nervous system that, in turn, can affect cardiac conduction.[119]

Mechanism of heart block Prolonged exposure to catecholamines in pheochromocytoma can lead to myocardial hypertrophy, ischemia, and eventually cardiomyopathy. The exact mechanism of heart block in pheochromocytoma is not known, and existing data are limited primarily to case reports; chronic ischemia leading to development of cardiomyopathy, along the lines of the inflammatory disorders discussed elsewhere in this article, may be mechanistic.[120–122] Additionally, AV block has been particularly noted during hypertensive paroxysms during which baroreceptor stimulation results in reflex vagal nerve stimulation that can lead owing to both sinus arrest as well as AV block.[120] Other mechanism include adrenergic receptor desensitization and particularly negative chronotropic effects of noradrenaline infusion.[122]

Primary Hyperaldosteronism

Primary hyperaldosteronism accounts for 5% to 15% of all hypertensive patients and is characterized by minerocorticoid (aldosterone) excess leading to hypertension and hypokalemia.[123] Patients with primary hyperaldosteronism have adverse cardiovascular effects that cannot just be explained by effects of hypertension.

Mechanism of heart block Data on AV block in primary hyperaldosteronism are limited and therefore the mechanism is not understood entirely. Besides hypertension, excess aldosterone leads to cardiac remodeling owing to cell proliferation and deposition of collagen fibers in the myocardium including the conduction system.[123] Fibrosis leads to reduced sodium current, reduced cell-to-cell coupling with connexin (CX43) downregulation, and microfibrosis-associated decreased transfer coupling.[124] Additionally conduction velocity across the AV node and His bundle is also adversely affected by hypokalemia. Effect of electrolyte abnormalities on membrane potential is discussed in Chiara Pavone and Gemma Pelargonio's article, "Reversible Causes of Atrioventricular Block," in this issue.

Salient features and treatment Progressive PR prolongation has been noted in patients with primary hyperaldosteronism. First-degree AV block was present in 16% of patients with primary hyperaldosteronism and correlated positively with interventricular septal wall thickness, left ventricular mass index, plasma aldosterone level, and degree of hypokalemia.[123,125] Patients with primary hyperaldosteronism with marked left ventricular hypertrophy, hypokalemia, and prominent aldosterone elevation are at risk for complete heart block when treated with beta blockers and nondyhydropyridine calcium channel blockers.[126]

With the treatment of underlying hyperaldosteronism with adrenalectomy, including judicious use of AV nodal blockers, PR interval prolongation and heart block have been noted to reverse completely in patients with primary hyperaldosteronism.[125]

Hereditary neuromuscular dystrophies

Myotonic dystrophy

Myotonic dystrophy is the most common autosomal-dominant adult-onset muscular dystrophy, particularly in adults of European ancestry. The prevalence of myotonic dystrophy ranges from 1 in 7400 to 1 in 10,700 in Europe.[127–129] It has 2 types: myotonic dystrophy type 1 and type 2. It is characterized by delayed skeletal muscle relaxation after contraction and systemic manifestations including cardiac arrhythmias, both AV block and ventricular arrhythmias that can lead to sudden cardiac death.[130] In a population-based study, the risk of cardiac conduction system disease was noted to be 60 times higher than in the general population.[131] Therefore, those meeting pacing indications are also recommended to undergo implantable cardioverter-defibrillator implantation if life expectancy exceeds a year.[132]

Mechanism of heart block The general mechanism is related to RNA toxicity. Myotonic dystrophy type 1 results from an expansion of a cytosine–thymine–guanine trinucleotide repeat in the 3'-untranslated region of the dystrophia myotonica protein kinase gene on chromosome 19q 13.3. Myotonic dystrophy type 2 results from expanded cytosine–cytosine–thymine–guanine tetranucleotide repeat expansion located on chromosome 3q 21.3. Although the exact cause of cardiac conduction involvement is unknown, multiple potential mechanisms exist. First, impaired function of the dystrophia myotonica protein kinase gene and/or protein encoded by a gene on a nearby locus result in abnormal cellular metabolism and cell damage by progressive interstitial fibrosis, fatty and lymphocyte infiltration, and myofiber disarray. On electron microscopy, myofibrillar degeneration and prominent I-bands have been identified to involve the sinoatrial node, AV node, and His bundle.[130,133] Additionally, abnormal glucose metabolism and phosphorylation in the myocardium, controlled by MMRGlu and κ3, respectively, can result from direct effects of abnormal protein serine–threonine protein kinase produced in myotonic dystrophy patients.[130]

Salient features Although there are limited data correlating histologic and EKG abnormalities in myotonic dystrophy, AV node fibrosis has been histologically confirmed in asymptomatic patients without EKG abnormalities, suggesting the relative inadequacy of EKG in identifying patients at risk for sudden cardiac death.[133] The risk of AV block is most significant in patients with myotonic dystrophy type 1. In a study of 406 patients, baseline EKG abnormalities including a PR interval of greater than 240 ms, second- or third-degree AV block, and a prolonged QRS interval were noted in 24%.[134] An increased PR interval has been noted in 21% to 40% of patients, and an increased HV interval in 56% of patients with myotonic dystrophy type 1.[130,135] Philips and colleagues compared studies that investigated the rate of change of conduction abnormalities and, although the data were mixed, the authors concluded that, although the rate of progression is gradual, it is occasionally rapid, and the rate of progression is not an accurate predictor of future sudden cardiac death risk.[130,136]

AV block has also been noted in myotonic dystrophy type 2, although with much less data compared with myotonic dystrophy type 1. In 2 studies, the risk of conduction abnormalities including AV block was noted to be 11% and 24%.[137,138]

Kearns–Sayre syndrome

Kearns–Sayre syndrome is a mitochondrial myopathy, with incidence of 1 in 125,000 live births, and results in a constellation of chronic progressive external ophthalmoplegia with pigmentary retinopathy and at least 1 other systemic manifestation, including AV block, usually before the age of 20 years.[139] Chronic progressive external ophthalmoplegia, which can also exist in isolation, is characterized by paresis of extraocular muscles and bilateral ptosis. Kearns–Sayre syndrome can be sporadic, autosomal dominant, autosomal recessive, or maternal owing to the involvement of either nuclear or mitochondrial DNA.[140]

Mechanism of heart block The exact reason for abnormal cardiac conduction is unknown. Cardiac biopsy of Kearns–Sayre syndrome patients have shown an absolute increase in the number and size of mitochondria in the cardiomyocytes owing to progressive mtDNA depletion leading to decreased mitochondrial enzyme activity that can, in turn, lead to cell death and conduction

system fibrosis.[139,141,142] The involvement of the His–Purkinje system compared with the rest of the myocardium is specifically thought to result from differences in its dedicated vascular supply and electrophysiologic characteristic of increased spontaneous (phase 4) depolarization that requires increased mitochondrial enzymatic activity.

Salient features Incident AV block was noted in 20 of 33 (61%) of patients with Kearns–Sayre syndrome and 8 of 78 (10%) of patients with chronic progressive external ophthalmoplegia in 1 study.[143] Another study reported the incidence of complete heart block to be 40%, and all patients progressed from left anterior fascicular block to bifascicular block.[139] Therefore, fascicular blocks in Kearns–Sayre syndrome carry a high, sudden, and often fatal risk of progression to complete heart block.[144]

Indications for permanent pacemaker implantation The 2018 American College of Cardiology/American Heart Association Task Force on Clinical Practice Guidelines, and the Heart Rhythm Society guideline recommendations for permanent pacing are summarized in **Fig. 8**. Notably, pacemaker implantation is recommended (Class I) among patients with myotonic dystrophy or Kearns–Sayre syndrome with second or third-degree AV block or an HV of more than 70 ms on electrophysiologic study.[132] Additionally, pacemaker implantation should be considered (Class IIa) among patients with Kearns–Sayre syndrome with other conduction abnormalities or among patients with myotonic dystrophy with a PR of greater than 240 ms and a left bundle branch block.[132] Patients with asymptomatic myotonic dystrophy or Kearns–Sayre syndrome without conduction abnormalities should be evaluated at least annually with an EKG, with consideration of electrophysiologic study for further risk stratification to identify patients with AV nodal disease and need for permanent pacing (**Fig. 9**).

There is also an increased risk of sudden cardiac death owing to ventricular arrhythmias in patients with myotonic dystrophy and Kearns–Sayre syndrome. In a prospective study, the overall sudden cardiac death risk was 33%.[134] Therefore, the guidelines also recommend implantable cardioverter-defibrillator implantation for any pacing indication in these patients if there is more than 1 year of meaningful expected survival.[132]

Duchenne and Becker muscular dystrophies

Duchenne muscular dystrophy (DMD) and Becker muscular dystrophy are X-linked disorders causing myopathy owing to dystrophin gene mutations on

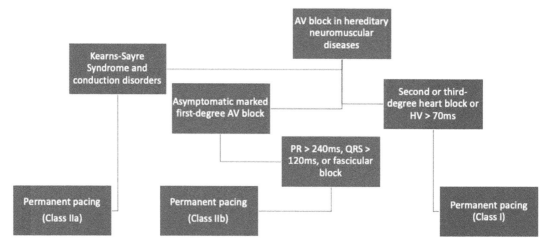

Fig. 8. Pacing indications for AV block in neuromuscular diseases. (*Data from* Kusumoto FM, Schoenfeld MH, Barrett C, et al. 2018 ACC/AHA/HRS Guideline on the Evaluation and Management of Patients With Bradycardia and Cardiac Conduction Delay: Executive Summary: A Report of the American College of Cardiology/American Heart Association Task Force on Clinical Practice Guidelines, and the Heart Rhythm Society. J Am Coll Cardiol. 2019;74(7):932-987)

chromosome Xp21.1 and primarily result in weakness of affected skeletal muscles. DMD is associated with earlier onset and most severe clinical symptoms, although cardiac involvement is a more predominant feature in Becker muscular dystrophy. AV block in DMD has been noted in a few case reports, particularly after the development of

cardiomyopathy, although it can be the first manifestation of cardiac involvement.[145,146] First-degree AV block is reported in 2% of patients with Becker muscular dystrophy, with complete AV block in both early and later decades of life reported as the initial manifestation of cardiac involvement.[147–149]

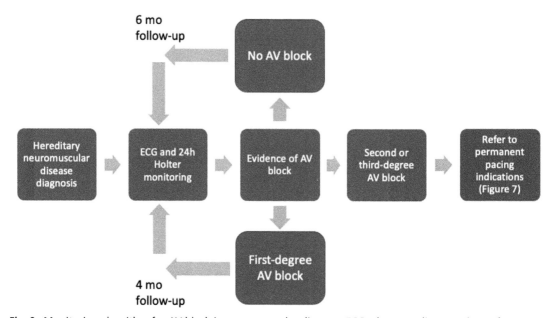

Fig. 9. Monitoring algorithm for AV block in neuromuscular diseases. ECG, electrocardiogram. (*Data from* Kusumoto FM, Schoenfeld MH, Barrett C, et al. 2018 ACC/AHA/HRS Guideline on the Evaluation and Management of Patients With Bradycardia and Cardiac Conduction Delay: Executive Summary: A Report of the American College of Cardiology/American Heart Association Task Force on Clinical Practice Guidelines, and the Heart Rhythm Society. J Am Coll Cardiol. 2019;74(7):932-987)

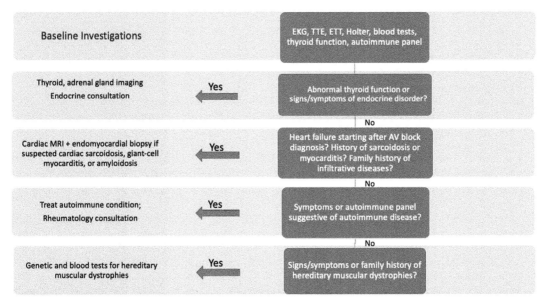

Fig. 10. Diagnostic algorithm for investigating high-grade AV block in young adults. ETT, exercise tolerance test; TTE, transthoracic echocardiogram. (*Data from* Barra SN, Providencia R, Paiva L, Nascimento J, Marques AL. A review on advanced atrioventricular block in young or middle-aged adults. Pacing Clin Electrophysiol. 2012;35(11):1395-1405)

Mechanism of heart block Dystrophin is a sarcolemmal protein that binds actin to extracellular matrix and is localized to the membrane surface of the His–Purkinje fibers.[150] The absence of dystrophin in His–Purkinje tissue, particularly in DMD, not only leads to abnormal conduction, but also to progressive replacement of cardiomyocytes by connective tissue or fat.[146,151] Electrophysiologic studies have shown conduction disturbance at the His and infra-Hisian levels.[145]

SUMMARY

Multiple systemic disease processes of widely varying etiology and clinical characteristics can result in cardiac infiltration that produces significant conduction system abnormalities, as well as increased risk of sudden cardiac death. Treatment of the underlying disease should be of primary focus, although adjunctive treatment with cardiac pacemaker or defibrillator implantation are also recommended in selected patients, particularly those with cardiac sarcoidosis or neuromuscular disorders.

CLINICS CARE POINTS

Fig. 10 summarizes a general diagnostic approach to evaluate for systemic diseases that can be adopted for young adults, mostly less than 60 years of age, presenting with high-grade AV block.

DISCLOSURE

Dr W.Z. Tzou is a consultant for or has received speaker honoraria, or research funding from Abbott, American Heart Association, Biosense Webster, Biotronik, Boston Scientific, and Medtronic. Dr S.R.A. Sabzwari has no relevant disclosures.

REFERENCES

1. Brenner DA, Jain M, Pimentel DR, et al. Human amyloidogenic light chains directly impair cardiomyocyte function through an increase in cellular oxidant stress. Circ Res 2004;94(8):1008–10.
2. Mishra S, Guan J, Plovie E, et al. Human amyloidogenic light chain proteins result in cardiac dysfunction, cell death, and early mortality in zebrafish. Am J Physiol Heart Circ Physiol 2013; 305(1):H95–103.
3. Coelho T, Maurer MS, Suhr OB. THAOS - the Transthyretin Amyloidosis Outcomes Survey: initial report on clinical manifestations in patients with hereditary and wild-type transthyretin amyloidosis. Curr Med Res Opin 2013;29(1):63–76.
4. Reisinger J, Dubrey SW, Lavalley M, et al. Electrophysiologic abnormalities in AL (primary) amyloidosis with cardiac involvement. J Am Coll Cardiol 1997;30(4):1046–51.
5. Barbhaiya CR, Kumar S, Baldinger SH, et al. Electrophysiologic assessment of conduction abnormalities and atrial arrhythmias associated with

amyloid cardiomyopathy. Heart Rhythm 2016; 13(2):383–90.

6. Donnellan E, Wazni OM, Saliba WI, et al. Prevalence, incidence, and impact on mortality of conduction system disease in transthyretin cardiac amyloidosis. Am J Cardiol 2020;128:140–6.

7. John RM. Arrhythmias in cardiac amyloidosis. J Innov Card Rhythm Manag 2018;9(3):3051–7.

8. Arkema EV, Cozier YC. Epidemiology of sarcoidosis: current findings and future directions. Ther Adv Chronic Dis 2018;9(11):227–40.

9. Patel N, Kalra R, Doshi R, et al. Hospitalization rates, prevalence of cardiovascular manifestations, and outcomes associated with sarcoidosis in the United States. J Am Heart Assoc 2018;7(2): e007844.

10. Swigris JJ, Olson AL, Huie TJ, et al. Sarcoidosis-related mortality in the United States from 1988 to 2007. Am J Respir Crit Care Med 2011;183(11): 1524–30.

11. Birnie DH, Kandolin R, Nery PB, et al. Cardiac manifestations of sarcoidosis: diagnosis and management. Eur Heart J 2017;38(35):2663–70.

12. Birnie DH, Nery PB, Ha AC, et al. Cardiac sarcoidosis. J Am Coll Cardiol 2016;68(4):411–21.

13. Patel B, Shah M, Gelaye A, et al. A complete heart block in a young male: a case report and review of literature of cardiac sarcoidosis. Heart Fail Rev 2017;22(1):55–64.

14. Sekhri V, Sanal S, Delorenzo LJ, et al. Cardiac sarcoidosis: a comprehensive review. Arch Med Sci 2011;7(4):546–54.

15. Rosenthal DG, Fang CD, Groh CA, et al. Heart failure, atrioventricular block, and ventricular tachycardia in sarcoidosis. J Am Heart Assoc 2021; 10(5):e017692.

16. Kandolin R, Lehtonen J, Airaksinen J, et al. Cardiac sarcoidosis: epidemiology, characteristics, and outcome over 25 years in a nationwide study. Circulation 2015;131(7):624–32. https://doi.org/10.1161/CIRCULATIONAHA.114.011522.

17. Birnie DH, Sauer WH, Bogun F, et al. HRS expert consensus statement on the diagnosis and management of arrhythmias associated with cardiac sarcoidosis. Heart Rhythm 2014;11(7):1305–23.

18. White JA, Rajchl M, Butler J, et al. Active cardiac sarcoidosis: first clinical experience of simultaneous positron emission tomography–magnetic resonance imaging for the diagnosis of cardiac disease. Circulation 2013;127(22):e639–41.

19. Sadek MM, Yung D, Birnie DH, et al. Corticosteroid therapy for cardiac sarcoidosis: a systematic review. Can J Cardiol 2013;29(9):1034–41.

20. Chim CS, Chan AC, Kwong YL, et al. Primary cardiac lymphoma. Am J Hematol 1997;54(1):79–83.

21. Reynen K. Frequency of primary tumors of the heart. Am J Cardiol 1996;77(1):107.

22. Tai CJ, Wang WS, Chung MT, et al. Complete atrio-ventricular block as a major clinical presentation of the primary cardiac lymphoma: a case report. Jpn J Clin Oncol 2001;31(5):217–20.

23. Curtsinger CR, Wilson MJ, Yoneda K. Primary cardiac lymphoma. Cancer 1989;64(2):521–5.

24. Montiel V, Maziers N, Dereme T. Primary cardiac lymphoma and complete atrio-ventricular block: case report and review of the literature. Acta Cardiol 2007;62(1):55–8.

25. Miguel CE, Bestetti RB. Primary cardiac lymphoma. Int J Cardiol 2011;149(3):358–63.

26. Shapiro LM. Cardiac tumours: diagnosis and management. Heart 2001;85(2):218–22.

27. Faganello G, Belham M, Thaman R, et al. A case of primary cardiac lymphoma: analysis of the role of echocardiography in early diagnosis. Echocardiography 2007;24(8):889–92.

28. Andrianto A, Mulia EPB, Suwanto D, et al. Case report: complete heart block as a manifestation of cardiac metastasis of oral cancer. F1000Res 2020;9:1243.

29. Ungprasert P, Wannarong T, Panichsillapakit T, et al. Cardiac involvement in mixed connective tissue disease: a systematic review. Int J Cardiol 2014;171(3):326–30.

30. Rebollar-Gonzalez V, Torre-Delgadillo A, Orea-Tejeda A, et al. Cardiac conduction disturbances in mixed connective tissue disease. Rev Invest Clin 2001;53(4):330–4.

31. Hajas A, Szodoray P, Nakken B, et al. Clinical course, prognosis, and causes of death in mixed connective tissue disease. J Rheumatol 2013; 40(7):1134–42.

32. Lash AD, Wittman AL, Quismorio FP Jr. Myocarditis in mixed connective tissue disease: clinical and pathologic study of three cases and review of the literature. Semin Arthritis Rheum 1986;15(4):288–96.

33. Love LA, Leff RL, Fraser DD, et al. A new approach to the classification of idiopathic inflammatory myopathy: myositis-specific autoantibodies define useful homogeneous patient groups. Medicine (Baltimore) 1991;70(6):360–74.

34. Brouwer R, Hengstman GJ, Vree Egberts W, et al. Autoantibody profiles in the sera of European patients with myositis. Ann Rheum Dis 2001;60(2): 116–23.

35. Alyan O, Ozdemir O, Geyik B, et al. Polymyositis complicated with complete atrioventricular block–a case report and review of the literature. Angiology 2003;54(6):729–31.

36. Denbow CE, Lie JT, Tancredi RG, et al. Cardiac involvement in polymyositis: a clinicopathologic study of 20 autopsied patients. Arthritis Rheum 1979;22(10):1088–92.

37. Haupt HM, Hutchins GM. The heart and cardiac conduction system in polymyositis-dermatomyositis: a

clinicopathologic study of 16 autopsied patients. Am J Cardiol 1982;50(5):998–1006.

38. Lightfoot PR, Bharati S, Lev M. Chronic dermatomyositis with intermittent trifascicular block. An electrophysiologic-conduction system correlation. Chest 1977;71(3):413–6.

39. Lynch PG. Cardiac involvement in chronic polymyositis. Br Heart J 1971;33(3):416–9.

40. Schaumburg HH, Nielsen SL, Yurchak PM. Heart block in polymyositis. N Engl J Med 1971;284(9): 480–1.

41. Reid JM, Murdoch R. Polymyositis and complete heart block. Br Heart J 1979;41(5):628–9.

42. Kandolin R, Lehtonen J, Salmenkivi K, et al. Diagnosis, treatment, and outcome of giant-cell myocarditis in the era of combined immunosuppression. Circ Heart Fail 2013;6(1):15–22.

43. Cooper LT Jr, Berry GJ, Shabetai R. Idiopathic giant-cell myocarditis–natural history and treatment. Multicenter giant cell myocarditis study Group investigators. N Engl J Med 1997;336(26):1860–6.

44. Barra SN, Providencia R, Paiva L, et al. A review on advanced atrioventricular block in young or middle-aged adults. Pacing Clin Electrophysiol 2012;35(11):1395–405.

45. Kandolin R, Lehtonen J, Kupari M. Cardiac sarcoidosis and giant cell myocarditis as causes of atrioventricular block in young and middle-aged adults. Circ Arrhythm Electrophysiol 2011; 4(3):303–9.

46. Davidoff R, Palacios I, Southern J, et al. Giant cell versus lymphocytic myocarditis. A comparison of their clinical features and long-term outcomes. Circulation 1991;83(3):953–61.

47. Ren H, Poston RS Jr, Hruban RH, et al. Long survival with giant cell myocarditis. Mod Pathol 1993; 6(4):402–7.

48. Davies RA, Veinot JP, Smith S, et al. Giant cell myocarditis: clinical presentation, bridge to transplantation with mechanical circulatory support, and long-term outcome. J Heart Lung Transpl 2002;21(6):674–9.

49. Menghini VV, Savcenko V, Olson LJ, et al. Combined immunosuppression for the treatment of idiopathic giant cell myocarditis. Mayo Clin Proc 1999; 74(12):1221–6.

50. Tselios K, Gladman DD, Harvey P, et al. Severe brady-arrhythmias in systemic lupus erythematosus: prevalence, etiology and associated factors. Lupus 2018;27(9):1415–23.

51. Natsheh A, Shimony D, Bogot N, et al. Complete heart block in lupus. Lupus 2019;28(13):1589–93.

52. Lazzerini PE, Capecchi PL, Laghi-Pasini F. Isolated atrioventricular block of unknown origin in adults and anti-Ro/SSA antibodies: clinical evidence, putative mechanisms, and therapeutic implications. Heart Rhythm 2015;12(2):449–54.

53. Lazzerini PE, Brucato A, Capecchi PL, et al. Isolated atrioventricular block of unknown origin in the adult and autoimmunity: diagnostic and therapeutic considerations exemplified by 3 anti-Ro/SSA-associated cases. HeartRhythm Case Rep 2015;1(5):293–9.

54. Behan WM, Behan PO, Gairns J. Cardiac damage in polymyositis associated with antibodies to tissue ribonucleoproteins. Br Heart J 1987;57(2):176–80.

55. Logar D, Kveder T, Rozman B, et al. Possible association between anti-Ro antibodies and myocarditis or cardiac conduction defects in adults with systemic lupus erythematosus. Ann Rheum Dis 1990; 49(8):627–9.

56. O'Neill TW, Mahmoud A, Tooke A, et al. Is there a relationship between subclinical myocardial abnormalities, conduction defects and Ro/La antibodies in adults with systemic lupus erythematosus? Clin Exp Rheumatol 1993;11(4):409–12.

57. Gordon PA, Rosenthal E, Khamashta MA, et al. Absence of conduction defects in the electrocardiograms [correction of echocardiograms] of mothers with children with congenital complete heart block. J Rheumatol 2001;28(2):366–9.

58. Lodde BM, Sankar V, Kok MR, et al. Adult heart block is associated with disease activity in primary Sjogren's syndrome. Scand J Rheumatol 2005;34(5):383–6.

59. Costa M, Gameiro Silva MB, Silva JA, et al. Anti-RO anti-LA anti-RNP antibodies and eletrocardiogram's PR interval in adult patients with systemic lupus erythematosus. Acta Reumatol Port 2008; 33(2):173–6.

60. Askanase AD, Friedman DM, Copel J, et al. Spectrum and progression of conduction abnormalities in infants born to mothers with anti-SSA/Ro-SSB/La antibodies. Lupus 2002;11(3):145–51.

61. Bergman G, Eliasson H, Mohlkert LA, et al. Progression to first-degree heart block in preschool children exposed in utero to maternal anti-SSA/Ro52 autoantibodies. Acta Paediatr 2012;101(5): 488–93.

62. Ambrosi A, Wahren-Herlenius M. Congenital heart block: evidence for a pathogenic role of maternal autoantibodies. Arthritis Res Ther 2012;14(2):208.

63. Bergman G, Skog A, Tingstrom J, et al. Late development of complete atrioventricular block may be immune mediated and congenital in origin. Acta Paediatr 2014;103(3):275–81.

64. Lo CH, Wei JCC, Tsai CF, et al. Syncope caused by complete heart block and ventricular arrhythmia as early manifestation of systemic lupus erythematosus in a pregnant patient: a case report. Lupus 2018;27(10):1729–31.

65. Prochaska MT, Bergl PA, Patel AR, et al. Atrioventricular heart block and syncope coincident with diagnosis of systemic lupus erythematosus. Can J Cardiol 2013;29(10):1330.e5–7.

66. Tselios K, Deeb M, Gladman DD, et al. Antimalarial-induced cardiomyopathy: a systematic review of the literature. Lupus 2018;27(4):591–9.

67. Jaeggi ET, Hamilton RM, Silverman ED, et al. Outcome of children with fetal, neonatal or childhood diagnosis of isolated congenital atrioventricular block. A single institution's experience of 30 years. J Am Coll Cardiol 2002;39(1):130–7.

68. Llanos C, Izmirly PM, Katholi M, et al. Recurrence rates of cardiac manifestations associated with neonatal lupus and maternal/fetal risk factors. Arthritis Rheum 2009;60(10):3091–7.

69. Waltuck J, Buyon JP. Autoantibody-associated congenital heart block: outcome in mothers and children. Ann Intern Med 1994;120(7):544–51.

70. Buyon JP, Clancy RM, Friedman DM. Cardiac manifestations of neonatal lupus erythematosus: guidelines to management, integrating clues from the bench and bedside. Nat Clin Pract Rheumatol 2009;5(3):139–48.

71. Brucato A, Cimaz R, Caporali R, et al. Pregnancy outcomes in patients with autoimmune diseases and anti-Ro/SSA antibodies. Clin Rev Allergy Immunol 2011;40(1):27–41.

72. Silverman ED, Buyon J, Laxer RM, et al. Autoantibody response to the Ro/La particle may predict outcome in neonatal lupus erythematosus. Clin Exp Immunol 1995;100(3):499–505.

73. Jaeggi E, Laskin C, Hamilton R, et al. The importance of the level of maternal anti-Ro/SSA antibodies as a prognostic marker of the development of cardiac neonatal lupus erythematosus a prospective study of 186 antibody-exposed fetuses and infants. J Am Coll Cardiol 2010;55(24):2778–84.

74. Gordon P, Khamashta MA, Rosenthal E, et al. Anti-52 kDa Ro, anti-60 kDa Ro, and anti-La antibody profiles in neonatal lupus. J Rheumatol 2004;31(12):2480–7.

75. Karnabi E, Boutjdir M. Role of calcium channels in congenital heart block. Scand J Immunol 2010;72(3):226–34.

76. Itzhaki I, Schiller J, Beyar R, et al. Calcium handling in embryonic stem cell-derived cardiac myocytes: of mice and men. Ann N Y Acad Sci 2006;1080:207–15.

77. Ciardulli A, D'Antonio F, Magro-Malosso ER, et al. Maternal steroid therapy for fetuses with second-degree immune-mediated congenital atrioventricular block: a systematic review and meta-analysis. Acta Obstet Gynecol Scand 2018;97(7):787–94.

78. Hickstein H, Kulz T, Claus R, et al. Autoimmune-associated congenital heart block: treatment of the mother with immunoadsorption. Ther Apher Dial 2005;9(2):148–53.

79. Maisch B, Ristic AD. Immunological basis of the cardiac conduction and rhythm disorders. Eur Heart J 2001;22(10):813–24.

80. Seferovic PM, Ristic AD, Maksimovic R, et al. Cardiac arrhythmias and conduction disturbances in autoimmune rheumatic diseases. Rheumatology (Oxford) 2006;45(Suppl 4):iv39–42.

81. Ahern M, Lever JV, Cosh J. Complete heart block in rheumatoid arthritis. Ann Rheum Dis 1983;42(4):389–97.

82. Rasker JJ, Cosh JA. Cause and age at death in a prospective study of 100 patients with rheumatoid arthritis. Ann Rheum Dis 1981;40(2):115–20.

83. Villecco AS, de Liberali E, Bianchi FB, et al. Antibodies to cardiac conducting tissue and abnormalities of cardiac conduction in rheumatoid arthritis. Clin Exp Immunol 1983;53(3):536–40.

84. Kemper JW, Baggenstoss AH, Slocumb CH. The relationship of therapy with cortisone to the incidence of vascular lesions in rheumatoid arthritis. Ann Intern Med 1957;46(5):831–51.

85. Janosik DL, Osborn TG, Moore TL, et al. Heart disease in systemic sclerosis. Semin Arthritis Rheum 1989;19(3):191–200.

86. Escudero J, Mc DE. The electrocardiogram in scleroderma: analysis of 60 cases and review of the literature. Am Heart J 1958;56(6):846–55.

87. Follansbee WP, Curtiss EI, Rahko PS, et al. The electrocardiogram in systemic sclerosis (scleroderma). Study of 102 consecutive cases with functional correlations and review of the literature. Am J Med 1985;79(2):183–92.

88. Roberts NK, Cabeen WR Jr, Moss J, et al. The prevalence of conduction defects and cardiac arrhythmias in progressive systemic sclerosis. Ann Intern Med 1981;94(1):38–40.

89. Ridolfi RL, Bulkley BH, Hutchins GM. The cardiac conduction system in progressive systemic sclerosis. Clinical and pathologic features of 35 patients. Am J Med 1976;61(3):361–6.

90. Volta U, Villecco AS, Bianchi FB, et al. Antibodies to cardiac conducting tissue in progressive systemic sclerosis. Clin Exp Rheumatol 1985;3(2):131–5.

91. Bulkley BH, Roberts WC. Ankylosing spondylitis and aortic regurgitation. Description of the characteristic cardiovascular lesion from study of eight necropsy patients. Circulation 1973;48(5):1014–27.

92. Davidson P, Baggenstoss AH, Slocumb CH, et al. Cardiac and aortic lesions in rheumatoid spondylitis. Proc Staff Meet Mayo Clin 1963;38:427–35.

93. Bergfeldt L, Moller E. Complete heart block–another HLA B27 associated disease manifestation. Tissue Antigens 1983;21(5):385–90.

94. Bergfeldt L, Vallin H, Edhag O. Complete heart block in HLA B27 associated disease. Electrophysiological and clinical characteristics. Br Heart J 1984;51(2):184–8.

95. Kinsella TD, Johnson LG, Ian R. Cardiovascular manifestations of ankylosing spondylitis. Can Med Assoc J 1974;111(12):1309–11.

96. Bergfeldt L, Edhag O, Vallin H. Cardiac conduction disturbances, an underestimated manifestation in ankylosing spondylitis. A 25-year follow-up study of 68 patients. Acta Med Scand 1982;212(4): 217–23.

97. Eom YS, Oh PC. Graves' disease presenting with complete atrioventricular block. Case Rep Endocrinol 2020;2020:6656875.

98. Kramer MR, Shilo S, Hershko C. Atrioventricular and sinoatrial block in thyrotoxic crisis. Br Heart J 1985;54(6):600–2.

99. Eraker SA, Wickamasekaran R, Goldman S. Complete heart block with hyperthyroidism. JAMA 1978;239(16):1644–6.

100. Stern MP, Jacobs RL, Duncan GW. Complete heart block complicating hyperthyroidism. JAMA 1970; 212(12):2117–9.

101. Sataline L, Donaghue G. Hypercalcemia, heart-block, and hyperthyroidism. JAMA 1970;213(8):1342.

102. Ortmann C, Du Chesne A, Brinkmann B. Inflammation of the cardiac conduction system in a case of hyperthyroidism. Int J Leg Med 1999;112(4):271–4.

103. Kim D, Smith TW. Effects of thyroid hormone on sodium pump sites, sodium content, and contractile responses to cardiac glycosides in cultured chick ventricular cells. J Clin Invest 1984;74(4):1481–8.

104. Haber RS, Loeb JN. Stimulation of potassium efflux in rat liver by a low dose of thyroid hormone: evidence for enhanced cation permeability in the absence of Na,K-ATPase induction. Endocrinology 1986;118(1):207–11.

105. Shirani J, Barron MM, Pierre-Louis ML, et al. Congestive heart failure, dilated cardiac ventricles, and sudden death in hyperthyroidism. Am J Cardiol 1993;72(3):365–8.

106. Toloune F, Boukili A, Ghafir D, et al. [Hyperthyroidism and atrioventricular block. Pathogenic hypothesis. Apropos of a case and review of the literature]. Arch Mal Coeur Vaiss 1988;81(9):1131–5.

107. Topaloglu S, Topaloglu OY, Ozdemir O, et al. Hyperthyroidism and complete atrioventricular block–a report of 2 cases with electrophysiologic assessment. Angiology 2005;56(2):217–20.

108. Schantz ET, Dubbs AW. Complete auriculoventricular block in myxedema with reversion to normal sinus rhythm on thyroid therapy. Am Heart J 1951; 41(4):613–9.

109. Lee JK, Lewis JA. Myxoedema with complete A-V block and Adams-Stokes disease abolished with thyroid medication. Br Heart J 1962;24:253–6.

110. Ohler WR. The heart in myxedema. Arch Intern Med 1934;53:165–87.

111. Davis JC. Myxedema heart with report of one case. Ann Intern Med 1930;4:733–41.

112. Luten D. Myxedema with partial heart block and severe anemia both of which disappeared under thyroid therapy. Mo Med 1929;26:73–7.

113. Aub JC, Stern SN. The influence of large doses of thyroid extract on the total metabolism and heart in a case of heart-block. Arch Intern Med 1918;21: 130–8.

114. Brewer DB. Myxoedema: an autopsy report with histochemical observations on the nature of the mucoid infiltrations. J Pathol Bacteriol 1951;63(3): 503–12.

115. Hamilton JD, Greenwood WF. Myxedema heart disease. Circulation 1957;15(3):442–7.

116. Zoll PM, Linenthal AJ, Gibson W, et al. Intravenous drug therapy of Stokes-Adams disease; effects of sympathomimetic amines on ventricular rhythmicity and atrioventricular conduction. Circulation 1958; 17(3):325–39.

117. Singh JB, Starobin OE, Guerrant RL, et al. Reversible atrioventricular block in myxedema. Chest 1973;63(4):582–5.

118. Beard CM, Sheps SG, Kurland LT, et al. Occurrence of pheochromocytoma in Rochester, Minnesota, 1950 through 1979. Mayo Clin Proc 1983; 58(12):802–4.

119. Zweiker R, Tiemann M, Eber B, et al. Bradydysrhythmia-related presyncope secondary to pheochromocytoma. J Intern Med 1997;242(3):249–53.

120. Paschalis-Purtak K, Pucilowska B, Prejbisz A, et al. Cardiac arrests, atrioventricular block, and pheochromocytoma. Am J Hypertens 2004;17(6):544–5.

121. McHirgui N, Rojbi I, Oueslati I, et al. Atrioventricular dissociation due to pheochromocytoma: a case report. Tunis Med 2014;92(10):645–6.

122. Haine SE, Miljoen HP, Blankoff I, et al. Atrioventricular dissociation due to pheochromocytoma in a young adult. Clin Cardiol 2010;33(12):E65–7.

123. Curione M, Petramala L, Savoriti C, et al. Electrical and myocardial remodeling in primary aldosteronism. Front Cardiovasc Med 2014;1:7.

124. de Jong S, van Veen TA, van Rijen HV, et al. Fibrosis and cardiac arrhythmias. J Cardiovasc Pharmacol 2011;57(6):630–8.

125. Rossi GP, Sacchetto A, Pavan E, et al. Remodeling of the left ventricle in primary aldosteronism due to Conn's adenoma. Circulation 1997;95(6):1471–8.

126. Rossi GP. Cardiac consequences of aldosterone excess in human hypertension. Am J Hypertens 2006;19(1):10–2.

127. Magee A, Nevin NC. The epidemiology of myotonic dystrophy in Northern Ireland. Community Genet 1999;2(4):179–83.

128. Siciliano G, Manca M, Gennarelli M, et al. Epidemiology of myotonic dystrophy in Italy: re-apprisal after genetic diagnosis. Clin Genet 2001;59(5): 344–9.

129. Norwood FL, Harling C, Chinnery PF, et al. Prevalence of genetic muscle disease in Northern England: in-depth analysis of a muscle clinic population. Brain 2009;132(Pt 11):3175–86.

130. Phillips MF, Harper PS. Cardiac disease in myotonic dystrophy. Cardiovasc Res 1997;33(1):13–22.

131. Johnson NE, Abbott D, Cannon-Albright LA. Relative risks for comorbidities associated with myotonic dystrophy: a population-based analysis. Muscle Nerve 2015;52(4):659–61.

132. Kusumoto FM, Schoenfeld MH, Barrett C, et al. 2018 ACC/AHA/HRS guideline on the evaluation and management of patients with bradycardia and cardiac conduction delay: executive summary: a report of the American College of Cardiology/American Heart Association Task Force on clinical practice guidelines, and the Heart Rhythm Society. J Am Coll Cardiol 2019;74(7):932–87.

133. Nguyen HH, Wolfe JT 3rd, Holmes DR Jr, et al. Pathology of the cardiac conduction system in myotonic dystrophy: a study of 12 cases. J Am Coll Cardiol 1988;11(3):662–71.

134. Groh WJ, Groh MR, Saha C, et al. Electrocardiographic abnormalities and sudden death in myotonic dystrophy type 1. N Engl J Med 2008;358(25):2688–97.

135. Olofsson BO, Forsberg H, Andersson S, et al. Electrocardiographic findings in myotonic dystrophy. Br Heart J 1988;59(1):47–52.

136. Prystowsky EN, Pritchett LC, Smith WM, et al. Electrophysiologic assessment of the atrioventricular conduction system after surgical correction of ventricular preexcitation. Circulation 1979;59(4):789–96.

137. Wahbi K, Meune C, Becane HM, et al. Left ventricular dysfunction and cardiac arrhythmias are frequent in type 2 myotonic dystrophy: a case control study. Neuromuscul Disord 2009;19(7):468–72.

138. Day JW, Ricker K, Jacobsen JF, et al. Myotonic dystrophy type 2: molecular, diagnostic and clinical spectrum. Neurology 2003;60(4):657–64.

139. Di Mambro C, Tamborrino PP, Silvetti MS, et al. Progressive involvement of cardiac conduction system in paediatric patients with Kearns-Sayre syndrome: how to predict occurrence of complete heart block and sudden cardiac death? Europace 2021;23(6):948–57.

140. DiMauro S, Schon EA, Carelli V, et al. The clinical maze of mitochondrial neurology. Nat Rev Neurol 2013;9(8):429–44.

141. Larsson NG, Holme E, Kristiansson B, et al. Progressive increase of the mutated mitochondrial DNA fraction in Kearns-Sayre syndrome. Pediatr Res 1990;28(2):131–6.

142. Polak PE, Zijlstra F, Roelandt JR. Indications for pacemaker implantation in the Kearns-Sayre syndrome. Eur Heart J 1989;10(3):281–2.

143. Yamashita S, Nishino I, Nonaka I, et al. Genotype and phenotype analyses in 136 patients with single large-scale mitochondrial DNA deletions. J Hum Genet 2008;53(7):598.

144. Welzing L, von Kleist-Retzow JC, Kribs A, et al. Rapid development of life-threatening complete atrioventricular block in Kearns-Sayre syndrome. Eur J Pediatr 2009;168(6):757–9.

145. Altekin RE, Yanikoglu A, Ucar M, et al. Complete AV block and cardiac syncope in a patient with Duchenne muscular dystrophy. J Cardiol Cases 2011;3(2):e68–70.

146. Fayssoil A, Orlikowski D, Nardi O, et al. Complete atrioventricular block in Duchenne muscular dystrophy. Europace 2008;10(11):1351–2.

147. Akdemir R, Ozhan H, Gunduz H, et al. Complete atrioventricular block in Becker muscular dystrophy. N Z Med J 2004;117(1194):U895.

148. Quinlivan R, Ball J, Dunckley M, et al. Becker muscular dystrophy presenting with complete heart block in the sixth decade. J Neurol 1995;242(6):398–400.

149. Angelini C, Fanin M, Freda MP, et al. Prognostic factors in mild dystrophinopathies. J Neurol Sci 1996;142(1–2):70–8.

150. Bies RD, Friedman D, Roberts R, et al. Expression and localization of dystrophin in human cardiac Purkinje fibers. Circulation 1992;86(1):147–53.

151. Finsterer J, Stollberger C. The heart in human dystrophinopathies. Cardiology 2003;99(1):1–19.

Pacing-Induced Cardiomyopathy

Shaan Khurshid, MD, MPH[a], David S. Frankel, MD[b],*

KEYWORDS

• Pacing-induced cardiomyopathy • Heart failure • Pacing

KEY POINTS

• Right ventricular (RV) pacing-induced cardiomyopathy (PICM) is typically defined as left ventricular systolic dysfunction resulting from electrical and mechanical dyssynchrony caused by chronic RV pacing.
• RV PICM is common, occurring in 10% to 20% of individuals exposed to frequent RV pacing.
• Several risk factors for PICM have been identified, yet the ability to accurately predict which individuals will develop PICM remains insufficient.
• Physiologic pacing, including biventricular and conduction system pacing, prevents the development of PICM and can reverse left ventricular systolic dysfunction after PICM has occurred.

INTRODUCTION

The potential for chronic right ventricular pacing (RVP) to cause an acquired cardiomyopathy, termed RV pacing-induced cardiomyopathy (PICM), has been clinically recognized for over 20 years.[1] Nevertheless, over one million pacemakers are currently implanted worldwide,[2] and most of the individuals who are exposed to RVP do not develop PICM.[3] Although more contemporary pacing strategies that can preserve ventricular synchrony (ie, physiologic pacing, such as biventricular pacing [BiV] or conduction system pacing [CSP]) decrease the risk of PICM, higher cost, difficulty of implantation, and increased rate of complications continue to favor traditional RVP in most cases.[4,5] As a result, RVP presently remains the standard of care for most patients who require pacing support in the absence of a pre-existing cardiomyopathy.[6] Such an approach is consistent with current guidelines from the European Society of Cardiology,[7] European Heart Rhythm Association,[8] and American Heart Association/American College of Cardiology/Heart Rhythm Society,[9]

which support physiologic pacing with BiV only in the presence of systolic dysfunction and ongoing requirement for ventricular pacing. Therefore, it is imperative for clinicians to understand which individuals are most likely to develop PICM, as well as the optimal strategies for surveillance and treatment after PICM is diagnosed, to minimize adverse outcomes related to RVP.

PATHOPHYSIOLOGY OF PICM

The potential for RVP to result in deleterious cardiovascular outcomes became apparent in the late 1990s and early 2000s. In a small randomized trial reported in 1994, Andersen and colleagues[1] found that individuals with sick sinus syndrome treated with atrial pacing, as opposed to RVP, had a lower incidence of atrial fibrillation (AF) and thromboembolic complications over 5 years of follow-up. Subsequently, the 2002 Dual Chamber and VVI Implantable Defibrillator (DAVID) trial[10] found that individuals randomized to DDD pacing with a lower rate limit of 70 beats per minute (mean RVP percentage 56%) had a 10% increase

This article originally appeared in *Cardiac Electrophysiology Clinics*, Volume 13 Issue 4, December 2021.
a Division of Cardiology and Cardiovascular Research Center, Massachusetts General Hospital, Yawkey 5B Heart Center, 55 Fruit Street, Boston, MA 02114, USA; b Cardiovascular Division, Perelman School of Medicine at the University of Pennsylvania, 3400 Spruce Street, 9 Founders Pavilion, Philadelphia, PA 19104, USA
* Corresponding author.
E-mail address: David.Frankel@pennmedicine.upenn.edu

in death or hospitalization when compared to those randomized to backup VVI pacing at 40 beats per minute (mean RVP percentage 3%). A subset analysis of the 2003 Mode Selection Trial (MOST), another randomized trial of VVI versus DDD pacing, similarly found that higher RVP percentage was a strong predictor of heart failure hospitalization.[11]

PICM is now recognized as an acquired cardiomyopathy caused by exposure to electrical and mechanical dyssynchrony resulting from RVP (**Fig. 1**). Animal studies suggest that dyssynchrony may lead to clinical cardiomyopathy by inducing alterations in myocardial perfusion, encouraging pathologic remodeling related to regional differences in wall stress, and promoting abnormalities in intracellular and extracellular regulation.[12] As many individuals are exposed to decades of RVP and never develop PICM, it is likely that substrate vulnerability plays an important role in PICM development, although the specific mechanisms underlying such vulnerability are not well-understood.

Although variable definitions exist in the literature, most commonly PICM is defined as a drop in left ventricular ejection fraction (LVEF) of ≥10% to a value <50%, without a clear alternative explanation, in the setting of significant RVP.[13] Some studies have additionally required the occurrence of heart failure symptoms, although such an approach inappropriately excludes the considerable proportion of individuals who develop an asymptomatic cardiomyopathy.[14] As individuals exposed to RVP frequently have competing potential causes of LVEF decline, PICM is most appropriately considered a diagnosis of exclusion, identified as the cause of

cardiomyopathy only after a reasonable search for alternative etiologies such as ischemia or uncontrolled hypertension is unrevealing.[13]

PICM FREQUENCY AND RISK FACTORS

Since the initial recognition of PICM as a clinical entity, several studies have examined the incidence of and clinical risk factors for developing PICM. An overview of retrospective observational studies describing PICM incidence and risk factors is compiled in **Table 1**. A summary of identified risk factors for developing PICM is depicted in **Fig. 1**.

In 2014, Khurshid and colleagues[13] reported a single-center experience of 257 individuals with normal baseline LVEF undergoing right ventricular pacemaker implantation. They observed an overall PICM incidence of 19% over a median follow-up of 3.5 years. Risk factors for PICM in multivariable models included male sex and wider native QRS duration. In 2016, Kiehl and colleagues[15] published a similarly designed study including 823 individuals and reported a PICM incidence of 12.3% over slightly longer follow-up. In multivariable models, increasing RV pacing percentage, and in particular RV pacing percentage ≥20%, was a strong risk factor for PICM. Notably, only individuals with RV pacing percentage ≥20% were included in the study by Khurshid and colleagues, and therefore both studies support the notion that 20% RV pacing is sufficient to cause PICM.

Several subsequent studies have suggested that postimplant surrogates of dyssynchrony may also identify risk for developing PICM. Lee and colleagues[16] performed a retrospective study of 234

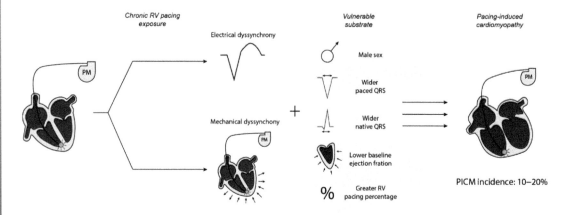

Fig. 1. Pathophysiology of PICM. An overview of the pathophysiology of PICM is depicted. Chronic exposure to RVP results in electrical dyssynchrony (manifested as a wide paced QRS complex) and mechanical dyssynchrony, including regional differences in myocardial contraction. Particularly in the presence of certain risk factors, electrical and mechanical dyssynchrony can lead to adverse remodeling and development of systolic dysfunction, manifesting in PICM. The prevalence of PICM is 10% to 20% over long-term follow-up.

Table 1

Summary of retrospective observational studies describing PICM incidence and risk factors

Study	Setting	N	Follow-up (y)	PICM Definition	PICM Incidence	PICM Risk Factors
Khurshid et al. 2014[13]	Single-center	257	3.3	LVEF decrease ≥10% to <50% No alternative cause of cardiomyopathy	19.5%	Native QRS duration (HR 1.03 per 1 ms increase) Male sex (HR 2.15)
Kiehl et al. 2016[15]	Single-center	823	4.3	Postimplant LVEF <40% or CRT upgrade	12.3%	Preimplant LVEF (HR 1.05 per 1% decrease) RVP percentage (HR 1.01 per 1% increase) >20% RVP (HR 6.76)
Lee et al. 2016[16]	Single-center	234	15.6	LVEF decrease >5% with HF symptoms No alternative cause of cardiomyopathy	20.5%	Old age (HR 1.62) Paced QRS duration (HR 1.54) Higher myocardial scar score (HR 1.23) Higher RVP percentage (HR 1.31)
Cho et al. 2018	Single-center	618	7.2	LVEF decrease ≥10% to <50% or new regional wall motion abnormality not attributable to coronary heart disease	14.1%	LBBB (HR 8.62) Paced QRS duration ≥ 155 ms (HR 2.61) ≥86% RVP (HR 2.42)
Kim et al. 2018[17]	Multi-center (3 sites)	130	4.5	LVEF decrease >10% to <50%	16.1%	Paced QRS duration (HR 1.05 per 1 ms increase)
Bansal et al. 2019[19]	Single-center	363	1.2	LVEF decrease >10%	13.8%	>60% RVP (HR 4.26) Interventricular dyssynchrony (HR 3.15)
Kaye et al. 2019[38]	Single-center	118	3.5	1. LVEF ≤40% if baseline LVEF >50% or absolute reduction ≥5% 2. LVEF ≤40% if baseline LVEF >50% or absolute reduction ≥10% 3. LVEF ≤40%	1. 9.3% 2. 5.9% 3. 39.0%	RVP percentage (effect size not reported)

individuals followed for over 15 years, reporting a PICM incidence of 20.5%. Risk factors for PICM included older age and wider paced QRS duration, as well as a greater electrocardiographic myocardial scar score. Kim and colleagues[17] also found that a wider paced QRS duration was associated with PICM. In a cross-sectional study comprising 184 individuals, Khurshid and colleagues[14] reported that paced QRS duration was associated with the presence of PICM at follow-up, with a paced QRS duration ≥150 ms demonstrating 95% sensitivity for the presence of PICM. Within 618 individuals followed for over 7 years, Cho and colleagues[18] found that PICM developed in 14.1%. A paced QRS duration ≥155 ms was again a strong risk factor for PICM, in addition to RVP percentage ≥86% and presence of LBBB before pacemaker implantation. Bansal and colleagues[19] found that echocardiographic evidence of interventricular dyssynchrony was an independent risk factor for PICM, with individuals demonstrating dyssynchrony having a 3-fold increased risk.

UPFRONT PHYSIOLOGIC PACING

Given the key role of electrical and mechanical dyssynchrony in the development of PICM, there has been increasing interest in upfront utilization of pacing strategies that preserve more physiologic ventricular activation (eg, BiV and CSP). The 2013 Biventricular versus Right Ventricular Pacing in Heart Failure Patients with Atrioventricular Block (BLOCK-HF[6]) study is the largest trial to date comparing RVP to physiologic pacing, randomizing 691 individuals with pre-existing heart failure (ie, New York Heart Association [NYHA] functional class I-III and LVEF ≤ 50%) to BiV or RVP. At 3 years follow-up (median RVP percentage >97% in both groups), BiV was associated with a 10% absolute reduction in the primary outcome of death, urgent heart failure care, and adverse LV remodeling. As a result, physiologic pacing is generally considered first-line therapy among individuals with pre-existing heart failure who have a substantial pacing requirement.

In contrast, the benefit of upfront physiologic pacing as compared to RVP is less clear among individuals without pre-existing heart failure. Several small studies have compared physiologic pacing to RVP as a means of preventing PICM (Table 2). Although larger studies are needed, available evidence supports the concept that PICM can essentially be prevented by use of physiologic pacing. At the same time, it is important to note that although physiologic pacing strategies

are becoming increasingly safe and effective, the rates of acute and chronic complications remain higher than those observed with RVP.[20,21]

Biventricular Pacing

Most of the studies investigating upfront physiologic pacing have assessed for echocardiographic evidence of adverse ventricular remodeling (eg, increasing LV volumes) as surrogates for PICM development. In 2011, Albertsen and colleagues[22] randomized 50 patients to BiV or RVP. At 3 years follow-up, the LVEF dropped from a mean of 59% to 53% in the RVP group, with no change in the BiV group. Notably, although sample size was limited, there were no differences in quality of life or NYHA functional class between the RVP and BiV groups. Similar results were observed in the comparably designed PACE trial,[23] which randomized 177 patients to RVP or BiV. After 2 years, individuals in the RVP group experienced a 10% drop in LVEF, whereas individuals in the BiV group had no change in LVEF. In total, 63% of individuals receiving RVP experienced a drop in LVEF ≥ 5%, as compared to 20% of individuals receiving BiV.

Multiple studies have compared the upfront use of BiV versus RVP following AV node ablation for refractory AF. In the 2005 PAVE trial,[24] 184 individuals undergoing AV node ablation were randomized to BiV or RVP. At 6 months, when compared to individuals receiving BiV, those receiving RVP had a lesser improvement in the 6-min walk test (24% vs 31%) and experienced a mean 5-point decrease in LVEF (no change in BiV group). In the AVAIL CLS/CRT trial,[25] 108 patients undergoing AV node ablation were randomized 4:1 to BiV or RVP. At 6 months, there was no difference in LVEF in the RVP group, but the BiV group had a statistically significant 3-point increase in LVEF.

Conduction System Pacing

More recently, several studies have assessed the use of upfront CSP (specifically His bundle pacing [HBP]) as compared to traditional RVP. In 2018, Vijayaraman and colleagues[21] reported a retrospective study in which individuals undergoing HBP were compared to individuals contemporaneously undergoing RVP at a sister hospital. HBP was attempted in 94 patients, but was successful only in 75 patients (80%). At 5 years, the primary outcome of death or hospitalization for heart failure occurred in 53% of the RVP group compared to 32% in the HBP group. They also reported the incidence of PICM, defined as a decline in LVEF greater than 10% resulting in an LVEF less than 50% among individuals receiving at least 40% RVP. PICM occurred in 22% of the RVP group

Table 2
Summary of studies comparing right ventricular versus physiologic pacing strategies among individuals with preserved preimplant left ventricular systolic function

Study	Setting	N	Mean Preimplant LVEF	Follow-up	Outcomes	Outcome Incidence	Risk Factors for Outcome
Non-randomized							
Abdelrahman et al., 2018[20]	Retrospective multi-center (2 sites)	433 (RVP) 304 (HBP)	54	2 y	Death, HF hospitalization, or upgrade to physiologic pacing	RVP: 32% HBP: 25%	Age (HR 1.02 per 1 y increase) Preimplant LVEF (HR 0.98 per 1% increase) Heart failure (HR 2.09) Chronic kidney disease (HR 1.75) HBP (vs RVP, HR 0.71) >20% RVP (effect size not reported)
Vijayaraman P et al., 2018[21]	Retrospective multi-center (2 sites)	98 (RVP) 75 (HBP)	55–57	5 y	Death or HF hospitalization PICM (LVEF decline >10% to <50% w/ RVP >40%)	RVP: 53% (PICM incidence 22%) HBP: 32% (PICM incidence 2%)	RVP (vs HBP, HR 1.9) >40% RVP (effect size not reported)
Randomized							
PAVE, 2005[24]	Multicenter	81 (RVP) 103 (BiV)	45–47	6 mo	LVEF, QoL scores, 6-min walk test	RVP: 24% improvement in 6-min walk, 5-pt decrease in LVEF, no change in QoL BiV: 31% improvement in 6-min walk, no change in LVEF, no change in QoL	Baseline LVEF ≤45%
Occhetta E et al., 2006[39]	Single-center, crossover	16 (RVP) 16 (BiV)	52	6 mo	NYHA class, QoL scores, 6-min walk test	RVP: no change in NYHA class, QoL, or 6-min walk BiV: 0.58-pt improvement in	None reported

(continued on next page)

Table 2
(continued)

Study	Setting	N	Mean Preimplant LVEF	Follow-up	Outcomes	Outcome Incidence	Risk Factors for Outcome
						NYHA class, 50% improvement in QoL score and 14% improvement in 6-min walk	
AVAIL CLS/CRT, 2010[25]	Multicenter (22 sites)	20 (RVP) 88 (BiV)	56–57	6 mo	LVEF	RVP: No significant change in LVEF BiV: 3.2-pt increase in LVEF	None reported
Albertsen et al., 2011[22]	Single-center	50 (RVP) 50 (BiV)	59–60	3 y	LVEF, dyssynchrony index	RVP: 6-pt decrease in LVEF; increase in dyssynchrony index BiV: No change in LVEF or dyssynchrony	None reported
PACE, 2011[23]	Multicenter (4 sites)	88 (RVP) 89 (BiV)	62	2 y	LVEF, LVESV	RVP: 9.5-pt decrease in LVEF; 9.9 mL increase in LVESV BiV: No difference in LVEF or LVESV	None reported
PREVENT-HF, 2011[40]	Multicenter (14 sites)	58 (RVP) 50 (BiV)	55–57	1 y	LVEDV	No difference in LVEDV at 12 mo	None reported

and only 2% of the HBP group. Of the 2 cases of LVEF decline in the HBP group, one was potentially attributable to myocardial infarction, while the other resolved with transition to BiV pacing, suggesting that conduction system activation may have been suboptimal in that individual. Notably, as compared to RVP, the incidence of lead revision (7% vs 3%) and generator change (9% vs 1%) were both higher with HBP.

A larger, similarly designed study was reported in 2018 by Abdelrahman and colleagues.[20] HBP was attempted in 332 consecutive patients, and successful in 302 (92%), whereas RVP was performed in 433 patients. At approximately 2 years, the primary endpoint of death, hospitalization for heart failure, or upgrade to BiV was significantly lower in the HBP group (25%) than in the RVP group (32%). Of note, improved outcomes with HBP were primarily observed in the subgroup of individuals receiving greater than 20% RVP, consistent with observational data suggesting that 20% RVP may represent a minimum threshold for PICM.[13,15] Again, the need for lead revision was substantially higher in the HBP group (4%) than in the RVP group (0.5%).

TREATMENT OF PICM

Given the increased costs, procedural complexity and complication rates associated with upfront physiologic pacing,[4,5] it is likely that most of the individuals who do not have pre-existing heart failure and require ventricular pacing will continue to receive RVP. As a result, it is important to understand whether PICM can be effectively treated (**Fig. 2**). Several recent studies have attempted to

characterize the response to provision of physiologic pacing among individuals with established PICM (**Table 3**). Consistent with dyssynchrony as the underlying mechanism of PICM development, studies generally demonstrate a robust response upon transitioning from RVP to physiologic pacing, even among individuals having had PICM for many years. Nevertheless, recovery of systolic dysfunction is not universally complete, and a minority of individuals with PICM do not respond to physiologic pacing. Further work is needed to assess whether nonresponse to physiologic pacing among individuals with PICM is related to irreversible myocardial injury and fibrosis, or misdiagnosis of PICM in the presence of an alternative cause of cardiomyopathy that is unrecognized (eg, Lamin A/C or sarcoidosis). Of note, as with any nonischemic cardiomyopathy, guideline-directed medical therapy should be provided to individuals with PICM, although the role of specific medical therapies has not been directly assessed in the PICM population.[26]

Biventricular Pacing

The first indication that BiV may effectively reverse PICM was a report by Nazeri and colleagues[27] including 21 patients with PICM. PICM was defined as a decline in LVEF from normal to ≤35% within 6 months of pacemaker implantation among individuals receiving ≥25% RVP and no evidence of an alternative cause of cardiomyopathy. Most individuals had PICM for only several months, with a mean time from PICM diagnosis to BiV upgrade of 5 months. Following upgrade to BiV, the mean LVEF improved from 31% to

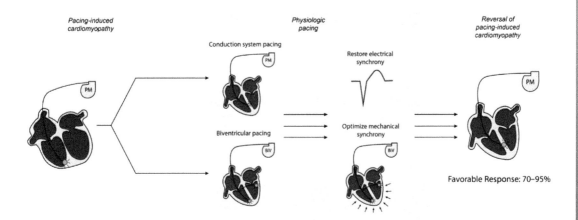

Fig. 2. Treatment of PICM. An overview of the treatment of PICM is depicted. PICM can be treated effectively with upgrade to a physiologic pacing strategy, either biventricular or conduction system pacing. Physiologic pacing leads to improvement of electrical synchrony (manifesting as narrowing of the paced QRS) and more synchronous intraventricular and interventricular contraction. Physiologic pacing leads to a substantial improvement in LVEF in 70% to 95% of individuals with PICM.

Table 3
Summary of studies of pacing-induced cardiomyopathy treatment

Study	Design	N	Mean Pretreatment LVEF (%)	PICM Definition	Response	Factors Predicting Response
Biventricular pacing						
Nazeri et al. 2010[*][,27]	Single-center retrospective	21	31.2	LVEF decrease to ≤35% No alternative cause of cardiomyopathy >25% RV pacing	Mean postupgrade LVEF: 37%	None found
Khurshid et al. 2018[28]	Single-center retrospective	69	29.3	LVEF decrease ≥10% to <50% No alternative cause of cardiomyopathy ≥20% RV pacing	Mean postupgrade LVEF: 45% Improvement in LVEF ≥5%: 86% Achievement of LVEF ≥35%: 72%	Native QRS duration (2-pt additional LVEF improvement per 10 ms decrease)
Conduction system pacing						
Shan et al. 2017[*][,31]	Single-center retrospective	11	36.1	LVEF decrease ≥10% to <50% No alternative cause of cardiomyopathy ≥20% RV pacing	Mean postupgrade LVEF: 53%	Not reported
Vijayaraman et al. 2019[4]	Single-center retrospective	60	34.3	LVEF decrease ≥10% to <50% No alternative cause of cardiomyopathy >20% RV pacing	Mean postupgrade LVEF: 48% LVEF ≥5%: 95% Achievement of LVEF ≥35%: 75%	Not reported

37%. Sixteen patients (76%) reported a significant improvement in heart failure symptoms. Among the 5 patients (24%) with no LVEF improvement, no risk factors could be identified for lack of response.

In 2018, Khurshid and colleagues[28] reported a sizable series of individuals with PICM undergoing upgrade to BiV. PICM was defined as a decline in LVEF $\geq$10% resulting in an LVEF less than 50% among individuals with $\geq$20% RVP at the time of PICM diagnosis. Among 69 individuals whose medical records were manually adjudicated for the presence of PICM (mean preupgrade LVEF 29%), upgrade to BiV resulted in substantial improvement in LVEF (mean postupgrade LVEF 45%). Notably, the diagnosis of PICM was fairly longstanding, with an average time from diagnosis to BiV upgrade of approximately 1.5 years. Fifty-nine patients undergoing upgrade experienced an improvement in LVEF $\geq$5% (86%), and 49 patients had an improvement in LVEF $\geq$10% (71%). Importantly, among individuals with a preupgrade LVEF at or below 35% (ie, the LVEF threshold used to determine candidacy for primary prevention implantable defibrillators[29]), the substantial majority (72%) achieved an improvement in LVEF to above 35%. In multivariable analysis, individuals with a narrower native QRS at the time of initial pacemaker implantation were more likely to respond to BiV upgrade (additional 2% LVEF improvement per 10 ms decrease). Importantly, the vast majority of LVEF improvement occurred within the year following BiV upgrade, and no malignant ventricular arrhythmias were observed in the PICM cohort during that time. Based on these observations, the authors proposed upgrade to physiologic pacing, with the addition of a defibrillator at 1 year in the minority of individuals in whom the LVEF remains $\leq$35% (see **Fig. 3**). Such an approach is supported by independent evidence suggesting a low risk of malignant ventricular arrhythmias in the PICM population.[30]

Conduction System Pacing

Recent studies suggest that HBP may also represent an effective treatment for established PICM. Shan and colleagues[31] reported a series of 18 patients referred for HBP. HBP was successful in 16 patients (89%). Of the 16 patients, 11 had a diagnosis of PICM. Of the PICM patients, the mean LVEF improved from 36% to 53% after HBP. Significant improvements in LV diastolic volume and mitral regurgitation were also observed. NYHA functional class decreased from 3.0 to 1.4 after HBP. No lead revisions were required within 2 years of follow-up.

Vijayaraman and colleagues[4] recently reported results of HBP among 60 individuals with PICM, defined as a decline in LVEF $\geq$10% resulting in an LVEF less than 50% among those exposed to greater than 20% RVP. HBP was successful in 57 patients (95%). The diagnosis of PICM was even more longstanding than the population reported by Khurshid and colleagues, with a mean time from diagnosis of PICM to upgrade over 6 years. After HBP, the paced QRS duration decreased from 177 ms to 114 ms. Among 55 PICM patients with echocardiographic follow-up, the mean LVEF increased from 34% preupgrade to 48% postupgrade. Improvement in LVEF $\geq$5% was observed in 52 patients (95%), and improvement $\geq$10% in 41 patients (75%). NYHA functional class decreased from 2.8 to 1.9 after HBP. Three patients (4%) required lead revision, all because of increased HBP capture thresholds.

AUTHORS' APPROACH

In the vast majority of patients with normal LVEF and high anticipated pacing burden, we initially deliver standard RVP, given simplicity of implantation and low rate of complications. Surveillance echocardiograms are performed every 1 to 2 years, and more frequently should heart failure symptoms develop. If the LVEF decreases $\geq$10% resulting in an LVEF less than 50%, guideline-directed medical therapy is initiated and a search for alternative etiologies, such as coronary artery disease or uncontrolled arrhythmias, is performed. If PICM is confirmed, upgrade to physiologic pacing is performed. Even if the LVEF is less than 35%, we typically upgrade to physiologic pacemaker only, as most PICM will substantially reverse following physiologic pacing. If the LVEF remains less than 35% after 1 year, consideration is given to further upgrade to a defibrillator (see **Fig. 3**).

FUTURE OUTLOOK

In recent years, PICM has become appropriately recognized as an important cause of heart failure-related morbidity among individuals undergoing RVP. Since the incidence of bradyarrhythmias appears to be increasing,[32] the public health burden attributable to PICM is likely to grow even further in the coming years. A better understanding of several aspects of PICM epidemiology and management will be critical to minimize the morbidity attributable to PICM.

First, improved methods of risk stratification for PICM development are needed to prioritize individuals for physiologic pacing. Although multiple studies have identified risk factors for PICM, no

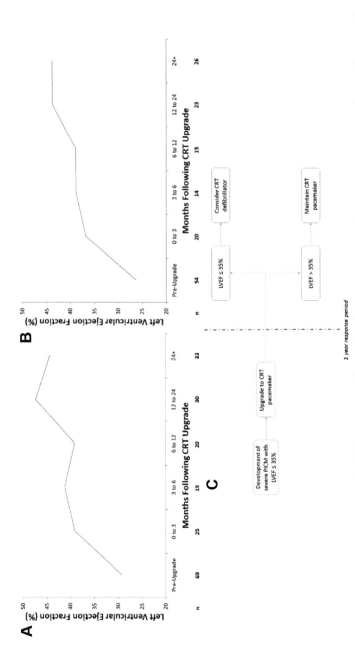

Fig. 3. Improvement of pacing-induced cardiomyopathy following upgrade to physiologic pacing. Mean improvement in LVEF after cardiac resynchronization therapy (CRT) upgrade is illustrated within the first 3 months, 3 to 6 months, 6 to 12 months, 12 to 24 months, and more than 24 months among (*A*) the entire pacing-induced cardiomyopathy (PICM) cohort and (*B*) the severe PICM cohort (nadir LVEF ≤35%). The number of patients undergoing an echocardiogram during each time range is indicated below the x-axis. A proposed CRT implantation strategy is depicted (*C*) in which patients with severe PICM undergo initial CRT pacemaker with upgrade to defibrillator to be considered among those with LVEF ≤35% after 1 year. LVEF = left ventricular ejection fraction. Reprinted with permission from Khurshid S, Obeng-Gyimah E, Supple GE, Schaller RD, Lin D, Owens AT, Epstein AE, Dixit S, Marchlinski FE, Frankel DS. Reversal of Pacing-Induced Cardiomyopathy Following Cardiac Resynchronization Therapy. JACC Clin Eletrophysiol. 2018 Feb;4(2):168-177.

individual factor or set of factors (outside of pre-existing systolic dysfunction[6]) has been shown to portend sufficiently high risk of PICM such that upfront physiologic pacing is considered first-line therapy. Small studies have implicated novel features, such as electrocardiographic scar score[16] or immediate post-implantation dyssynchrony,[19] as potential additional PICM risk factors. It is possible that the ability to predict the development of PICM can be improved further through the development of composite prediction models comprising a multitude of features, potentially including imaging or biomarker data. Prospective validation of such scores would be needed before they could be used to select individuals most likely to benefit from upfront physiologic pacing.

Second, future work is needed to assess the chronic effects of RV pacing beyond decrease in systolic function. After initiation of RVP, the incidence of HF hospitalization and worsening HF-related symptoms appears to increase out of proportion to the degree of LV systolic dysfunction observed.[10,21] Therefore, it is likely that RVP may result in HF symptoms through mechanisms other than induction of LV systolic dysfunction, such as adverse effects on diastolic function,[33] increased risk of incident AF,[34] and worsening of mitral regurgitation.[13,31] A more comprehensive understanding of the mechanisms underlying worsening HF after exposure to RVP may improve our ability to detect individuals earlier in the course of PICM development and facilitate prompt upgrade to physiologic pacing.

Third, continued development of improved methods for delivering physiologic pacing may lead to more opportunities to prevent exposure to RVP in the first place. Although evidence suggests that upfront physiologic pacing using methods such as BiV or HBP can avert the development of PICM, both techniques continue to be associated with greater complication rates and lower long-term durability as compared to traditional RVP.[5,20] Early evidence suggests that left bundle pacing is easier to perform and results in lower capture thresholds than HBP,[35–37] but further work is needed to assess the role of this technique in preventing and treating PICM. In the future, it is conceivable that certain methods of physiologic pacing may become sufficiently safe and effective as to become first-line therapy for most individuals requiring ventricular pacing.

SUMMARY

PICM is a common cause of LV systolic dysfunction, affecting 10% to 20% of individuals exposed to frequent RVP. Factors associated with increased PICM risk include male sex, older age, lower pre-implantation LVEF, wider native QRS, wider paced QRS, higher electrocardiographic scar score, and post-implantation dyssynchrony. Physiologic pacing (eg, BiV or CSP) is an effective method to prevent PICM in at-risk individuals, as well as to reverse systolic dysfunction among individuals with established PICM. Future work is needed to improve the delivery of physiologic pacing, and to develop more accurate methods of prioritizing individuals at highest risk for RVP-related morbidity in whom physiologic pacing strategies may be preferred.

DISCLOSURE

The authors have nothing to disclose.

REFERENCES

1. Andersen HR, Thuesen L, Bagger JP, et al. Prospective randomised trial of atrial versus ventricular pacing in sick-sinus syndrome. Lancet 1994;344(8936): 1523–8.
2. Mond HG, Proclemer A. The 11th world survey of cardiac pacing and implantable cardioverter-defibrillators: calendar year 2009–a World Society of Arrhythmia's project. Pacing Clin Electrophysiol 2011;34(8):1013–27.
3. Yu C-M, Chan JY-S, Zhang Q, et al. Biventricular pacing in patients with bradycardia and normal ejection fraction. N Engl J Med 2009;361(22): 2123–34.
4. Vijayaraman P, Herweg B, Dandamudi G, et al. Outcomes of His-bundle pacing upgrade after long-term right ventricular pacing and/or pacing-induced cardiomyopathy: insights into disease progression. Heart Rhythm 2019;16(10):1554–61.
5. Chung ES, St John Sutton MG, Mealing S, et al. Economic value and cost-effectiveness of biventricular versus right ventricular pacing: results from the BLOCK-HF study. J Med Econ 2019;22(10): 1088–95.
6. Curtis AB, Worley SJ, Adamson PB, et al. Biventricular pacing for atrioventricular block and systolic dysfunction. N Engl J Med 2013;368(17):1585–93.
7. Ponikowski P, Voors AA, Anker SD, et al. 2016 ESC guidelines for the diagnosis and treatment of acute and chronic heart failure: the task force for the diagnosis and treatment of acute and chronic heart failure of the European Society of Cardiology (ESC) developed with the special contribution of the Heart Failure Association (HFA) of the ESC. Eur Heart J 2016;37(27):2129–200.
8. European Society of Cardiology (ESC), European Heart Rhythm Association (EHRA), Brignole M, et al. 2013 ESC guidelines on cardiac pacing and

cardiac resynchronization therapy: the task force on cardiac pacing and resynchronization therapy of the European Society of Cardiology (ESC). Developed in collaboration with the European Heart Rhythm Association (EHRA). Europace 2013;15(8):1070–118.

9. Tracy CM, Epstein AE, Darbar D, et al. 2012 ACCF/AHA/HRS focused update of the 2008 guidelines for device-based therapy of cardiac rhythm abnormalities: a report of the American College of Cardiology Foundation/American Heart Association task force on practice guidelines and the Heart Rhythm Society. [corrected]. Circulation 2012;126(14):1784–800.

10. Wilkoff BL, Cook JR, Epstein AE, et al. Dual-chamber pacing or ventricular backup pacing in patients with an implantable defibrillator: the Dual Chamber and VVI Implantable Defibrillator (DAVID) Trial. JAMA 2002;288(24):3115–23.

11. Sweeney MO, Hellkamp AS, Ellenbogen KA, et al. Adverse effect of ventricular pacing on heart failure and atrial fibrillation among patients with normal baseline QRS duration in a clinical trial of pacemaker therapy for sinus node dysfunction. Circulation 2003;107(23):2932–7.

12. Ahmed FZ, Khattar RS, Zaidi AM, et al. Pacing-induced cardiomyopathy: pathophysiological insights through matrix metalloproteinases. Heart Fail Rev 2014;19(5):669–80.

13. Khurshid S, Epstein AE, Verdino RJ, et al. Incidence and predictors of right ventricular pacing-induced cardiomyopathy. Heart Rhythm 2014;11(9):1619–25.

14. Khurshid S, Liang JJ, Owens A, et al. Longer paced QRS duration is associated with increased prevalence of right ventricular pacing-induced cardiomyopathy. J Cardiovasc Electrophysiol 2016;27(10):1174–9.

15. Kiehl EL, Makki T, Kumar R, et al. Incidence and predictors of right ventricular pacing-induced cardiomyopathy in patients with complete atrioventricular block and preserved left ventricular systolic function. Heart Rhythm 2016;13(12):2272–8.

16. Lee S-A, Cha M-J, Cho Y, et al. Paced QRS duration and myocardial scar amount: predictors of long-term outcome of right ventricular apical pacing. Heart Vessels 2016;31(7):1131–9.

17. Kim JH, Kang K-W, Chin JY, et al. Major determinant of the occurrence of pacing-induced cardiomyopathy in complete atrioventricular block: a multicentre, retrospective analysis over a 15-year period in South Korea. BMJ Open 2018;8(2):e019048.

18. Cho SW, Gwag HB, Hwang JK, et al. Clinical features, predictors, and long-term prognosis of pacing-induced cardiomyopathy. Eur J Heart Fail 2019;21(5):643–51.

19. Bansal R, Parakh N, Gupta A, et al. Incidence and predictors of pacemaker-induced cardiomyopathy with comparison between apical and non-apical

right ventricular pacing sites. J Interv Card Electrophysiol 2019;56(1):63–70.

20. Abdelrahman M, Subzposh FA, Beer D, et al. Clinical outcomes of His bundle pacing compared to right ventricular pacing. J Am Coll Cardiol 2018;71(20):2319–30.

21. Vijayaraman P, Naperkowski A, Subzposh FA, et al. Permanent His-bundle pacing: long-term lead performance and clinical outcomes. Heart Rhythm 2018;15(5):696–702.

22. Albertsen AE, Mortensen PT, Jensen HK, et al. Adverse effect of right ventricular pacing prevented by biventricular pacing during long-term follow-up: a randomized comparison. Eur J Echocardiogr 2011;12(10):767–72.

23. Chan JY-S, Fang F, Zhang Q, et al. Biventricular pacing is superior to right ventricular pacing in bradycardia patients with preserved systolic function: 2-year results of the PACE trial. Eur Heart J 2011;32(20):2533–40.

24. Doshi RN, Daoud EG, Fellows C, et al. Left ventricular-based cardiac stimulation post AV nodal ablation evaluation (the PAVE study). J Cardiovasc Electrophysiol 2005;16(11):1160–5.

25. Orlov MV, Gardin JM, Slawsky M, et al. Biventricular pacing improves cardiac function and prevents further left atrial remodeling in patients with symptomatic atrial fibrillation after atrioventricular node ablation. Am Heart J 2010;159(2):264–70.

26. Yancy CW, Jessup M, Bozkurt B, et al. 2017 ACC/AHA/HFSA focused update of the 2013 ACCF/AHA guideline for the management of heart failure: a report of the American College of Cardiology/American Heart Association task force on clinical practice guidelines and the Heart Failure Society of America. Circulation 2017;136(6):e137–61.

27. Nazeri A, Massumi A, Rasekh A, et al. Cardiac resynchronization therapy in patients with right ventricular pacing-induced cardiomyopathy. Pacing Clin Electrophysiol 2010;33(1):37–40.

28. Khurshid S, Obeng-Gyimah E, Supple GE, et al. Reversal of pacing-induced cardiomyopathy following cardiac resynchronization therapy. JACC Clin Electrophysiol 2018;4(2):168–77.

29. Al-Khatib SM, Stevenson WG, Ackerman MJ, et al. 2017 AHA/ACC/HRS guideline for management of patients with ventricular arrhythmias and the prevention of sudden cardiac death: executive summary. Circulation 2018;138(13):e210–71.

30. Barra S, Duehmke R, Providencia R, et al. Patients upgraded to cardiac resynchronization therapy due to pacing-induced cardiomyopathy are at low risk of life-threatening ventricular arrhythmias: a long-term cause-of-death analysis. Europace 2018;20(1):89–96.

31. Shan P, Su L, Zhou X, et al. Beneficial effects of upgrading to His bundle pacing in chronically paced

patients with left ventricular ejection fraction <50. Heart Rhythm 2018;15(3):405–12.

32. Virani SS, Alonso A, Benjamin EJ, et al. Heart disease and stroke statistics-2020 update: a report from the American Heart Association. Circulation 2020;141(9):e139–596.

33. Egnaczyk GF, Chung ES. The relationship between cardiac resynchronization therapy and diastolic function. Curr Heart Fail Rep 2014;11(1):64–9.

34. Nielsen JC, Kristensen L, Andersen HR, et al. A randomized comparison of atrial and dual-chamber pacing in 177 consecutive patients with sick sinus syndrome: echocardiographic and clinical outcome. J Am Coll Cardiol 2003;42(4):614–23.

35. Vijayaraman P, Subzposh FA, Naperkowski A, et al. Prospective evaluation of feasibility and electrophysiologic and echocardiographic characteristics of left bundle branch area pacing. Heart Rhythm 2019;16(12):1774–82.

36. Li X, Li H, Ma W, et al. Permanent left bundle branch area pacing for atrioventricular block: feasibility, safety, and acute effect. Heart Rhythm 2019; 16(12):1766–73.

37. Hanley A, Heist EK. Left ventricular endocardial pacing/leadless pacing. Card Electrophysiol Clin 2019; 11(1):155–64.

38. Kaye G, Ng JY, Ahmed S, et al. The prevalence of pacing-induced cardiomyopathy (PICM) in patients with long term right ventricular pacing - is it a matter of definition? Heart Lung Circ 2019;28(7):1027–33.

39. Occhetta E, Bortnik M, Magnani A, et al. Prevention of ventricular desynchronization by permanent para-Hisian pacing after atrioventricular node ablation in chronic atrial fibrillation: a crossover, blinded, randomized study versus apical right ventricular pacing. J Am Coll Cardiol 2006;47(10):1938–45.

40. Stockburger M, Gómez-Doblas JJ, Lamas G, et al. Preventing ventricular dysfunction in pacemaker patients without advanced heart failure: results from a multicentre international randomized trial (PREVENT-HF). Eur J Heart Fail 2011;13(6):633–41.

Pacing of Specialized Conduction System

Santosh K. Padala, MD, Kenneth A. Ellenbogen, MD*

KEYWORDS

- Ventricular pacing • Physiologic pacing • His bundle pacing • Left bundle branch area pacing
- Cardiac resynchronization therapy • Cardiomyopathy

KEY POINTS

- Conduction system pacing in the form of His bundle pacing or left bundle branch area pacing maintains electrical and mechanical synchrony of the left ventricle.
- Conduction system pacing prevents the untoward effects of nonphysiological, chronic right ventricular pacing.
- His bundle pacing is the most ideal form of physiologic pacing but technical challenges lead to premature battery depletion and lead revisions are the major impediments.
- Left bundle branch area pacing is an attractive alternative to His bundle pacing for providing physiologic pacing in patients with bradycardia and heart failure.
- Cardiac resynchronization therapy with His bundle pacing or left bundle branch area pacing holds a tremendous promise and may provide better resynchronization than traditional biventricular pacing.

INTRODUCTION

Pacing has been the mainstay therapy for management of symptomatic bradyarrhythmias for decades. Historically, cardiac pacing was achieved using large, external, alternating current powered devices in 1950s which subsequently evolved to "wearable" battery-powered external devices.[1] With significant technological evolution implantable pacemakers with transvenous leads were introduced in early 1960s. Right ventricular (RV) apical pacing has been primary strategy to improve survival and quality of life in patients requiring permanent ventricular pacing. It was not until early 2000, when reports on the detrimental effects of chronic RV apical pacing on left ventricular (LV) systolic function (pacing-induced cardiomyopathy [PICMP]) surfaced and caught the attention of cardiac electrophysiologists.

In the MOde Selection Trial (MOST) substudy published in 2003, more than 40% of RV apical pacing in patients with sinus node dysfunction and normal LV ejection fraction (LVEF) was associated with a significant increase in incidence of heart failure hospitalizations and atrial fibrillation (AF) despite maintaining atrioventricular (AV) synchrony.[2] Similar findings were reported subsequently in the Pacing to Avoid Cardiac Enlargement (PACE) study in 2009, which randomized patients with bradycardia and a normal LVEF to RV apical pacing versus biventricular pacing.[3] During a mean follow-up of 4.8 years, patients with RV apical pacing were more likely to have deterioration in systolic function and heart failure hospitalization compared with those with biventricular pacing.[4]

Chronic RV pacing can be even more detrimental in patients with an impaired LVEF at

This article originally appeared in *Cardiac Electrophysiology Clinics*, Volume 13 Issue 4, December 2021.
Conflicts of Interest: Dr Padala is a consultant for Medtronic. Dr Ellenbogen received honoraria from Atricure, Biosense Webster, Medtronic, Boston Scientific, and Biotronik, and Abbott.
Department of Cardiac Electrophysiology, Virginia Commonwealth University, Gateway Building, 3 Road Floor, 3-216, 1200 East Marshall Street, Richmond, VA, USA
* Corresponding author.
E-mail address: kenneth.ellenbogen@vcuhealth.org

baseline and can result in the worsening of preexisting cardiomyopathy. In the Dual Chamber and VVI Implantable Defibrillator (DAVID) Trial published in 2002, patients with a LVEF of 40% or less who were randomized to a dual-chamber pacing mode with a baseline pacing rate of 70 bpm had a significantly higher primary composite end point of death or heart failure hospitalization compared with patients randomized to a single-chamber ventricular pacing mode with backup pacing at 40 bpm.[5] These findings were further reinforced in a larger randomized study of Biventricular versus Right Ventricular Pacing in Heart Failure Patients with AV Block (BLOCK-HF) study that enrolled patients with anticipated high ventricular pacing burden and a LVEF of 50% or less.[6] Over a mean follow-up of 3 years, the primary composite end point of death from any cause, heart failure hospitalization, and increase in LV end-systolic volume index occurred significantly more in patients with RV pacing compared with the biventricular pacing group. Patients in the biventricular pacing group also had significant improvements in the quality of life and New York Heart Association functional class symptoms.[6]

MAGNITUDE AND PATHOPHYSIOLOGY OF PACING-INDUCED CARDIOMYOPATHY

The incidence of PICMP varies widely based on the definition (a decrease in EF of <50% vs <40%, absolute decrease in EF by 5% vs 10%, and or development of HF symptoms) and ranges between 10% and 20% over a 3- to 4-year period of chronic RV apical pacing.[7,8] PICMP may develop as soon as 6 months after the institution of chronic RV apical pacing in patients with AV block as noted in a large study using MarketScan database.[9] Recent studies have reported RV apical pacing burden threshold as low as 20% may suffice to cause PICMP in patients with an AV block.[10] Studies have examined the role of RV nonapical pacing sites (RV outflow tract and RV septal pacing), however, with conflicting data on the potential benefits of mitigating LV dysfunction.[11,12]

RV apical pacing results in slow, myocyte–myocyte propagation between the ventricles, as opposed to the rapid physiologic activation of ventricles when propagation occurs via the His–Purkinje conduction system. The exact pathophysiologic mechanism of PICMP has not been fully elucidated, but it is thought to be due to the intraventricular and interventricular dyssynchrony created by nonphysiological activation of the ventricles resulting in impaired mechanical contraction, abnormal myocardial metabolism, altered regional perfusion, increased fibrosis, functional mitral regurgitation, decreased cardiac output, and increased filling pressures.[8] In addition, chronic RV apical pacing can result in left atrial remodeling and impair atrial function, predisposing to atrial arrhythmias.[13–15]

INCEPTION OF CONDUCTION SYSTEM PACING

The quest for an optimal ventricular pacing site provided an impetus to pace the His–Purkinje conduction system directly to preserve the physiologic activation of the ventricles, thereby mitigating the untoward effects of chronic RV apical pacing. First attempt at temporary His bundle pacing (HBP) was reported by Narula and colleagues in 1970.[16] Deshmukh and colleagues[17] in 2000 reported successful implantation of an active fixation lead at the His bundle location in 12 of 18 patients (67%) with permanent AF, a narrow QRS, and a LVEF of less than 40% after an AV junction ablation. Early studies on HBP implantation were cumbersome because they implanted standard pacing leads by reshaping stylets, used a mapping catheter from the groin to identify the His bundle signals to assist with HBP lead implantation, and frequently implanted a back-up RV pacing lead.[18–21]

It was not until 2014 when HBP gained significant momentum after Sharma and colleagues[22] reported 80% permanent HBP success rate with a lumenless, exposed helix lead delivered through a specialized sheath and without using a mapping catheter or a back-up RV lead. The study also showed significant decrease in heart failure hospitalization in patients requiring more than 40% ventricular pacing in the HBP group compared with the RV pacing group (2% vs 15%; $P = .02$). Subsequently, several investigators from around the world reported the safety, feasibility, and superiority of HBP over RV pacing. His bundle pacemakers have been implanted successfully in patients with normal His–Purkinje conduction, bundle branch block (BBB), AV block, and in selected patients as an alternative to cardiac resynchronization therapy (CRT) (**Table 1**). Based on these studies, the 2018 American College of Cardiology/American Heart Association/Heart Rhythm Society guideline on the management of bradycardia endorsed a class IIa indication for HBP in patients with AV block and a LVEF between 36% and 50%, and a class IIb in patients with AV block at the level of AV node.[23]

With time, the technical challenges and chronic HBP lead performance issues surfaced that tempered the initial enthusiasm with HBP implantation and limited its widespread adoption in routine

Table 1
Selected studies published on HBP

Author/Year (Ref)	Study Type	Indication for HBP	No. of Patients	Success Rate	Follow-up (mo)	CO and LO
Deshmukh et al,[17] 2000	Single-center, retrospective	AV nodal ablation, chronic AF, LVEF of <40%, narrow QRS,	18	12 (66%)	23	CO: Improvement in LV end-systolic dimension, LVEF, functional status, and decrease in cardiothoracic ratio LO: 2 (16.6%); 1 high threshold and 1 lead dislodgement
Deshmukh and Romanyshyn,[18] 2004	Single-center, retrospective	Persistent AF, systolic heart failure, narrow QRS	54	39 (72%)	42	CO: Improvement in LVEF, functional status, dp/dt, exercise time, oxygen uptake and anaerobic threshold
Occhetta et al,[21] 2006	Prospective, crossover, blinded, randomized	AV nodal ablation, chronic AF, narrow QRS Randomized to 6 mo of RV pacing vs NS-HBP	18	17 (94%)	12	CO: Improvement in NYHA functional class, 6-min walk test, quality of life and hemodynamic parameters
Kronborg et al,[44] 2014	Prospective, crossover, double-blinded, randomized	AV block, narrow QRS, LVEF of >40% Randomized to 12 mo of HBP vs RV pacing	38	32 (84%)	24	CO: Improvement in LVEF and mechanical synchrony No improvement in NYHA functional class, 6-min walk test or quality of life
Sharma et al,[22] 2015	Multicenter, retrospective	SSS, AV block, AF Compared HBP vs RV pacing	94	75 (80%)	24	CO: Improvement in HF hospitalization outcomes No improvement in mortality or AF LO: 3 lead revisions (4%)
Vijayaraman et al,[45] 2015	Single-center, retrospective	AV block (nodal and infranodal) AV nodal ablation	100	84 (84%) [93% AV nodal, 76% infranodal]	19	CO: NR LO: 5 (6%) patients required lead revision for increased thresholds or exit block

(continued on next page)

Table 1
(continued)

Author/Year (Ref)	Study Type	Indication for HBP	No. of Patients	Success Rate	Follow-up (mo)	CO and LO
Pastore et al,[15] 2016	Single-enter, retrospective	AV block Compared HBP vs RV pacing	148	NR	58	CO: HBP associated with lower risk of AF occurrence compared with RV pacing
Huang et al,[71] 2017	Single-center, prospective	AV nodal ablation, persistent AF, HF, narrow QRS	52	50 (96%)	21	CO: Improved LVEF, LV volumes, functional class. Reduced diuretic use LO: Acute increase in HBP threshold in 5 patients; failed AV nodal ablation in 6 and His bundle injury in 2 patients
Vijayaraman et al,[70] 2017	Single-center, retrospective	AV nodal ablation, narrow QRS	42	40 (95%)	19	CO: Improved LVEF and functional class LO: Acute increase in HBP threshold in 7 patients; 1 required lead revision
Vijayaraman et al,[46] 2018	Multicenter, retrospective	SSS, AV block, AF Compared HBP vs RV pacing	94	75 (80%)	60	CO: Stable LVEF, reduced incidence of PICMP and HF hospitalizations in HBP group. LO: Higher lead revisions (6.7%) and generator changes (9%) in the HBP group Mean battery longevity 4.2 ± 0.4 y
Abdelrehman et al,[47] 2018	Multicenter, retrospective	SSS, AV block, AF Compared HBP vs RV pacing	332	304 (92%)	24	CO: Decrease in composite end point of all-cause mortality, HF hospitalization, and or upgrade to BiV with HBP LO: 14% had HBP capture thresholds ≥2.5 V; lead revision in 14 patients (4.2%)

Study	Design	Indication	N	Success	Follow-up (mo)	Outcomes
Bhatt et al,[24] 2018	Single-center, retrospective	SSS, AV block, CRT	101	76 (75%)	24	CO: NR; LO: Increasing threshold (≥2.5 V) in 32% and lead revision in 8%
Sarkar et al,[48] 2019	Single-center, retrospective	SSS, AV block, AF, CRT	22	19 (86%)	12	CO: Improved LVEF
Keene et al,[49] 2019	Multicenter, observational	SSS, AV block, AF, CRT	529	81%	7.2	LO: 8.5% had threshold increase of >3 V; 7.5% patients had His lead revision or lead deactivation
Zanon et al,[25] 2019	Multicenter, retrospective	SSS, AV block, AF, CRT	844	NR	36	LO: 28% had HBP capture thresholds of ≥2.5 V; 9% had loss of His bundle capture; HBP interrupted in 64 patients (7.6%); Mean battery longevity 5.9 ± 2.1 y
Ravi et al,[50] 2020	Single-center, prospective HBP vs RVP	SSS, AV block	105 HBP 120 RVP	NR	23	CO: HBP was associated with lowered risk of new-onset AF in patients with >20% pacing and a trend toward a decreased risk of AF progression in patients with pacing of >40%
De Pooter et al,[51] 2020	Multicenter	AV block after TAVR	16	81% 69% in LBBB patients	11	LO: Stable lead parameters; 1 patient had significant increase in threshold >2 V
Teigeler et al,[26] 2021	Single-center, retrospective	SSS, AV block, AF, CRT	295	274 (93%)	23	LO: 24% had HBP capture thresholds of ≥2.5 V; 28% had HBP threshold increase by ≥1 V; 17% had loss of His bundle capture; 11% required lead revision

Abbreviations: AVN, atrioventricular node; AVB, atrioventricular block; BIV, biventricular; CO, clinical outcomes; CRT, cardiac resynchronization therapy; dp/dt, ratio of pressure change in the ventricular cavity during the isovolemic contraction period; HF, heart failure; LBB, left bundle branch; LBBB, left BBB; LO, lead outcomes; NR, not reported; RVP, right ventricular pacing; RBBB, right BBB; SSS, sick sinus syndrome; TAVR, transcatheter aortic valve replacement.

clinical practice.[24–26] This opportunely has led to the advent of left bundle branch area pacing (LBBAP) by Huang and colleagues[27] in 2017 as an alternative site for conduction system pacing (CSP) in a patient with heart failure and LBBB. Since its original description, several studies have demonstrated the safety and feasibility of LBBAP (**Table 2**). LBBAP is rapidly emerging as a reliable, physiologic alternative to HBP.

MECHANISMS OF CORRECTION OF BUNDLE BRANCH BLOCKS WITH CONDUCTION SYSTEM PACING

The ability of CSP to preserve the coordinated and synchronous ventricular contractions by activation of the His–Purkinje system is very appealing. Several mechanisms have been proposed by which CSP normalizes the QRS in patients with BBB. The concept of functional longitudinal dissociation within the His bundle was first postulated by Kaufmann and Rothberger in 1919.[28] James and Sherf[29] later supported this theory in 1971 by confirming the longitudinally arranged cells separated by fine collagen within the His bundle using light microscopy and electron microscopy. These findings were confirmed clinically by Narula and colleagues[30] in 1977 by demonstrating QRS narrowing with pacing slightly distal to the presumed site of block in proximal His bundle in patients with left BBB (LBBB). The authors hypothesized that the BBBs are likely due to a delay within fibers in the proximal His bundle that are predestined to become either the right bundle branch (RBB) or LBB and hence can be recruited by pacing distal to the site of the block (**Fig. 1**A). The evidence for proximal disease was elegantly proved recently by Upadhyay and colleagues[31] by detailed intracardiac mapping of the LV septum in patients with LBBB by placing a linear multielectrode catheter. The authors reported complete conduction block in 64% of the patients (72% at left His and 28% at proximal LBB) and intact Purkinje activation without conduction block in 36% of cases. Based on these findings, it became apparent why in some patients we are able to correct the BBB by pacing distal to the site of the block (proximal disease) and why in some patients we fail to correct the conduction disease (intact Purkinje activation).

The other plausible explanation is the virtual electrode effect. This effect was demonstrated in another recent elegant study by Niri and colleagues[32] in the ovine heart preparations. Increasing the pacing pulse width not only increased the distance an electrode could be from the LBB and still capture it, but also overcame conduction slowing or conduction block created with an ethanol-cooled needle or surgical incision. This consequence of increased pulse width is due to the virtual electrode effect and likely explains correction of conduction system disease in cases with pacing lead implanted proximal to the site of the block or in cases with extensive disease where correction is seen only at higher output (see **Fig. 1**B). Other unproved mechanisms that may also play a role include transverse connections between the bundles, and retrograde activation of His and RBB, especially with LBBAP.

CONDUCTION SYSTEM PACING IMPLANTATION TECHNIQUES

The step-by-step approach to HBP and LBBAP has been described previously.[33–36] In brief, we perform CSP using a SelectSecure 3830-69 cm pacing lead (Medtronic, Minneapolis, MN) which is a 4.1F, isodiametric, lumen-less, exposed helix lead. It is delivered either via the 7F fixed curve sheath (C315 HIS, Medtronic) or a 9F deflectable sheath (SelectSite C304-HIS, Medtronic). The 12-lead electrocardiogram (ECG) recordings and the intracardiac electrograms from the pacing lead were simultaneously displayed and continuously recorded on an electrophysiology recording system (Prucka Cardiolab, GE Healthcare, Waukesha, WI). After obtaining axillary access, the delivery sheath is advanced to the peri-Hisian area over a guidewire that is later replaced by the pacing lead.

For HBP, the His bundle region is mapped for a unipolar His recording. Attempts are made to identify the distal His potential without atrial electrogram before lead fixation. When His bundle potentials are not recorded, pace mapping is performed. Once His bundle capture is confirmed, the lead is rotated 5 to 10 times for fixation (**Fig. 2**).

For LBBAP, the first step is to identify the distal His signal and save it as a reference. If His signals are not identified, tricuspid annulus or annular signal (small a, large V) can be used as a reference. The pacing lead is advance about 1.5 to 2.0 cm distal to this reference point. Pace mapping is performed to identify the ideal site for fixation (inferior lead and avR/avL discordance).[36] The lead is then rotated deep into the septum toward the LV subendocardium with close monitoring of the impedance and QRS morphology changes. Careful attention should also be paid to the occurrence of ectopic beats with qR or rsR′ morphology (fixation beats) that suggest the pacing lead is in close proximity to the left conduction system and avoid further rotations to prevent trans-septal perforation.[37] LBBA capture is confirmed by the previously published criteria.[35] If the LBBAP criteria

Table 2
Selected studies published on LBBAP

Author/Year (Ref)	Study Type	Indication for LBBAP	No. of Patients	Success Rate	Follow-up (mo)	CO and LO
Chen et al,[52] 2018	Prospective LBBAP vs RVP	SSS, 75% AV/infranodal block, 20%	20	NR	3	LO: Stable lead parameters
Zhang et al,[53] 2019	Prospective LBBAP vs RVP	SSS, 48% AVB, 38%	23	87%	NR	LO: Stable lead parameters at implant
Hou et al,[54] 2019	Prospective	SSS, 29% AVB, 37% AF with SVR, 34%	56	NR	4.5	CO: LBBAP patients with LBB potential had similar LV mechanical synchrony to that of HBP based on phase analysis of gated SPECT myocardial perfusion imaging Stable LVEF LO: Stable lead parameters 1 acute lead dislodgement intraoperatively
Li et al,[55] 2019	Retrospective	AVB, 100%	33	91%	3	CO: Stable LVEF LO: Stable lead parameters 1 acute septal perforation intraoperatively
Li et al,[56] 2019	Prospective	SSS, 68% AVB, 32%	87	80%	3	LO: Stable lead parameters
Vijayaraman et al,[57] 2019	Prospective	SSS, 23% AVB, 54% AVN ablation, 7% CRT, 11% HBP failure, 7%	100	93%	3	LO: Stable lead parameters 3 lead dislodgements within 24 h requiring revision 3 acute septal perforations intraoperatively
Hasumi et al,[58] 2019	Retrospective	Advanced AVB, 100% Failed HBP	21	81%	6	LO: Stable lead parameters
Cai et al,[59] 2020	Prospective Observational LBBAP vs RVP	SSS, 100%	40	90%	Echocardiogram on day 3	CO: LBBAP preserved mechanical synchrony similar to native conduction LBBAP lead to favorable hemodynamic effects RVp resulted in electrical and mechanical dyssynchrony and worse hemodynamic effects

(continued on next page)

Table 2
(continued)

Author/Year (Ref)	Study Type	Indication for LBBAP	No. of Patients	Success Rate	Follow-up (mo)	CO and LO
Jiang et al,[60] 2020	Retrospective	BBB with QRSd of >130 ms Atypical BBB, 13.6% 5 LBBB and 5 RBBB Typical BBB, 86.4% 30 LBBB and 33 RBBB	73	30.0% 82.5%	NR	CO: Typical BBB morphology (Strauss criteria) predicts successful QRS correction with LBBAP LO: 4 acute septal perforations intraoperatively
Wang et al,[61] 2020	Prospective Randomized LBBAP vs RVP	SSS, 32% AVB, 54% AF with SVR, 14%	66	94%	6	CO: LBBAP resulted in narrower QRSd, shorter QT and QTc interval, lower QTD and QTcD, and shorter $T_{peak-end}$ interval compared with RVp, suggesting better depolarization–repolarization reserve LO: Stable lead parameters 1 septal perforation at 1 mo requiring revision 2 lead dislodgements: one at 2 mo and the other at 4 mo
Li et al,[62] 2020	Prospective	BBB, EF of ≥40%	55	83.6% RBBB 93% LBBB 73%	6	CO: Improved LV synchrony, RV synchrony and LVEF LO: Stable lead parameters 1 acute septal perforation intraoperatively
Vijayaraman et al,[63] 2020	Multicenter retrospective	AVB after TAVR	28	93%	12	CO: Stable LVEF LO: Stable lead parameters
Lin et al,[64] 2020	Prospective	SSS, 33% AVB, 67%	39	92%	3	LO: Stable lead parameters

Study	Design	Patient characteristics	No. of patients	Success rate	Follow-up (mo)	Outcomes
Wang et al,[65] 2020	Prospective	Included only patients with a QRSd of <120 ms; SSS, 30%; AVB, 64%; AF, 6%	70	NR	12	CO: No difference in echocardiographic parameters in patients with or without LBB potential; LO: Stable lead parameters in patients with or without LBB potential; 1 chronic septal perforation at 6 mo
Ravi et al,[66] 2020	Prospective	SSS, 14.0%; AVB, 49.1%; AVN ablation, 10.5%; CRT, 24.6%	59	97%	6	CO: LVEF improved from 30 ± 11% to 42 ± 15% in 21 patients with cardiomyopathy; HF hospitalizations in 7 patients (12.3%); Deaths, 4; LO: Stable lead parameters; 3 (5.3%) required lead revision: 2 macrodislodgements at days 4 and 34, and 1 chronic septal perforation at day 98; 4 patients with loss of LBB capture
Padala et al,[67] 2020	Multicenter Prospective	SSS, 28.7%; AVB, 52.5%; AVN ablation, 10.0%; CRT, 8.8%	341	89%	4	LO: Stable lead parameters; 3 lead dislodgements, 2 within 24 h and 1 at 2 wk; 15 acute septal perforations intraoperatively
Qian et al,[68] 2020	Observational HBP vs LBBAP	SSS, 29.2%; AVB, 42.7%; AF with SVR, 10.3%; AVN Ablation, 4.9%; CRT, 13%	185 LBBAP, 64 HBP	96% LBBAP, 87.6% HBP	8.8, 19.6	CO: Patients with a baseline EF of >50% had preserved EF at follow-up both with HBP and LBBAP; Patients with an EF of <50% had improvement in EF; LBBAP: EF improved from 31.6 ± 8.7% to 43.3 ± 10% (P<.001); HBP: EF improved from 33.8 ± 9.3% to 45.3 ± 14.4% (P = .002)

(continued on next page)

Table 2
(continued)

Author/Year (Ref)	Study Type	Indication for LBBAP	No. of Patients	Success Rate	Follow-up (mo)	CO and LO
						LO: Stable LBBAP lead parameters 12.5% had >1 V threshold increase in HBP group, none in LBBAP group
De Pooter et al,[39] 2021	Prospective	SSS, 16% AVB, 60% CRT, 24%	50 (25 with stylet-driven leads and 25 with lumenless leads)	87% (stylet driven) 89% (lumenless)	3	CO: In patients with LBBB and HF, the EF improved from $37 \pm 11\%$ to $45 \pm 14\%$ at 1 mo follow-up echo Septal coronary artery fistula in 1 patient on postprocedural echo with stylet driven lead without any clinical significance LO: Stable lead parameters 3 acute septal perforations intraoperatively
Su et al,[69] 2021	Prospective	SSS, 25.7% AVB/AF with AVN ablation, 60% LBBB with HF, 14.2%	632	97.8%	18.6	CO: LVEF was preserved in overall group In patients with a QRSd of $\geq$120 ms: EF improved from 48.82 $\pm$ 17.78% to 58.12 $\pm$ 13.04% (P<.001) LO: Stable lead parameters 2 patients had acute lead dislodgement within 24 h and required lead revision 2 acute (intraoperative) and 1 chronic septal perforation 39 patients (8.9%) had permanent RBB injury 11 patients had LBB capture threshold increase by >1 V 6 patients had LBB capture threshold of >3 V at 0.5 ms 2 had loss of LBB capture

Abbreviations: AVN, atrioventricular node; AVB, atrioventricular block; AF with SVR, AF with slow ventricular rate; CO, clinical outcomes; CRT, cardiac resynchronization therapy; HF, heart failure; LO, lead outcomes; NR, not reported; QRSd; QRS duration; QTc, corrected QT interval; QTD, QT dispersion; RVp, right ventricular pacing; SSS, sick sinus syndrome; SPECT MPI, single photon emission computed tomography myocardial perfusion imaging.

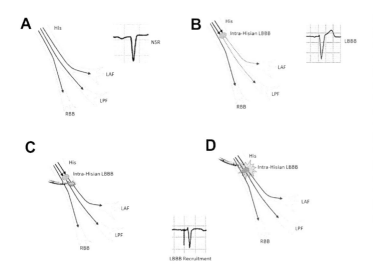

Fig. 1. Mechanisms of correction of BBBs with conduction system pacing. (A–C) depicting longitudinal dissociation theory with predestined RBB and LBB fibers in the proximal His. (A) Normal His–Purkinje system (HPS) activation. (B) HPS activation in the setting of intra-Hisian LBBB. (C) Pacing distal to the site of block leading to normal HPS activation. (D) Pacing proximal to the site of the block but still with normal HPS activation owing to virtual electrode effect. LAF, left anterior fascicle; LPF, left posterior fascicle; LBB, left bundle branch; NSR, normal sinus rhythm.

are not met despite adequate lead depth in the septum or if the lead would not penetrate deep into septum, the lead is repositioned to a more apical location on the septum. In cases where the nondeflectable sheath did not provide enough reach to get to the ideal location on the RV septum, a C304 His deflectable sheath can be used. LBBAP is considered unsuccessful if at least 2 or more LBBAP criteria were not met despite 4 or more attempts ate lead fixation (**Fig. 3**).

Recent studies have used stylet-driven leads (SDL) to perform CSP.[38,39] Orlov and colleagues[38] reported comparable HBP success rates with SDL and lumenless leads (89% vs 88%). However, the acute HBP thresholds were significantly higher with SDL than with the lumenless lead (2.6 ± 1.5 V vs 1.5 ± 1.2 V; P = .02) and remained stable at 8 months. De Pooter and colleagues[39] reported similar LBBAP success rates (87% vs 89%) and similar acute thresholds (0.5 ± 0.15 V vs

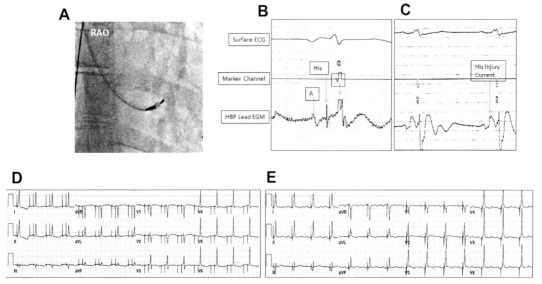

Fig. 2. Approach to HBP lead implantation. (A) Right anterior oblique view showing the pacing lead at the His bundle area. (B) Unipolar electrogram recordings from the HBP lead displayed on the analyzer. Gain settings of 0.05 mV/mm and sweep speed of 50 mm/s. Note the atrial, His and ventricular electrograms before lead fixation. (C) After lead fixation, note the His bundle injury on the electrogram recording signifying adequate fixation. (D) 12-lead ECG demonstrating selective HBP morphology with isoelectric interval between the pacing spike and QRS onset. (E) A 12-lead ECG demonstrating NS HBP morphology with delta wave between the pacing spike and QRS complex.

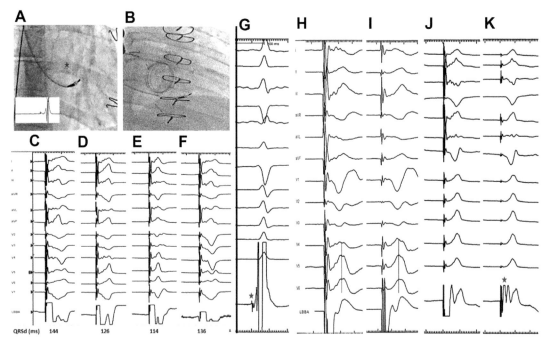

Fig. 3. Step-by-step approach to LBBAP lead implantation. (*A*) Fluoroscopic RAO view. * he distal His bundle position. Insert shows distal His bundle electrogram. The sheath and 3830 lead are advanced about 2 cm distal to the distal His bundle electrogram. (*B*) The sheath and 3830 lead are advanced about 2 cm distal using the bioprosthetic aortic valve as a reference. (*C*) Ideal site for lead fixation showing LBB QRS morphology with inferior lead and avR/avL discordance. (*D*) After 4 turns, notice the narrowing of QRS and V1 morphology. (*E*) After 2 more turns, unipolar tip pacing revealed a stim-QRS latency of 20 ms, a RBB morphology with rsR' in V1, and a QRSd of 114 ms, suggesting LBB capture. (*F*) Unipolar ring pacing reveals RV basal septal capture with LBB morphology and QRSd of 136 ms. (*G*) *The LBB potential. The LBB potential to QRS duration was 20 ms. (*H* and *I*) stimulus to peak of R wave in V5 (LVAT) at 5V and 1V respectively, was short and constant at 65 ms. (*J* and *K*) Threshold testing during unipolar tip pacing showing transition from NS LBBAP to selective LBBAP at 0.6 V at 0.4 ms. * The discrete EGM with selective LBBA capture. (Modified from Padala SK, Ellenbogen KA. Left bundle branch pacing is the best approach to physiological pacing. Heart Rhythm O2. 2020;1(1):59-67. Published 2020 Apr 27. https://doi.org/10.1016/j.hroo.2020.03.002; with permission)

0.4 ± 0.17 V; *P* = .25) with SDL and lumenless leads, respectively. Although SDLs are reported to provide better stability, it is our opinion that SDLs theoretically have several disadvantages over the lumenless leads and these include larger caliber leads (5.1F–5.8F), a nonisodiametric design, the need for adequate preparation before lead fixation and extraction/repositioning, and the risk for large bore septal perforation, especially during LBBAP. Future studies are required to further assess these differences between the SDLs and lumenless leads.

CONFIRMATION OF CONDUCTION SYSTEM CAPTURE AND DEFINITIONS

When CSP is intended, it is critical to demonstrate capture of the conduction system. In our experience, His bundle capture is easier to establish than LBBA capture. For HBP, the procedure is deemed successful if selective (S) or nonselective (NS) His bundle capture is demonstrated. HBP is considered when the surface ECG has an isoelectric interval between the pacing spike and the onset of a QRS complex identical to the native conduction and a discrete local electrogram on unipolar recordings. NS-HBP is considered when there is a delta wave between the pacing spike and the QRS complex and no discrete local electrogram on unipolar recordings.[33,34] S-HBP can also be confirmed using device electrograms. A near field electrogram with time to peak of more than 40 ms, a near field initial positive deflection after the pacing spike, or a far field QRS duration of less than 120 ms was consistent with S-HBP.[40] The absence of His bundle capture at implant or a loss of His bundle capture during follow-up (septal capture only) can be confirmed by QRS notching or slurring in ECG leads I, V1, V4 to V6, and a prolonged R-wave peak time (RWPT) of greater than 110 ms in V6.[41]

Successful LBBAP is considered when 2 or more of the following criteria are met, as published previously[35]:

1. Paced morphology of RBBB pattern.
2. Presence of LBB potential.
3. LV activation time: measured from the stimulus to the peak of the R wave in V5/V6.
   a. Short and constant at high (5V) and low (1V) output pacing.
4. Determination of S and NS LBB pacing.
   a. S-LBB: Stim-QRS latency and discrete local EGM separate from stimulus artifact seen.
   b. NS-LBB: No stim-QRS latency. No discrete local EGM separate from stimulus artifact.
5. Evidence for direct LBB capture.

Unlike HBP, LBBAP almost always results in simultaneous capture of the LBB and the surrounding myocardium owing to its anatomic location in the muscular septum. Jastrzębski and colleagues[42] described programmed extrastimulus to differentiate LBB capture versus LV septal myocardial capture based on their differential effective refractory periods. Response to premature beats was categorized as myocardial when the paced QRS morphology changed to myocardial only capture (broader QRS, with a slur/notch/plateau and/or with change in amplitude/polarity in several leads), or S-LBB when the paced QRS morphology changed to a typical RBB morphology preceded by a latency. Either myocardial or S-LBB was considered diagnostic of LBB capture and was noted in 80% of the patients with LBBAP. Jastrzębski and colleagues[43] recently described another electrocardiographic criterion to confirm LBB capture. They demonstrated that the capture of LBB in patients with non-LBBB rhythm can be confirmed when the paced V6 RWPT, measured from the QRS onset, equals the native nonpaced V6 RWPT or when the stim to V6 RWPT equals the LBB potential to the native nonpaced V6 RWPT. In patients with LBBB at baseline, capture of the LBB can be confirmed when the paced V6 RWPT is shorter than the native V6 intrinsicoid deflection by more than the trans-septal conduction time.[43] These criteria need to be validated in future studies.

CONDUCTION SYSTEM PACING FOR ATRIOVENTRICULAR BLOCK

Patients with AV block are anticipated to have a high burden of ventricular pacing, because such would be most ideal candidates for CSP. The reported HBP success rates in patients with AV block in literature are variable depending on the experience of the center and degree of underlying conduction system disease.15,18,22,24–26,44–51 In an experienced electrophysiology center implementing HBP for the first time, the overall success rate was 75%.[24] However, when stratified based on the indication, the success rates in patients with Mobitz I versus Mobitz II versus complete heart block were 92% versus 81% versus 56%, respectively. In an experienced center for HBP, the success rates in patients with AV block was reported as 84%.[45] However, when stratified based on the site of AV block, patients with AV nodal block had significantly higher success rates compared with infranodal AV block (93% vs 76%; $P<.05$). By contrast, studies have consistently reported higher success rates with LBBAP ranging between 80% and 95% regardless of presence of BBB. Approximately two-thirds of patients with LBBB will have some narrowing of their QRS (**Fig. 4**).[39,52–69] **Tables 1 and 2** show selected studies of HBP and LBBAP for all bradycardia indications.

Several observational studies have reported improved clinical outcomes with CSP compared with RV pacing (see **Tables 1 and 2**). In one of the largest series, Abdelrahman and colleagues[47] compared 332 patients who received HBP (92% success) with 440 patients who received RV pacing and demonstrated a significant decrease in the primary end point of HF hospitalization, all-cause mortality, and need for upgrade to biventricular CRT among all comers with HBP (25% vs 32%; $P = .02$; hazard ratio, 0.71). This difference was primarily seen among patients requiring a more than 20% ventricular pacing burden (HBP vs RV pacing: 25% vs 36%; $P = .02$; hazard ratio, 0.65).

CONDUCTION SYSTEM PACING FOR REFRACTORY ATRIAL FIBRILLATION BEFORE ATRIOVENTRICULAR JUNCTION ABLATION

Among patients with symptomatic drug and catheter ablation refractory AF pace and ablate strategy has shown to improve cardiac symptoms, exercise duration, quality of life, and health care use (Wood 2000). CSP is an ideal choice in such patients because it preserves physiologic ventricular activation after AV junction ablation. The safety and feasibility of HBP and subsequent AV junction ablation has been shown in multiple studies with success rates of HBP implantation as high as 96% in this cohort in recent studies.[17,21,70–72] Owing to the close proximity of HBP lead to the AV junction, extreme caution should be exercised to avoid unintentional damage to the HBP lead. In a study by Vijayaraman and colleagues,[70] 7 of 37 patients (19%) had an acute increase in HBP threshold from 0.5 to 1.5 V when ablation had to be performed

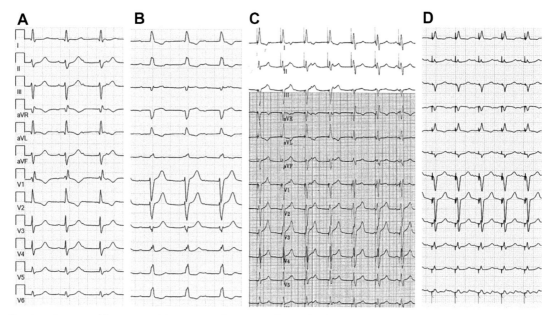

Fig. 4. A 21-year-old woman with congenital aortic and mitral valve stenosis underwent mechanical aortic and mitral valve replacement complicated by complete heart block. (*A, B*) ECGs showing complete heart block with alternating RBBB/LAFB and LBBB escape rhythm. (*C*) ECG rhythm strip after LBBAP lead implant during single-chamber ventricular pacing mode bipolar pacing. Note the change in the QRS morphology in V1 from QS to rsr' at 1.5 V at 0.4 ms. This is due to the loss of ring/anodal capture. (*D*) Follow-up ECG of presenting rhythm 1 month later in device clinic at 2V at 0.4 ms. This was the final pacing configuration with QRSd of 110 ms and QS in V1, suggesting anodal capture. The threshold was 0.7 V at 0.4 ms. An echocardiogram 9 months later showed a normal LVEF despite 100% ventricular pacing. (From Padala SK, Ellenbogen KA. Left bundle branch pacing is the best approach to physiological pacing. Heart Rhythm O2. 2020;1(1):59-67. Published 2020 Apr 27. https://doi.org/10.1016/j.hroo.2020.03.002; with permission)

at the tip electrode or between the ring and tip electrodes, and one required lead revision owing to significant rise in threshold at 2-week follow-up. In another study by Huang and colleagues,[71] successful AV junction ablation was achieved in 42 of 50 patients (81%) with HBP leads. The reasons for failure of permanent HBP in this study was failed AV junction ablation in 2, His bundle injury by ablation in 2, and resumption of AV nodal conduction after initial acute AV junction ablation in 4 patients. Recently, LBBAP has also shown to be an effective alternative strategy to provide physiologic pacing in this cohort.[67,69,73] AV junction ablation in patients with LBBAP leads is likely to be more successful and technically less challenging, because the lead is distal to the site of ablation. Future studies are needed to compare HBP versus LBBAP in patients with refractory AF planned for AV junction ablation.

CONDUCTION SYSTEM PACING FOR CARDIAC RESYNCHRONIZATION THERAPY

CSP has gained an enormous prominence for resynchronization therapy in patients with BBB and heart failure. Although traditional biventricular

pacing has been the gold standard for decades and has been shown to improve clinical outcomes in multiple studies, resynchronization with biventricular pacing results owing to a fusion of 2 non-physiological wavefronts resulting in only a modest ventricular resynchronization.[74] Furthermore, the success rates of biventricular pacing are limited by coronary venous anatomy and phrenic nerve stimulation, and about 30% of the patients are nonresponders. CSP on the other hand results in complete HBP[20,75-81] or near complete LBBAP[82-88] resynchronization and is likely to provide the greatest benefit in patients with BBB and heart failure (**Tables 3 and 4**) (**Figs. 5 and 6**).

In a small, head-to-head, acute crossover comparison study, Arnold and colleagues[89] demonstrated that HBP delivered better resynchronization (a greater decrease in QRS duration, LV activation time, and LV dyssynchrony index) and greater acute hemodynamic response (improvement in systolic blood pressure) than biventricular pacing in patients with heat failure with LBBB referred for traditional biventricular CRT. In a nonrandomized observational study of 137 patients with LBBB and an EF of 40% or less (predominantly nonischemic cardiomyopathy)

Table 3
Selected studies on HBP for cardiac resynchronization therapy

Author/Year (Ref)	Study Type	Indication	No. of Patients	Success Rate	Follow-up (mo)	CO and LO
Barba-Pichardo et al,[20] 2013	Prospective	Rescue HBP in pts with failed LV leads	16	56%	31	CO: Improvement in LVEF, LV dimensions and NYHA functional class LO: No capture loss or lead displacements
Lustgarten et al,[75] 2015	Randomized Crossover	CRT Indications: HBP and LV leads in all patients	29	72%	12	CO: Significant improvements in LVEF (26% to 32%, $P = .04$ in HBP; 26% to 31%, $P = .02$ in BIV), functional status, 6-min walk distance with both HBP and BIV CRT in 12 pts who completed the crossover LO: HBP thresholds required for maximal electrical resynchronization were higher compared with BIV CRT
Ajijola et al,[76] 2017	Retrospective	Rescue HBP in pts with failed LV leads	21	76%	12	CO: Improvement in LVEF 27 ± 10% to 41 ± 13%, $P<.001$, LV dimensions LO: 1 patient with rise in HBP threshold. No dislodgements
Sharma et al,[77] 2018	Multicenter Retrospective	All comers for CRT: Group 1: Rescue HBP (rescue CRT); Group 2: Primary HBP	106	90%	14	CO: Improvement in NYHA functional class and LVEF from 30 ± 10% to 43 ± 13%, $P = .0001$ Overall response rate = 73%, Super responders = 38% LO: Increase in HBP capture threshold >2V or >5V at 1 ms in 7 patients Loss of BBB recruitment in 3

(continued on next page)

Table 3
(continued)

Author/Year (Ref)	Study Type	Indication	No. of Patients	Success Rate	Follow-up (mo)	CO and LO
Sharma et al,[78] 2018	Multicenter Retrospective	HBP in pts with RBBB and indication for CRT: primary or rescue strategy	39	95%	15	CO: Improvement in NYHA functional class and LVEF from 31 ± 10% to 39 ± 13%, $P = .0001$ Overall response rate = 76%, Super responders = 20% LO: Increase in HBP capture threshold >1V in 3 patients Loss of BBB recruitment in 1
Upadhyay et al,[79] 2019	Randomized Multicenter HIS CRT vs BIV CRT HIS-SYNC trial	HF, wide QRS and CRT indication	40	48% crossover in HIS CRT 26% crossover in BIV CRT	6	CO: Improved LVEF with both HIS CRT (26.3% to 31.9%, $P<.001$) and BIV CRT (30.5% to 34%, $P<.001$) HIS CRT was not superior to BIV CRT with regards to LVEF improvement or echocardiographic response LO: No lead dislodgements. Higher pacing thresholds with HBP compared with BIV pacing
Huang et al,[80] 2019	Prospective	HBP in patients with LBBB and indication for CRT	74	76%	37	CO: Improvement in LVEF from 32.4 ± 8.9% to 55.9 ± 10.7% [$P<.001$], LV dimensions and NYHA functional class LO: Stable HBP thresholds
Singh et al,[81] 2020	Multicenter Retrospective	LBBB and cardiomyopathy	7	NR	14.5	CO: LVEF improved from 25% to 50% ($P = .003$) LV end-systolic dimension and end-diastolic dimensions decreased NYHA functional class improved

Abbreviations: BIV, biventricular; CO, clinical outcomes; CRT, cardiac resynchronization therapy; LO, lead outcomes; LV, left ventricular; NYHA, New York Heart Association; RBBB, right BBB; RV, right ventricle.

Table 4
Selected studies on LBBAP for cardiac resynchronization therapy

Author/Year (Ref)	Study Type	Indication for LBBAP	No. of Patients	Success Rate	Follow-up (mo)	CO and LO
Zhang et al,[82] 2019	Prospective	HF, reduced EF, LBBB NICMP, 82% ICMP, 18%	11	NR	6.7	CO: Improvement in LVEF by >5% from baseline in all, >20% from baseline in 7 patients Improvement in LV synchrony by pulsed-wave Doppler and tissue synchronization imaging LO: Stable lead parameters
Li et al,[83] 2020	Prospective	HF, NYHA functional class II–IV, EF of <50% and CRT indications NICMP, 76% ICMP, 16% PICMP, 8%	25 5 as rescue strategy		9	CO: LVEF improved from 35.2 ± 7% to 46.9 ± 10.2% (P<.001) LO: Stable lead parameters
Li et al,[84] 2020	Multicenter Prospective	LBBB, LVEF of ≤35%, NYHA functional class II–IV NICMP, 80.6% ICMP, 19.4%	37 12 as rescue strategy	81%	6	CO: LVEF improved from 28.8 ± 4.5% to 44.3 ± 8.7% (P<.001) In propensity matching, LBBAP resulted in a greater decrease in QRSd, greater improvement in LVEF, and super response rate compared with biventricular CRT LO: Stable lead parameters
Guo et al,[85] 2020	Prospective LBBAP vs BIV CRT (propensity matching)	LBBB, LVEF of ≤35%, NYHA functional class II–IV NICMP, 90.5% ICMP, 9.5%	24	87.5%	14.3	CO: LVEF improved from 26.8 ± 3.8% to 45.6 ± 9.2% (P<.0001) at 6 mo follow-up echo in LBBAP group Significant improvement in NYHA functional class; no HFH CRT response rate and super response rate was higher in LBBAP compared with BIV CRT LO: Stable lead parameters

(continued on next page)

Table 4
(continued)

Author/Year (Ref)	Study Type	Indication for LBBAP	No. of Patients	Success Rate	Follow-up (mo)	CO and LO
Wang et al,[86] 2020	Prospective LBBAP vs BIV CRT (propensity matching)	NSR, LBBB, LVEF of ≤ 35%, QRSd of >140 ms (men), QRSd of >130 ms (women), NYHA functional class II–IV NICMP, 90% ICMP, 10%	10	100%	6	CO: LVEF improved from 30 ± 5% to 50.9 ± 10.7% (*P*<.0001) in the LBBAP group The improvement in LVESD, LVEDD, LVEF, and CRT response rate was higher in the LBBAP group compared with the BIV CRT group LO: Stable lead parameters; lower capture thresholds with LBBAP compared with BIV CRT
Huang et al,[87] 2020	Multicenter Prospective	LBBB, EF of <50%, HF, failure to achieve LBB correction with HBP NICMP, 100%	63	97%	18	CO: LVEF improved from 33 ± 8% to 55 ± 10% (*P*<.001) at 1 y LVEF normalized ≥50% in 75% of patients at 1 y NYHA functional class improved significantly No deaths or HFH LO: Stable lead parameters
Vijayaraman et al,[88] 2021	Multicenter Retrospective	HF, NYHA functional class II–IV and CRT or pacing indications NICMP, 56% ICMP, 44%	325	85%	6	CO: LVEF improved from 33 ± 10% to 44 ± 11% (*P*<.01) Echocardiographic response (≥5 EF improvement) in 73% Clinical response (improvement by 1 NYHA functional class and no HFH) in 72% LO: Stable lead parameters 5 lead dislodgements: 3 in 24 h, 2 at 2-wk follow-up 2 loss of conduction system capture 10 acute septal perforations intraoperatively

Abbreviations: BIV, biventricular; CRT, cardiac resynchronization therapy; HF, heart failure; HFH, heart failure hospitalization; ICMP, ischemic cardiomyopathy; LV, left ventricular; LVESD, left ventricular end-systolic dimension; LVEDD, left ventricular end-diastolic dimension; NICMP, nonischemic cardiomyopathy; NYHA, New York Heart Association; QRSd, QRS duration; PICMP, pacing induced cardiomyopathy; RBBB, right BBB.

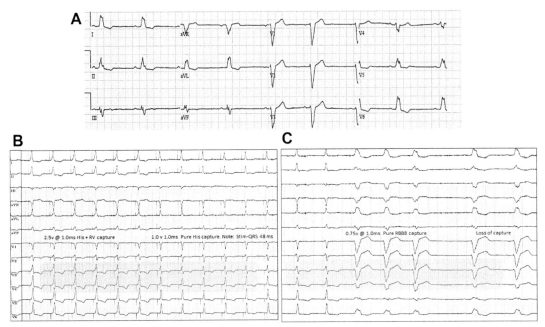

Fig. 5. An 81-year-old man with ischemic cardiomyopathy, an EF of 30%, and LBBB was referred for CRT-D implantation. An HBP lead was implanted as a bail-out strategy after CS lead implantation failed. (*A*) Baseline 12-lead ECG showing typical LBB morphology with a QRSd o 168 ms. (*B*) After successful HBP lead implantation, threshold testing was performed in a unipolar tip pacing configuration. Note the transition from NS-HBP to S-HBP at 1V@1 ms with complete LBBB recruitment with a QRSd of 90 ms. Note the delta wave between the pacing spike and QRS complex during NS-HBP and the isoelectric interval between the pacing spike and the QRS onset during S-HBP (*blue box*). (*C*) As the output was further decreased, note the last 3 paced beats with typical LBBB morphology (similar to baseline QRS morphology) before loss of capture. This is because of selective capture of predestined RBB fibers at low output in the His bundle region. An echocardiogram 12 months later showed improvement in the LVEF to 40% to 45%. The patient reported improvement in symptoms (NYHA functional class I). HBP lead parameters remained stable at 1 year: R waves 2.2 mV, S-HBP capture threshold 2.0V@1ms.

referred for CRT, patients who received HBP or LBBAP demonstrated similar improvements in symptoms and LV function, but significantly greater than those seen in patients treated with biventricular pacing suggesting that CSP outperforms traditional biventricular pacing.[90]

In the first randomized, multicenter His-SYNC trial (His Bundle Pacing vs Coronary Sinus Pacing for Cardiac Resynchronization Therapy), 41 patients were randomized to His CRT versus biventricular CRT.[79] In the intention-to-treat analysis, although His CRT resulted in a significant decrease in QRS duration, it was not superior to biventricular CRT with regards to LVEF improvement or rate of echocardiographic response over a median follow-up of 6.2 months.[79] The study was heavily criticized for being underpowered and for improper patient selection that resulted in high crossover rates (48% in the His CRT group and 26% in the biventricular CRT group).

Although HBP provides the most ideal cardiac resynchronization in patients with BBB, higher capture thresholds and an inability to correct the underlying BBB have been the major impediments. Even in experienced hands, permanent HBP with LBBB correction could be achieved in only 76% of the patients with heat failure with LBBB referred for CRT.[80] A novel concept of sequential HBP followed by LV pacing (His Optimized CRT, HOT CRT) to maximize electrical resynchronization was tested by Vijayaraman and colleagues[91] among 27 patients with advanced heart failure and conduction disturbances (LBBB 17, intraventricular conduction defect 5, RV pacing 5) only partially corrected by HBP. During a mean follow-up of 14 months, HOT CRT resulted in significant reduction in QRS duration, 84% clinical response rate, and 92% echocardiographic response rate ($\geq$5% increase in the LVEF).

Recently, studies have shown feasibility and improved clinical outcomes with LBBAP for CRT (see **Table 4**). In a prospective, multicenter study, Huang and colleagues[87] reported a very high LBBAP success rate of 97% among 63 patients with LBBB and nonischemic cardiomyopathy. During a mean follow-up of 1 year, the LVEF

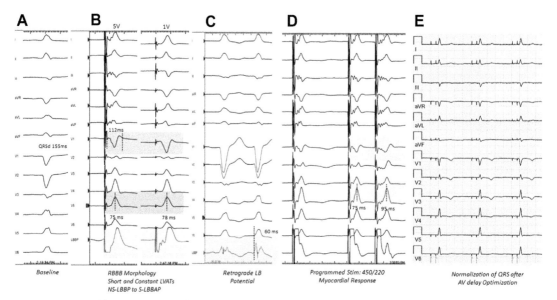

Fig. 6. A 46-year-old woman with sick sinus syndrome, LBBB, an EF of 40% to 45%, NICMP, and New York Heart Association functional class II symptoms received a dual chamber pacemaker with LBBAP lead for CRT. (*A*) Baseline rhythm strip showing typical LBB morphology with a QRSd of 155 ms. (*B*) After successful implantation of LBBAP lead, unipolar tip pacing at high (5V) and low (1V) output showed an rsR′ pattern in V1 with a QRSd of 112 ms (*purple box*), short and constant stimulus to LV activation time (LVAT) at high and low output pacing (*gray box*), and NS- to S-LBBAP transition (*orange box*). (*C*) During intrinsic rhythm, a consistent high-frequency potential was noted 60 ms from the surface QRS (*green box*) on the pacing lead in the LBBA. This is likely a retrograde LBB potential. (*D*) Programmed electrical stimulation from the LBBAP lead at 450/220 shows widening of the QRS (*yellow box*) and lengthening of the LVAT (*blue box*) during the extrastimulus, suggestive of transition from NS-LBBA capture to myocardial capture. All of these features are suggestive of LBBA capture. (*E*) A 12-lead ECG shows complete normalization of the QRS after AV delay optimization to allow intrinsic conduction down the RBB with simultaneous pacing of the LBB. Anechocardiogram 6 months later showed improvement in the LVEF from 50% to 55%. The patient reported improvement in symptoms (New York Heart Association functional class I). The LBBAP lead parameters remained stable at 1 year: R waves 12 mV, threshold 0.625V@0.4 ms.

increased significantly from 33 ± 8% to 55 ± 10% (*P*<.001) and there were no deaths or heart failure hospitalizations. Strikingly, LVEF normalized in 75% of the patients. Vijayaraman and colleagues[88] in a multicenter study reported 85% LBBAP success rate among 325 patients with LVEF less than 50% referred for CRT for heterogenous indications. During a mean follow-up of 6 months, there was a significant decrease in QRS duration, as well as an improvement in clinical and echocardiographic response with LBBAP. The LBBAP thresholds remained low and stable during follow-up in both of these studies.[87,88]

CONDUCTION SYSTEM PACING FOR PACING-INDUCED CARDIOMYOPATHY

CSP is a reliable alternative to biventricular pacing and has shown to restore the LV systolic dysfunction in patients with PICMP.[92–94] In a study by Vijayaraman and colleagues,[93] HBP was successful in 57 of 60 patients (95%) with PICMP and showed significant improvement in LVEF from

34 ± 9.6% to 48 ± 9.8% (*P*<.001) during the follow-up. In a smaller study of 13 patients with PICMP by Qian and colleagues,[94] LBBAP upgrade was associated with a significant improvement in LVEF from 40 ± 5% to 48 ± 9.5% during a mean follow-up of 10.4 months. This study also assessed the usefulness of LBBAP upgrade in 14 patients with heart failure with a preserved LVEF of 50% or greater presumed to be due to chronic RV pacing. The authors found that LBBAP was associated with improvement in serum *N*-terminal B-type natriuretic protein levels and New York Heart Association functional class symptoms.[94] The results of these studies suggest that the electrical and structural changes induced by chronic RV apical pacing can be reversed effectively by institution of CSP.

CONDUCTION SYSTEM PACING FOR PAINFUL LEFT BUNDLE BRANCH SYNDROME

Painful LBBB syndrome is a rare but under-recognized entity and should be suspected in patients with chest pain and LBBB in the absence of ischemia. Historically, these patients have been treated with limited efficacy using exercise regimens, atrioventricular nodal blockers, or RV or biventricular pacemakers. CSP via HBP or LBBAP should be the ideal pacing strategy in these cases because it can result in complete resolution of LBBB and associated symptoms. HBP has been reported to successfully treat patients with painful LBBB syndrome,[95–99] but may require high thresholds for LBB correction.[95,97] We reported the first 2 cases in literature of painful LBBB syndrome successfully treated with LBBAP with complete resolution of LBBB and symptoms.[100] The first report of pacing (cardiac resynchronization therapy) to eliminate severe dyspnea caused by rate-dependent LBBB was reported by Prystowsky and colleagues.[101]

CHRONIC LEAD PERFORMANCE AND COMPLICATIONS

There are limited data on the long-term performance of CSP leads with only 3 reports published on HBP leads and 1 report on a LBBAP lead to date.[25,26,46,69] In the largest, observational, 2-center study, Zanon and colleagues[25] reported the long-term performance of HBP leads among 844 patients. The HBP thresholds at a median follow-up of 36 months were 2.5 V or more at 1 ms in 28% of the patients. ECG during follow-up showed septal pacing (loss of His bundle capture) in 9% of

patients. HBP interruption (lead revision/deactivation) was seen in 7.6% of patients. The median time for battery replacement was 5.8 years. In another single-center study assessing HBP lead outcomes at 60 months, lead revision was required in 6.7% of patients and generator change in 9% of patients with a mean battery longevity of 4.2 ± 0.4 years.[46] In a recently published single-center retrospective study, Teigeler and colleagues[26] reported intermediate-term HBP lead outcomes among 274 patients. During a median follow-up of 19 months, the mean capture threshold increased significantly to 1.7 V from 1.1 V at implantation (P<.001). About 28% of patients had a threshold increase of 1 V or more compared with the implant threshold, 24% of patients had capture thresholds of 2.5 V or more, and 7% had 3.5 V or more at 1 ms during chronic follow-up. ECG during follow-up showed septal pacing in 17% of patients. Compared with prior studies, the percentage of patients requiring lead revision was much higher at 11%. This was in part due to inclusion of 5 patients in the present study who had a significant increase in the threshold or loss of His bundle capture after AV junction ablation (**Fig. 7**).[26] High thresholds at implant, a delayed increase in thresholds necessitating frequent generator replacements, and high lead revision rates are major drawbacks of HBP leads.

Su and colleagues[69] reported on the long-term performance of LBBAP leads among 618 patients in a single-center study with a mean follow-up

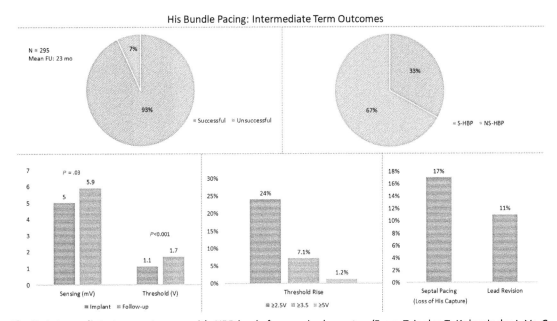

Fig. 7. Intermediate-term outcomes with HBP leads from a single center. (From Teigeler T, Kolominsky J, Vo C, et al. Intermediate-term performance and safety of His-bundle pacing leads: A single-center experience. Heart Rhythm. 2021;18(5):743-749. https://doi.org/10.1016/j.hrthm.2020.12.031; with permission)

period of 18 months. The mean LBBAP threshold at implant was 0.65 V at 0.5 ms and remained stable at 0.68 V and 0.69 V at the 1-year and 2-year follow-ups, respectively. The R waves remained stable and there were no sensing issues. During follow-up, 2 patients had acute lead dislodgement (0.3%), 2 had loss of LBB capture (0.3%), 6 patients had a LBB capture threshold of more than 3 V at 0.5 ms (1%), and 1 had septal perforation (0.16%). Persistent RBB injury was noted in 9% of patients. There were no strokes or coronary artery injuries.

ANATOMY AND HISTOLOGY OF THE CONDUCTION SYSTEM

The anatomy of the conduction system is discussed elsewhere in this issue. The following paragraphs focus on the differences between the HBP and LBBAP acutely with regard to success

rates and chronically with regard to the lead performance can be explained by the anatomy and histology of the conduction system.[101] The His bundle is a thin cylindrical structure and can be divided anatomically into 3 portions: (1) the penetrating bundle of His, which penetrates the fibrous membranous septum or central fibrous body and emerges beneath the right and noncoronary cusp, (2) the nonbranching portion, which runs a variable course on the crest of the muscular ventricular septum, and (3) the branching portion that branches off to give left and RBBs. Implantation of an HBP lead requires greater precision and a longer learning curve and can be technically challenging owing to a narrow target zone. By contrast, LBBAP lead implantation is technically less challenging and requires less precision and a shorter learning curve owing to wider target zone.[67] LBBAP can be achieved by implantation of the lead at the left bundle main trunk or at the

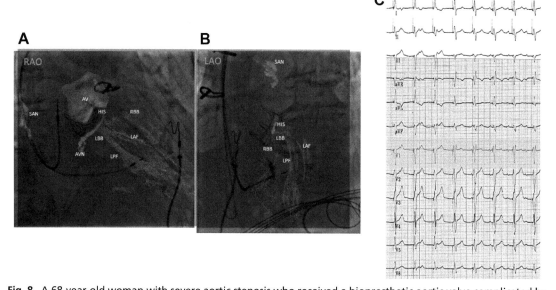

Fig. 8. A 68-year-old woman with severe aortic stenosis who received a bioprosthetic aortic valve complicated by complete heart block. The ECG showed sinus rhythm with complete heart block and RBBB morphology escape rhythm with a QRSd of 142 ms. She received a dual chamber pacemaker with LBBAP lead. Initial attempts to place the lead 1 to 2 cm below the bioprosthetic aortic valve as a marker for His region failed owing to possible septal fibrosis. The lead was then placed deep in the midposterior septum to engage the left posterior fascicle (LPF). (*A* and *B*) Right anterior oblique (RAO) and left anterior oblique (LAO) views of the LBBAP lead. The RAO and LAO images of the conduction system are superimposed on the fluoroscopic images: sinus node (*blue*), paranodal area (*turquoise*), atrioventricular conduction axis (*green*), right (*red*), and left (*purple*) Purkinje networks. Note the proximity of the LBBAP lead to the LPF. An LAO fluoroscopic image also shows a septogram with the lead depth up to ring electrode in the septum. (*C*) ECG rhythm strip after LBBAP lead implant during single-chamber ventricular pacing mode bipolar pacing shows change in QRS morphology in V1 from QS to Qr at 2.5 V at 0.4 ms (*blue box*). This is due to the loss of ring/anodal capture. Pacing shows rsR' in V1 with left axis deviation suggestive of LPF capture with a relatively narrow QRSd of 120 ms. AVN, atrioventricular node; AV, aortic valve; LAF, left anterior fascicle; LBB, left bundle branch; LPF, left posterior fascicle; SAN, sinoatrial node. (Modified from Stephenson RS, Atkinson A, Kottas P, et al. High resolution 3-Dimensional imaging of the human cardiac conduction system from microanatomy to mathematical modeling. Sci Rep. 2017;7(1):7188. Published 2017 Aug 3. https://doi.org/10.1038/s41598-017-07694-8; Creative Commons Attribution 4.0 International License)

fascicles in the basal-mid septum (**Fig. 8**). The narrow QRS duration with LBBAP is likely due to the dense arborization of the left bundle branch and Purkinje network allowing rapid conduction and simultaneous capture of a greater part of the LV.

Additionally, the His bundle is surrounded by dense fibrous tissue and limited myocardium. This nature likely explains the high pacing thresholds required to capture the conduction system, the delayed increase in thresholds owing to local fibrosis, and the low-amplitude R waves resulting in sensing issues. By contrast, LBB is surrounded by thin fibrous tissue and dense myocardium. As such, pacing thresholds are low and stable, and yield a large R wave amplitude similar to RV apical pacing.[102]

FUTURE DIRECTIONS

New, dedicated sheaths from different manufacturers have improved the success rates of CSP. The success rates of HBP may further be improved by refining the lead design (a steroid-eluting tip, a longer helix). Unlike HBP, where the QRS morphology changes during pacing are relatively simple and are standardized, LBBAP is associated with varied QRS morphologies and can be challenging to differentiate from LV septal pacing only. The criteria for LBBA capture need to be refined and validated. The long-term safety profile, lead integrity and the risk of extraction of LBBAP leads needs to be determined. Risk of RV cardiomyopathy with LBBAP needs to be assessed. The role of CSP in patients requiring CRT needs to be investigated in large prospective randomized clinical trials with long-term follow-up.

SUMMARY

CSP in the form of HBP and LBBAP allows normal LV activation, thereby preventing the adverse consequences of RV pacing. CSP is associated with favorable clinical and echocardiographic outcomes in patients with AV block, refractory AF, and PICM, as well as in patients referred for cardiac resynchronization therapy. HBP is the most ideal form of physiologic pacing, but technical challenges during the procedure, high thresholds at implantation, a delayed increase in thresholds, high rates of lead revision, and premature battery replacements are the major barriers. LBBAP has emerged as an attractive alternative and has shown to provide adequate electrical and mechanical resynchronization with stable long-term lead parameters.

FUNDING

No funding was received for this project.

REFERENCES

1. Mulpuru SK, Madhavan M, McLeod CJ, et al. Cardiac pacemakers: function, troubleshooting, and management: part 1 of a 2-part series. J Am Coll Cardiol 2017;69(2):189–210.
2. Sweeney MO, Hellkamp AS, Ellenbogen KA, et al. Adverse effect of ventricular pacing on heart failure and atrial fibrillation among patients with normal baseline QRS duration in a clinical trial of pacemaker therapy for sinus node dysfunction. Circulation 2003;107(23):2932–7.
3. Yu C-M, Chan JY-S, Zhang Q, et al. Biventricular pacing in patients with bradycardia and normal ejection fraction. N Engl J Med 2009;361(22): 2123–34.
4. Yu C-M, Fang F, Luo X-X, et al. Long-term follow-up results of the pacing to avoid cardiac enlargement (PACE) trial. Eur J Heart Fail 2014;16(9):1016–25.
5. Wilkoff BL, Cook JR, Epstein AE, et al. Dual-chamber pacing or ventricular backup pacing in patients with an implantable defibrillator: the Dual Chamber and VVI Implantable Defibrillator (DAVID) Trial. JAMA 2002;288(24):3115–23.
6. Curtis AB, Worley SJ, Adamson PB, et al. Biventricular pacing for atrioventricular block and systolic dysfunction. N Engl J Med 2013;368(17):1585–93.
7. Kaye G, Ng JY, Ahmed S, et al. The prevalence of pacing-induced cardiomyopathy (PICM) in patients with long term right ventricular pacing - is it a matter of definition? Heart Lung Circ 2019; 28(7):1027–33.
8. Merchant FM, Mittal S. Pacing induced cardiomyopathy. J Cardiovasc Electrophysiol 2020;31(1): 286–92.
9. Merchant FM, Hoskins MH, Musat DL, et al. Incidence and time course for developing heart failure with high-burden right ventricular pacing. Circ Cardiovasc Qual Outcomes 2017;10(6):e003564.
10. Kiehl EL, Makki T, Kumar R, et al. Incidence and predictors of right ventricular pacing-induced cardiomyopathy in patients with complete atrioventricular block and preserved left ventricular systolic function. Heart Rhythm 2016;13(12):2272–8.
11. Kaye GC, Linker NJ, Marwick TH, et al. Effect of right ventricular pacing lead site on left ventricular function in patients with high-grade atrioventricular block: results of the protect-pace study. Eur Heart J 2015;36(14):856–62.
12. Hussain MA, Furuya-Kanamori L, Kaye G, et al. The effect of right ventricular apical and nonapical pacing on the short- and long-term changes in left ventricular ejection fraction: a systematic review and meta-analysis of randomized-controlled trials. Pacing Clin Electrophysiol 2015;38(9):1121–36.
13. Xie J-M, Fang F, Zhang Q, et al. Left atrial remodeling and reduced atrial pump function after chronic

right ventricular apical pacing in patients with preserved ejection fraction. Int J Cardiol 2012;157(3): 364–9.

14. Xie J-M, Fang F, Zhang Q, et al. Acute effects of right ventricular apical pacing on left atrial remodeling and function. Pacing Clin Electrophysiol 2012;35(7):856–62.

15. Pastore G, Zanon F, Baracca E, et al. The risk of atrial fibrillation during right ventricular pacing. Europace 2016;18(3):353–8.

16. Narula OS, Scherlag BJ, Samet P. Pervenous pacing of the specialized conducting system in man. His bundle and A-V nodal stimulation. Circulation 1970;41(1):77–87.

17. Deshmukh P, Casavant DA, Romanyshyn M, et al. Permanent, direct his-bundle pacing: a novel approach to cardiac pacing in patients with normal His-Purkinje activation. Circulation 2000;101(8): 869–77.

18. Deshmukh PM, Romanyshyn M. Direct his-bundle pacing: present and future. Pacing Clin Electrophysiol 2004;27(6 Pt 2):862–70.

19. Barba-Pichardo R, Moriña-Vázquez P, Fernández-Gómez JM, et al. Permanent his-bundle pacing: seeking physiological ventricular pacing. Europace 2010;12(4):527–33.

20. Barba-Pichardo R, Manovel Sánchez A, Fernández-Gómez JM, et al. Ventricular resynchronization therapy by direct His-bundle pacing using an internal cardioverter defibrillator. Europace 2013;15(1): 83–8.

21. Occhetta E, Bortnik M, Magnani A, et al. Prevention of ventricular desynchronization by permanent para-Hisian pacing after atrioventricular node ablation in chronic atrial fibrillation: a crossover, blinded, randomized study versus apical right ventricular pacing. J Am Coll Cardiol 2006;47(10): 1938–45.

22. Sharma PS, Dandamudi G, Naperkowski A, et al. Permanent His-bundle pacing is feasible, safe, and superior to right ventricular pacing in routine clinical practice. Heart Rhythm 2015;12(2):305–12.

23. Kusumoto FM, Schoenfeld MH, Barrett C, et al. 2018 ACC/AHA/HRS guideline on the evaluation and management of patients with bradycardia and cardiac conduction delay: a report of the American Ccollege of Cardiology/American Heart Association Task Force on Clinical Practice Guidelines and the Heart Rhythm Society. Circulation 2019;140(8):e382–482.

24. Bhatt AG, Musat DL, Milstein N, et al. The efficacy of His bundle pacing: lessons learned from implementation for the first time at an experienced electrophysiology center. JACC Clin Electrophysiol 2018;4(11):1397–406.

25. Zanon F, Abdelrahman M, Marcantoni L, et al. Long term performance and safety of His bundle pacing: a multicenter experience. J Cardiovasc Electrophysiol 2019;30(9):1594–601.

26. Teigeler T, Kolominsky J, Vo C, et al. Intermediate-term performance and safety of His-bundle pacing leads: a single-center experience. Heart Rhythm 2021. https://doi.org/10.1016/j.hrthm.2020.12.031.

27. Huang W, Su L, Wu S, et al. A novel pacing strategy with low and stable output: pacing the left bundle branch immediately beyond the conduction block. Can J Cardiol 2017;33(12):1736.e1–3.

28. Kaufmann R, Rothberger C. Beiträge zur Entstehungsweise extrasystolischer allorhythmien. Z Ges Exp Med 1919;9:104–22.

29. James TN, Sherf L. Fine structure of the his bundle. Circulation 1971;44(1):9–28.

30. Narula OS. Longitudinal dissociation in the his bundle. Bundle branch block due to asynchronous conduction within the his bundle in man. Circulation 1977;56(6):996–1006.

31. Upadhyay GA, Cherian T, Shatz DY, et al. Intracardiac delineation of septal conduction in left bundle-branch block patterns. Circulation 2019;139(16): 1876–88.

32. Niri A, Bhaskaran A, Asta J, et al. Stimulation and propagation of activation in conduction tissue: implications for left bundle branch area pacing. Heart Rhythm 2021. https://doi.org/10.1016/j.hrthm.2020.12.030.

33. Dandamudi G, Vijayaraman P. How to perform permanent His bundle pacing in routine clinical practice. Heart Rhythm 2016;13(6):1362–6.

34. Vijayaraman P, Chung MK, Dandamudi G, et al. His bundle pacing. J Am Coll Cardiol 2018;72(8): 927–47.

35. Huang W, Chen X, Su L, et al. A beginner's guide to permanent left bundle branch pacing. Heart Rhythm 2019;16(12):1791–6.

36. Padala SK, Ellenbogen KA. Left bundle branch pacing is the best approach for physiologic pacing. Heart Rhythm O2. 2020;1(1):59–67.

37. Jastrzębski M, Kiełbasa G, Moskal P, et al. Fixation beats: a novel marker for reaching the left bundle branch area during deep septal lead implantation. Heart Rhythm 2021;18(4):562–9.

38. Orlov MV, Casavant D, Koulouridis I, et al. Permanent his-bundle pacing using stylet-directed, active-fixation leads placed via coronary sinus sheaths compared to conventional lumen-less system. Heart Rhythm 2019;16(12):1825–31.

39. De Pooter J, Calle S, Timmermans F, et al. Left bundle branch area pacing using stylet-driven pacing leads with a new delivery sheath: a comparison with lumen-less leads. J Cardiovasc Electrophysiol 2021;32(2):439–48.

40. Saini A, Serafini NJ, Campbell S, et al. Novel method for assessment of His bundle pacing morphology using near field and far field device

electrograms. Circ Arrhythm Electrophysiol 2019; 12(2):e006878.

41. Jastrzębski M, Moskal P, Curila K, et al. Electrocardiographic characterization of non-selective His-bundle pacing: validation of novel diagnostic criteria. Europace 2019;21(12):1857–64.

42. Jastrzębski M, Moskal P, Bednarek A, et al. Programmed deep septal stimulation: a novel maneuver for the diagnosis of left bundle branch capture during permanent pacing. J Cardiovasc Electrophysiol 2020;31(2):485–93.

43. Jastrzębski M, Kiełbasa G, Curila K, et al. Physiology-based electrocardiographic criteria for left bundle branch capture. Heart Rhythm 2021. https://doi.org/10.1016/j.hrthm.2021.02.021.

44. Kronborg MB, Mortensen PT, Poulsen SH, et al. His or para-His pacing preserves left ventricular function in atrioventricular block: a double-blind, randomized, crossover study. Europace 2014;16(8): 1189–96.

45. Vijayaraman P, Naperkowski A, Ellenbogen KA, et al. Electrophysiologic insights into site of atrioventricular block: lessons from permanent His bundle pacing. JACC Clin Electrophysiol 2015;1(6):571–81.

46. Vijayaraman P, Naperkowski A, Subzposh FA, et al. Permanent his-bundle pacing: long-term lead performance and clinical outcomes. Heart Rhythm 2018;15(5):696–702.

47. Abdelrahman M, Subzposh FA, Beer D, et al. Clinical outcomes of His bundle pacing compared to right ventricular pacing. J Am Coll Cardiol 2018; 71(20):2319–30.

48. Sarkar R, Kaur D, Subramanian M, et al. Permanent HIS bundle pacing feasibility in routine clinical practice: experience from an Indian center. Indian Heart J 2019;71(4):360–3.

49. Keene D, Arnold AD, Jastrzębski M, et al. His bundle pacing, learning curve, procedure characteristics, safety, and feasibility: insights from a large international observational study. J Cardiovasc Electrophysiol 2019;30(10):1984–93.

50. Ravi V, Beer D, Pietrasik GM, et al. Development of new-onset or progressive atrial fibrillation in patients with permanent HIS bundle pacing versus right ventricular pacing: results from the RUSH HBP registry. J Am Heart Assoc 2020;9(22): e018478.

51. De Pooter J, Gauthey A, Calle S, et al. Feasibility of His-bundle pacing in patients with conduction disorders following transcatheter aortic valve replacement. J Cardiovasc Electrophysiol 2020;31(4): 813–21.

52. Chen K, Li Y, Dai Y, et al. Comparison of electrocardiogram characteristics and pacing parameters between left bundle branch pacing and right ventricular pacing in patients receiving pacemaker therapy. Europace 2019;21(4):673–80.

53. Zhang J, Wang Z, Cheng L, et al. Immediate clinical outcomes of left bundle branch area pacing vs conventional right ventricular pacing. Clin Cardiol 2019;42(8):768–73.

54. Hou X, Qian Z, Wang Y, et al. Feasibility and cardiac synchrony of permanent left bundle branch pacing through the interventricular septum. Europace 2019;21(11):1694–702.

55. Li X, Li H, Ma W, et al. Permanent left bundle branch area pacing for atrioventricular block: feasibility, safety, and acute effect. Heart Rhythm 2019; 16(12):1766–73.

56. Li Y, Chen K, Dai Y, et al. Left bundle branch pacing for symptomatic bradycardia: implant success rate, safety, and pacing characteristics. Heart Rhythm 2019;16(12):1758–65.

57. Vijayaraman P, Subzposh FA, Naperkowski A, et al. Prospective evaluation of feasibility and electrophysiologic and echocardiographic characteristics of left bundle branch area pacing. Heart Rhythm 2019;16(12):1774–82.

58. Hasumi E, Fujiu K, Nakanishi K, et al. Impacts of left bundle/peri-left bundle pacing on left ventricular contraction. Circ J 2019;83(9):1965–7.

59. Cai B, Huang X, Li L, et al. Evaluation of cardiac synchrony in left bundle branch pacing: insights from echocardiographic research. J Cardiovasc Electrophysiol 2020. https://doi.org/10.1111/jce. 14342.

60. Jiang Z, Chang Q, Wu Y, et al. Typical BBB morphology and implantation depth of 3830 electrode predict QRS correction by left bundle branch area pacing. Pacing Clin Electrophysiol 2020; 43(1):110–7.

61. Wang J, Liang Y, Wang W, et al. Left bundle branch area pacing is superior to right ventricular septum pacing concerning depolarization-repolarization reserve. J Cardiovasc Electrophysiol 2020;31(1): 313–22.

62. Li X, Fan X, Li H, et al. ECG patterns of successful permanent left bundle branch area pacing in bradycardia patients with typical bundle branch block. Pacing Clin Electrophysiol 2020;43(8):781–90.

63. Vijayaraman P, Cano Ó, Koruth JS, et al. His-Purkinje conduction system pacing following transcatheter aortic valve replacement: feasibility and safety. JACC Clin Electrophysiol 2020;6(6):649–57.

64. Lin J, Chen K, Dai Y, et al. Bilateral bundle branch area pacing to achieve physiological conduction system activation. Circ Arrhythm Electrophysiol 2020;13(8):e008267.

65. Wang S, Lan R, Zhang N, et al. LBBAP in patients with normal intrinsic QRS duration: electrical and mechanical characteristics. Pacing Clin Electrophysiol 2021;44(1):82–92.

66. Ravi V, Hanifin JL, Larsen T, et al. Pros and cons of left bundle branch pacing: a single-center

experience. Circ Arrhythm Electrophysiol 2020; 13(12):e008874.

67. Padala SK, Master VM, Terricabras M, et al. Initial experience, safety, and feasibility of left bundle branch area pacing: a multicenter prospective study. JACC Clin Electrophysiol 2020;6(14):1773–82.

68. Qian Z, Qiu Y, Wang Y, et al. Lead performance and clinical outcomes of patients with permanent His-Purkinje system pacing: a single-centre experience. Europace 2020;22(Suppl_2):ii45–53.

69. Su L, Wang S, Wu S, et al. Long-term safety and feasibility of left bundle branch pacing in a large single-center study. Circ Arrhythm Electrophysiol 2021;14(2):e009261.

70. Vijayaraman P, Subzposh FA, Naperkowski A. Atrioventricular node ablation and His bundle pacing. Europace 2017;19(suppl_4):iv10–6.

71. Huang W, Su L, Wu S, et al. Benefits of permanent His bundle pacing combined with atrioventricular node ablation in atrial fibrillation patients with heart failure with both preserved and reduced left ventricular ejection fraction. J Am Heart Assoc 2017; 6(4):e005309.

72. Su L, Cai M, Wu S, et al. Long-term performance and risk factors analysis after permanent His-bundle pacing and atrioventricular node ablation in patients with atrial fibrillation and heart failure. Europace 2020;22(Suppl_2):ii19–26.

73. Wang S, Wu S, Xu L, et al. Feasibility and efficacy of His bundle pacing or left bundle pacing combined with atrioventricular node ablation in patients with persistent atrial fibrillation and implantable cardioverter-defibrillator therapy. J Am Heart Assoc 2019;8(24):e014253.

74. Cleland JG, Abraham WT, Linde C, et al. An individual patient meta-analysis of five randomized trials assessing the effects of cardiac resynchronization therapy on morbidity and mortality in patients with symptomatic heart failure. Eur Heart J 2013;34(46):3547–56.

75. Lustgarten DL, Crespo EM, Arkhipova-Jenkins I, et al. His-bundle pacing versus biventricular pacing in cardiac resynchronization therapy patients: a crossover design comparison. Heart Rhythm 2015;12(7):1548–57.

76. Ajijola OA, Upadhyay GA, Macias C, et al. Permanent his-bundle pacing for cardiac resynchronization therapy: initial feasibility study in lieu of left ventricular lead. Heart Rhythm 2017;14(9):1353–61.

77. Sharma PS, Dandamudi G, Herweg B, et al. Permanent His-bundle pacing as an alternative to biventricular pacing for cardiac resynchronization therapy: a multicenter experience. Heart Rhythm 2018;15(3):413–20.

78. Sharma PS, Naperkowski A, Bauch TD, et al. Permanent His bundle pacing for cardiac resynchronization therapy in patients with heart failure and

right bundle branch block. Circ Arrhythm Electrophysiol 2018;11(9):e006613.

79. Upadhyay GA, Vijayaraman P, Nayak HM, et al. His corrective pacing or biventricular pacing for cardiac resynchronization in heart failure. J Am Coll Cardiol 2019;74(1):157–9.

80. Huang W, Su L, Wu S, et al. Long-term outcomes of His bundle pacing in patients with heart failure with left bundle branch block. Heart 2019;105(2): 137–43.

81. Singh R, Devabhaktuni S, Ezzeddine F, et al. His-bundle pacing: a novel treatment for left bundle branch block-mediated cardiomyopathy. J Cardiovasc Electrophysiol 2020;31(10):2730–6.

82. Zhang W, Huang J, Qi Y, et al. Cardiac resynchronization therapy by left bundle branch area pacing in patients with heart failure and left bundle branch block. Heart Rhythm 2019;16(12):1783–90.

83. Li X, Qiu C, Xie R, et al. Left bundle branch area pacing delivery of cardiac resynchronization therapy and comparison with biventricular pacing. ESC Heart Fail 2020;7(4):1711–22.

84. Li Y, Yan L, Dai Y, et al. Feasibility and efficacy of left bundle branch area pacing in patients indicated for cardiac resynchronization therapy. Europace 2020;22(Suppl_2):ii54–60.

85. Guo J, Li L, Xiao G, et al. Remarkable response to cardiac resynchronization therapy via left bundle branch pacing in patients with true left bundle branch block. Clin Cardiol 2020;43(12):1460–8.

86. Wang Y, Gu K, Qian Z, et al. The efficacy of left bundle branch area pacing compared with biventricular pacing in patients with heart failure: a matched case-control study. J Cardiovasc Electrophysiol 2020;31(8):2068–77.

87. Huang W, Wu S, Vijayaraman P, et al. Cardiac resynchronization therapy in patients with nonischemic cardiomyopathy using left bundle branch pacing. JACC Clin Electrophysiol 2020;6(7): 849–58.

88. Vijayaraman P, Ponnusamy S, Cano Ó, et al. Left bundle branch area pacing for cardiac resynchronization therapy: results from the international LBBAP collaborative study group. JACC Clin Electrophysiol 2021;7(2):135–47.

89. Arnold AD, Shun-Shin MJ, Keene D, et al. His resynchronization versus biventricular pacing in patients with heart failure and left bundle branch block. J Am Coll Cardiol 2018;72(24):3112–22.

90. Wu S, Su L, Vijayaraman P, et al. Left bundle branch pacing for cardiac resynchronization therapy: nonrandomized on-treatment comparison with His bundle pacing and biventricular pacing. Can J Cardiol 2021;37(2):319–28.

91. Vijayaraman P, Herweg B, Ellenbogen KA, et al. His-optimized cardiac resynchronization therapy to maximize electrical resynchronization: a feasibility

study. Circ Arrhythm Electrophysiol 2019;12(2): e006934.

92. Shan P, Su L, Zhou X, et al. Beneficial effects of upgrading to His bundle pacing in chronically paced patients with left ventricular ejection fraction <50. Heart Rhythm 2018;15(3):405–12.

93. Vijayaraman P, Herweg B, Dandamudi G, et al. Outcomes of His-bundle pacing upgrade after long-term right ventricular pacing and/or pacing-induced cardiomyopathy: insights into disease progression. Heart Rhythm 2019;16(10):1554–61.

94. Qian Z, Wang Y, Hou X, et al. Efficacy of upgrading to left bundle branch pacing in patients with heart failure after right ventricular pacing. Pacing Clin Electrophysiol 2021;44(3):472–80.

95. Suryanarayana PG, Frankel DS, Marchlinski FE, et al. Painful left bundle branch block syndrome treated successfully with permanent His bundle pacing. Heartrhythm Case Rep 2018;4(10):439–43.

96. Viles-Gonzalez JF, Mahata I, Anter E, et al. Painful left bundle branch block syndrome treated with His bundle pacing. J Electrocardiol 2018;51(6): 1019–22.

97. Ferrara MG, Cappucci RV, Wang DY. Chest pain resolution with His-bundle pacing in a patient with left bundle branch block-related nonischemic left ventricular dysfunction. J Innov Card Rhythm Manag 2019;10(9):3810–4.

98. Oladunjoye OO, Oladunjoye AO, Oladiran O, et al. Persistent exertional chest pain in a marathon runner: exercise-induced, painful, left bundle branch block syndrome treated with his-bundle pacing. Mayo Clin Proc Innov Qual Outcomes 2019;3(2): 226–30.

99. Smith KA, Frey J, McKenzie A, et al. The use of His bundle pacing for the treatment of painful left bundle branch block syndrome. Clin Case Rep 2020;8(6):1025–9.

100. Garg A, Master V, Ellenbogen KA, et al. Painful left bundle branch block syndrome successfully treated with left bundle branch area pacing. JACC Case Rep 2020;2(4):568–71.

101. Prystowsky EN, Padanilam BJ. Cardiac resynchronization therapy reverses severe dyspnea associated with acceleration-dependent left bundle branch block in a patient with structurally normal heart. J Cardiovasc Electrophysiol 2019;30(4): 517–9.

102. Padala SK, Cabrera JA, Ellenbogen KA. Anatomy of the cardiac conduction system. Pacing Clin Electrophysiol 2021;44(1):15–25.

Moving?

Make sure your subscription moves with you!

To notify us of your new address, find your **Clinics Account Number** (located on your mailing label above your name), and contact customer service at:

Email: journalscustomerservice-usa@elsevier.com

800-654-2452 (subscribers in the U.S. & Canada)
314-447-8871 (subscribers outside of the U.S. & Canada)

Fax number: 314-447-8029

**Elsevier Health Sciences Division
Subscription Customer Service
3251 Riverport Lane
Maryland Heights, MO 63043**

*To ensure uninterrupted delivery of your subscription, please notify us at least 4 weeks in advance of move.